Paediatric Surgical Diagnosis

Atlas of Disorders of Surgical Significance

SECOND EDITION

Paediatric Surgical Diagnosis

Atlas of Disorders of Surgical Significance

SECOND EDITION

Spencer W. Beasley
Paediatric Surgeon, Christchurch Hospital
Professor of Paediatric Surgery, Departments of Paediatrics and Surgery, University of Otago
Christchurch, New Zealand

John Hutson
Paediatric Urologist, The Royal Children's Hospital
Chair of Paediatric Surgery, Department of Paediatrics, University of Melbourne
Melbourne, Australia

Mark Stringer
Paediatric Surgeon, Wellington Hospital
Honorary Professor, Department of Paediatrics & Child Health, University of Otago
Wellington, New Zealand

Sebastian K. King
Paediatric Surgeon, The Royal Children's Hospital
Clinical Associate Professor, Department of Paediatrics, University of Melbourne
Melbourne, Australia

Warwick J. Teague
Paediatric Surgeon & Director of Trauma Services, The Royal Children's Hospital
Clinical Associate Professor, Department of Paediatrics, University of Melbourne
Melbourne, Australia

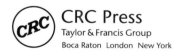
CRC Press
Taylor & Francis Group
Boca Raton London New York

CRC Press is an imprint of the
Taylor & Francis Group, an **informa** business

CRC Press
Taylor & Francis Group
6000 Broken Sound Parkway NW, Suite 300
Boca Raton, FL 33487-2742

© 2018 by Taylor & Francis Group, LLC
CRC Press is an imprint of Taylor & Francis Group, an Informa business

No claim to original U.S. Government works

Printed on acid-free paper

Printed and bound in India by Replika Press Pvt. Ltd.

International Standard Book Number-13: 978-1-1381-9732-9 (Paperback)

Library of Congress Cataloging-in-Publication Data

Names: Beasley, Spencer W., author. | Hutson, John M., author. | Stringer,
Mark D., author. | King, Sebastian, author. | Teague, Warwick J., author.
Title: Pediatric diagnosis : atlas of disorders of surgical significance /
Spencer Beasley, John Hutson, Mark D. Stringer, Sebastian King, Warwick
Teague.
Description: Second edition. | Boca Raton : CRC Press, [2018] | Includes
bibliographical references and index. |
Identifiers: LCCN 2017052034 (print) | LCCN 2017052272 (ebook) | ISBN
9781315279978 (eBook General) | ISBN 9781315279961 (eBook PDF) | ISBN
9781315279954 (eBook ePub3) | ISBN 9781315279947 (eBook Mobipocket) |
ISBN 9781138197329 (pbk. : alk. paper)
Subjects: | MESH: Diagnostic Techniques, Surgical | Child | Infant | Atlases
Classification: LCC RD137.3 (ebook) | LCC RD137.3 (print) | NLM WO 517 | DDC
617.9/8--dc23
LC record available at https://lccn.loc.gov/2017052034

Visit the Taylor & Francis Web site at
http://www.taylorandfrancis.com

and the CRC Press Web site at
http://www.crcpress.com

Contents

Foreword to the first edition

Paediatric surgery is age-related general surgery in a broad sense, involving many specialty fields. This book represents the essential elements of the multifaceted nature of the surgery of infancy and childhood.

Three very experienced individuals with well-recognised expertise in clinical care, education and research wrote this book. They have worked their entire careers in one of the most important children's centres in the world, so this book brings with it a level of authority which is unmatched.

The authors' goal was to develop an illustrated guide to diagnosis of the important paediatric surgical conditions. The common, the occasional and some rare conditions are all here. Although it would be virtually impossible to include every conceivable rare disorder, the authors come close; and certainly every condition likely to be encountered in a practitioner's professional life time is presented including entities seen mainly in third world countries. There is a great need for a book of this nature, which teaches the basics that trainees are frequently not taught today as high-tech medicine is emphasised. The emphasis is on primary care and additional management geared for medical students, trainees and practitioners in paediatrics, obstetrics and various surgical specialities, as well as nurses who might need a quick reference for diagnosis.

The particularly valuable aspect of this pictorial text is that it stresses physical diagnosis illustrated by beautiful photographs, x-rays and other imaging studies. In addition to marvellous illustrations, good descriptive legends and a concise text present a list of differential diagnoses and at least one reliable approach to confirmatory studies where appropriate.

No attempt is made to be exhaustive in the treatment of any disorder, which makes this book particularly useful for the intended audience around the world. The authors advise their readers to use this book in conjunction with a standard text for comprehensive coverage, but it would certainly stand alone as a visual guide to rapid diagnosis of almost any paediatric surgical condition likely to be seen in routine practice. This book is well organised into sections, which are comprehensively treated. In addition to conditions usually treated by general paediatric surgeons, those treated by ophthalmologists, neurosurgeons, urologists, otolaryngologists, orthopaedists and plastic surgeons are covered. Neonatal as well as acquired disorders are included. A book like this could only have come from the life's work of three such experienced paediatric surgeons.

James A. O'Neill, Jr, MD
C. Everett Koop Professor of Paediatric Surgery
University of Pennsylvania, School of Medicine
Surgeon-in-Chief, Children's Hospital of Philadelphia
Philadelphia, PA, USA

Foreword to the first edition

Foreword to the second edition

This second edition of *Atlas of Paediatric Surgery,* now titled *Paediatric Surgical Diagnosis: Atlas of Disorders of Surgical Significance*, is a superbly illustrated and well-organized guide to most common anomalies in children's surgery as well as many that are uncommon. While this text is not intended to be encyclopaedic in scope, it does present in considerable depth the broad spectrum of general and thoracic paediatric surgery, as well as offer an important perspective to any children's provider in paediatric urology, head and neck surgery, ophthalmology, orthopaedics, neurosurgery and, indeed, all of children's surgery. The emphasis is on providing photographs and illustrations to assist in the recognition, clinical understanding and multidisciplinary management of the various abnormalities. This edition builds on the first; it is not only beautifully photographed and illustrated, but it is improved in the organization and clarity of the supporting text. Taken together, the succinct narratives and lucid visual presentations make the text useful to a broad audience. Children's surgery encompasses such diverse pathology that collection of this information, and particularly these photographs, would take most individuals several careers to compile. The authors have done this for the reader with emphasis on diagnostic information including radiographic and other imaging, as well as intraoperative photographs. The presentation is uniquely informative in aggregate.

The atlas is edited by five of the most senior and well recognized children's surgeons in the world. All are experts and bring a wealth of clinical experience to this work. The authors have added new information in this edition, particularly related to antenatal diagnosis and treatment. While *in-utero* assessment and intervention were possible previously, these have become a standard aspect of care in the time interval since the first edition was published. These areas are addressed in chapter one, while the second chapter is dedicated to major congenital anomalies which would be symptomatic or apparent in the neonatal period. Together these chapters will be quite useful to any who wish to understand newborn surgical anomalies. The introductory chapters are followed by anatomical and organ system presentations, concluding with trauma and gynaecological conditions. The overall focus is on visual clarity and a pragmatic bedside clinical approach to these children with surgical needs. The atlas is designed not as a comprehensive surgical reference text or operating atlas, but as a companion or adjunct to such standard presentations, adding a depth of understanding and visual diagnostic clarity that is unique. It will be a valuable addition to the libraries of institutions and individuals who care for children with surgical needs. This includes not just general and thoracic paediatric surgeons but all children's surgeons, as well as other allied health professionals, those who are learning about these patients, including residents, fellows and students, and indeed anyone with an interest in the surgical problems of infants and children.

Keith T. Oldham, MD
Professor of Surgery, Division of Pediatric Surgery
Medical College of Wisconsin
Marie Z. Uihlein Chair of Pediatric Surgery
and Surgeon-in-Chief
Children's Hospital of Wisconsin
Milwaukee, WI, USA

Acknowledgements

ACKNOWLEDGEMENTS FOR THE FIRST EDITION

No one surgeon, not even one in the busiest clinical practice, could collect the range and variety of conditions displayed in this atlas within a lifetime. Therefore, despite fairly extensive collections of our own, we have been heavily reliant on the contributions of a number of colleagues. Many of these have gone to considerable effort to provide us with as comprehensive a coverage of the specialty as possible, and to them we are extremely grateful. They include: Alex Auldist, John Barnett, Don Cameron, Tony Catto-Smith, Bill Cole, David Croaker, Paddy Dewan, Bob Dickens, James Elder, Roger Hall, David James, Peter Jones, Anne Kosloske, Julian Keogh, Geoff Klug, Neil McMullin, Azad Najmaldin, Kevin Pringle, T.M. Ramanaujam, Barry Shandling, Errol Simpson, Arnold Smith, Durham Smith, John Solomon, Douglas Stephens, Keith Stokes, Russell Taylor, Roger Voigt, Alan and Susie Woodward. Ramanujam, in particular went to extraordinary lengths to provide us with a fine series of slides of the most bizarre and rare conditions. We are grateful to our many registrars who have had to organise the photography of many of the lesions.

Slides of interesting cases often are passed between colleagues and, with time, their origin may become obscure. It is quite possible that a number of illustrations included in this atlas have not been acknowledged appropriately. To those who have the original source of these illustrations, we are truly grateful, despite their anonymity.

An enormous contribution has been made by staff of the Educational Resource Centre of The Royal Children' Hospital, Melbourne, who have been happy to bear the burden of copying (and maintaining in order) a large number of slides, and to produce a number of line drawings. Their full cooperation in this project over many months has made the editors' task much easier.

The secretarial staff of the Department of Surgery, Elizabeth Vorrath and Judith Hayes, now well used to the rigours of medical manuscripts, have confirmed their mastery of complex, numerous and ever-changing legends. Their efficiency and good humour has obscured any frustrations they might have had.

Our ever-patient families have provided the support that has allowed us to devote consecutive long weekends to the project. We are happy to return the time to them in full now it is completed.

Finally, we are grateful to Peter Altman who encouraged us to embark on the project and who has provided helpful guidance throughout. The professional work of Chapman and Hall has been a major factor contributing to this work, which we hope will be of use to paediatric surgical aspirants and teachers for many years to come.

ACKNOWLEDGEMENTS FOR THE SECOND EDITION

Once again we are indebted to The Royal Children's Hospital Creative Studio (previously Educational Resource Centre) for their expert assistance in taking many of the clinical photographs as well as dealing with the artwork and digital file management.

We thank Shirley D'Cruz, Personal Assistant to Professor John Hutson, who worked tirelessly to prepare the base texts and image legends for revision. Shirley then shouldered the

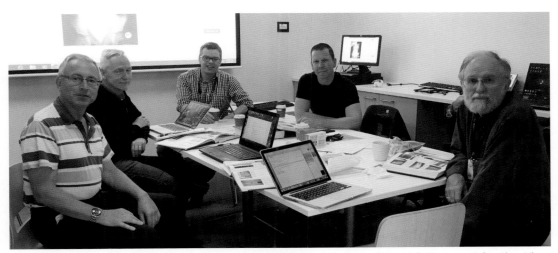

Fig. 1 The authors (from left to right): Spencer Beasley, Mark Stringer, Warwick Teague, Sebastian King and John Hutson.

lion's share of the responsibility for ensuring version control throughout the complex task of revising the text and legends, and managing the nuances and needs of five editors and a publisher across three time zones.

Many of the original photographs provided in the first edition have been retained. In addition, we have included photographs and images provided by the listed contributors to this edition.

The staff of CRC Press throughout have been wonderfully patient and understanding of us, particularly in the final stages where the actual layout and accuracy of the figures and their legends has become important. From Cherry Allen, to Peter Beynon and Paul Bennett, the meticulous care they have taken assembling a substantial file of figures, and their detailed understanding of what we have tried to achieve, has made our work so much easier.

Creating an atlas of this magnitude takes an enormous amount of time: this time is often at the end of an already long day, and it is time that otherwise would have been spent with our wives and families. So it is to Christy, Susan, Alice, Charlotte and Kirsty, and our respective children, who have had to tolerate and forgive us our absences during the preparation of this book, that we are so grateful.

Contributors

Raimah Ahmed
Urology Resident
The Royal Children's Hospital
Melbourne, Australia

Keith Amarakone
Trauma Fellow
The Royal Children's Hospital
Melbourne, Australia

Katherine Baguley
Otorhinolaryngologist
Wellington Regional Hospital
Wellington, New Zealand

Elhamy Bekhit
Radiologist
The Royal Children's Hospital
Melbourne, Australia

Aurore Bouty
Urologist
The Royal Children's Hospital
Melbourne, Australia

Brendon Bowkett
Paediatric Surgeon
Wellington Children's Hospital
Wellington, New Zealand

Chris Coombs
Plastic and Reconstructive Surgeon
The Royal Children's Hospital
Melbourne, Australia

Charles Davis
Craniofacial Surgeon
Wellington Regional Hospital
Wellington, New Zealand

Jan de Faber
Ophthalamologist
Rotterdam Eye Hospital
Rotterdam, The Netherlands

Phillipa Depree
Paediatric Radiologist
Christchurch Hospital
Christchurch, New Zealand

Aniruddh Deshpande
Paediatric Surgeon
John Hunter Children's Hospital
Newcastle, Australia

Andrew Dobson
Paediatric Surgical Registrar
Christchurch Hospital
Christchurch, New Zealand

Leo Donnan
Orthopaedic Surgeon
The Royal Children's Hospital
Melbourne, Australia

Charlotte Elder
Adolescent Gynaecologist
The Royal Children's Hospital
Melbourne, Australia

James Elder
Ophthalmologist
The Royal Children's Hospital
Melbourne, Australia

Louise Goossens
Senior Medical Photographer
Wellington Regional Hospital
Wellington, New Zealand

Mary-Louise Greer
Radiologist
Hospital for Sick Children
Toronto, Canada

Sonia Grover
Adolescent Gynaecologist
The Royal Children's Hospital
Melbourne, Australia

Haytham Kubba
Paediatric Otorhinolaryngologist
The Royal Children's Hospital
Melbourne, Australia

Simon John
Paediatric Neurosurgeon
Christchurch Hospital
Christchurch, New Zealand

Michael Johnson
Orthopaedic Surgeon
The Royal Children's Hospital
Melbourne, Australia

Basil Leodoro
General Surgeon
Ministry of Health
Port Vila, Vanuatu

Parkash Mandhan
Paediatric Surgeon
Christchurch Hospital
Christchurch, New Zealand

Kiki Maoate
Paediatric Surgeon
Christchurch Hospital
Christchurch, New Zealand

Jay Marlow
Maternal and Fetal Medicine Specialist
Wellington Regional Hospital
Wellington, New Zealand

Stephen McInally
Medical Photographer
University of Newcastle
Newcastle, Australia

Randal Morton
Otorhinolaryngologist
Auckland, New Zealand

Cameron Palmer
Trauma Data Manager
The Royal Children's Hospital
Melbourne, Australia

Tony Penington
Plastic and Reconstructive Surgeon
The Royal Children's Hospital
Melbourne, Australia

Rod Phillips
General Paediatrician
The Royal Children's Hospital
Melbourne, Australia

TM Ramanajum
Paediatric Surgeon
University of Malaya
Kuala Lumpur, Malaysia

Elizabeth Rose
Otorhinolaryngologist
The Royal Children's Hospital
Melbourne, Australia

Victoria Scott
Paediatric Surgeon
Christchurch Hospital
Christchurch, New Zealand

Anne Smith
Forensic Paediatrician
Victorian Forensic Paediatric Medical
    Service
Melbourne, Australia

Alice Stringer
Otorhinolaryngologist
Wellington Regional Hospital
Wellington, New Zealand

Prue Weigall
Physiotherapist
The Royal Children's Hospital
Melbourne, Australia

Jonathan Wells
Paediatric Surgeon
Christchurch Hospital
Christchurch, New Zealand

Toni-Maree Wilson
Paediatric Surgeon
Wellington Hospital
Wellington, New Zealand

Zacharias Zachariou
Paediatric Surgeon
University of Nicosia
Nicosia, Cyprus

Augusto Zani
Paediatric Surgeon
Hospital for Sick Children
Toronto, Canada

Introduction

More than any other specialty, with the possible exception of dermatology, paediatric surgery lends itself to an illustrated guide to diagnosis. In the neonate, the dramatic appearance of exomphalos, gastroschisis, bladder exstrophy and prune belly syndrome is obvious. Anorectal malformations present with a spectrum of features, some of which are quite subtle, but which can be demonstrated with careful clinical examination. Even some internal lesions, such as volvulus, meconium ileus and bowel atresia, have external features, such as abdominal distension. The majority of orthopaedic deformities and inguinoscrotal lesions are diagnosed entirely on clinical grounds, most of which can be illustrated clearly on photography. Likewise, abnormalities and lesions of the head and neck, which are common in this age group, are usually superficial or structural, enabling easy clinical diagnosis. The relatively obscure areas of the thorax and urinary tract may have few or vague clinical features, but become apparent on appropriate radiological or other types of imaging.

This illustrated guide to the diagnosis of paediatric surgical disorders sets out to cover the broad spectrum of abnormalities encountered in this specialty. Although we have concentrated on the common lesions, we have deliberately included some extremely rare conditions to highlight the enormous variation that one may encounter in a specialty that includes bizarre congenital abnormalities.

The first chapter focuses on antenatal diagnosis, in recognition of the fact that nowadays most structural congenital abnormalities are diagnosed antenatally, and the paediatric surgeon becomes involved in the care of the unborn infant and its family well before birth. In this chapter we have deliberately included the type of ultrasound images encountered by paediatric surgeons in their everyday practice rather than concentrating on some of the recently introduced but not always widely available 'state of the art' imaging techniques. The second chapter deals with major neonatal abnormalities that are apparent at, or shortly after, birth; some will have been diagnosed several months prior to birth. Chapters 3 to 9 deal with the regions of the body sequentially, working from the head and neck, through the trunk, to the limbs. Abnormalities of the respiratory, gastrointestinal and urinary systems may be associated with a variety of external clinical manifestations but, more often than not, the definitive diagnosis is made only after specialised radiological investigation or at operation. Consequently, the operative views illustrate those conditions in which a diagnosis is made at surgery, or where the operative appearance is characteristic and clarifies the diagnosis. No attempt has been made to include details of operative technique. In the chapter on trauma, which covers all systems, special emphasis is given to non-accidental injury and in particular sexual abuse, as this is an area of considerable importance, and the clinician must be aware of the relevant features.

There are three major limitations to any pictorial guide to diagnosis. First, given the limitations of length, it is impossible to include all conditions or their variations. For example, the sections on anorectal malformations or disorders of sexual differentiation are extensive but not comprehensive: they could be vastly expanded, but for the sake of a relatively concise book this is not feasible. Second, many well-recognised conditions occur extremely rarely and, even in a large institution, certain conditions may be seen only once every decade or so. If they are not captured on film at the time of presentation, and before their operative correction, it may take some time before another similar case presents. In this regard, the editors are grateful to the many contributors who have helped 'fill the gaps'. Third, some conditions have no external clinical or radiological features that lend themselves to photography, which means that they tend to be 'down-played' in a pictorial book of this type. This is not to ignore or deny their importance, but obviously those conditions that are easily demonstrated photographically will tend to gain greater prominence. For this reason, it is important that this book should be read in conjunction with a standard paediatric surgery text if comprehensive coverage of the specialty is required.

Antenatal diagnosis | CHAPTER 1

Antenatal diagnosis of major congenital abnormalities in the fetus has become commonplace as a result of the increasing use and sophistication of antenatal ultrasonographic equipment. Initially, it was thought that the antenatal diagnosis of fetal abnormalities would lead to better treatment and an improved outcome, but so far, this expectation has only been partly fulfilled. Nevertheless, there is little doubt that perinatal treatment of several abnormalities is improved by their foreknowledge.

Between 18 and 21 weeks of gestation is regarded as the best time for the early detection of most fetal abnormalities, although if there is a previous history of fetal abnormalities (e.g. spina bifida) an ultrasound examination earlier in pregnancy may be indicated, with either repetition of the ultrasound scan at suitable intervals throughout the pregnancy or progression to more invasive tests, such as amniocentesis, chorionic villus and fetal blood sampling. Antenatal diagnosis of fetal abnormalities has identified a group of severely affected fetuses with complex lethal abnormalities which in the past never survived the pregnancy. Those with abnormalities that are less severe and who survive long enough to reach birth – and surgical attention – are already a selected group in whom good surgical results would be expected. The range of abnormalities detectable by antenatal ultrasound scanning includes anencephaly, spina bifida, hydrocephalus, encephalocele, cardiac abnormalities, urinary tract obstruction, congenital lung malformations, congenital diaphragmatic hernia, ovarian cysts, ventral abdominal wall defects, duodenal atresia and gross skeletal abnormalities.

For a time it was hoped that early antenatal recognition of some of these conditions (e.g. congenital diaphragmatic hernia, hydrocephalus and urinary tract obstruction) would allow intrauterine fetal surgery to prevent ongoing or secondary injury to the fetus, but so far the results of fetal surgery in all but a few highly selected conditions have been disappointing. Perhaps the main value of antenatal diagnosis is that the affected infant can be delivered at a tertiary institution and the appropriate treatment initiated at birth. This may avoid some of the problems of neonatal transport and of delayed diagnosis.

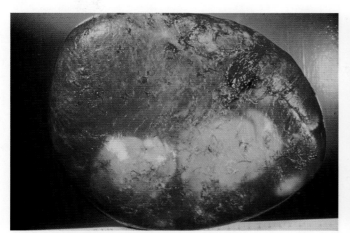

Fig. 1.1 An abortus with an intact amniotic sac containing a fetus within it. At least 10% of pregnancies abort in the embryonic stage (the first 8 weeks of gestation), mostly from chromosomal anomalies or gross malformations.

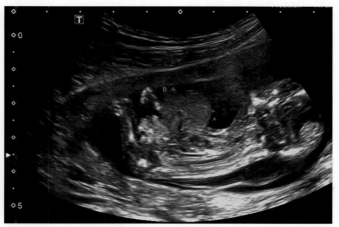

Fig. 1.2 Exomphalos in a 12-week fetus showing prolapse of the liver into the sac.

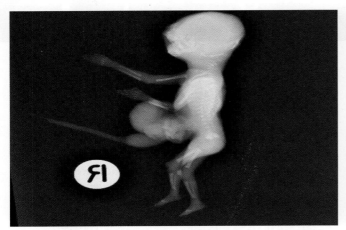

Fig. 1.3 Exomphalos in an aborted fetus demonstrated on postmortem babygram. It displays the relatively small size of the abdomen compared with the volume of bowel and liver in the sac. This illustrates why return of the sac contents into the abdominal cavity after birth can be difficult.

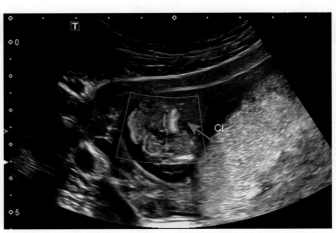

Fig. 1.4 Exomphalos in a fetus with trisomy 13. Doppler flow is seen in the umbilical cord vessels (arrow).

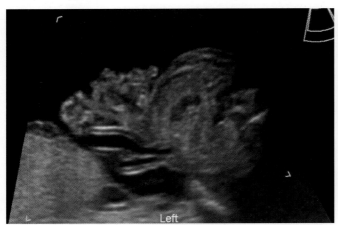

Fig. 1.5 Gastroschisis. Multiple loops of bowel have extruded through a defect in the anterior abdominal wall.

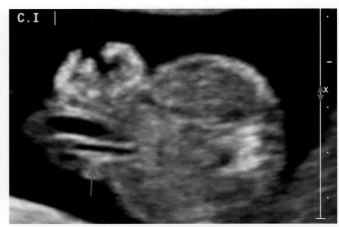

Fig. 1.6 Antenatal scan at 16 weeks' gestation showing trunk and umbilical cord (arrow) with bowel loops protruding just to the right of the attachment of the umbilical cord.

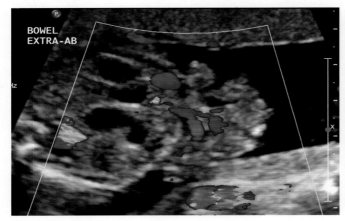

Fig. 1.7 Colour Doppler ultrasound scan in a 32-week gestation fetus with gastroschisis showing blood flow in the extra-abdominal mesenteric vessels.

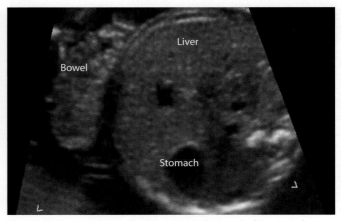

Fig. 1.8 Gastroschisis. Transverse abdominal ultrasound scan of a 19-week gestation fetus showing stomach and liver in the abdomen and extruded bowel.

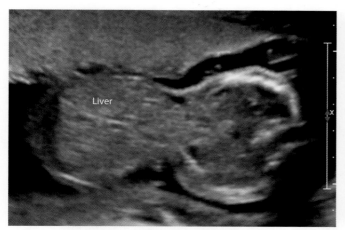

Fig. 1.9 A giant exomphalos containing the liver in a 16-week gestation fetus. Note the size of the exomphalos in comparison to the abdominal circumference.

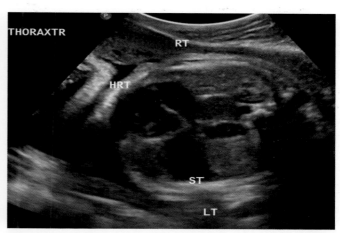

Fig. 1.10 Scan at 24 weeks' gestation showing a congenital diaphragmatic hernia with a fluid-filled cavity (stomach, ST) beside the heart (HRT).

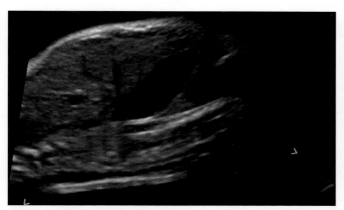

Fig. 1.11 Left-sided diaphragmatic hernia. Longitudinal scan of thorax showing a fluid-filled stomach in the thorax.

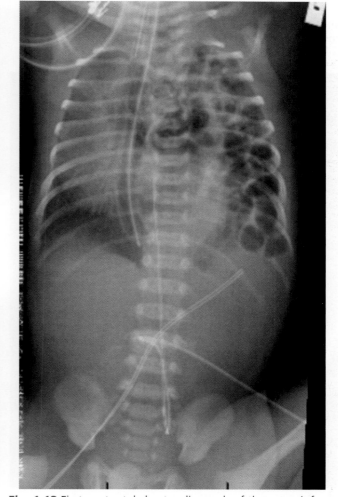

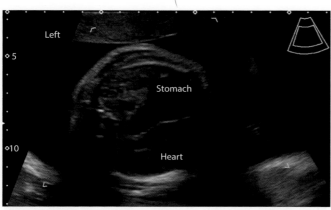

Fig. 1.12 Antenatal scan at 29 weeks' gestation showing a fluid-filled stomach beside the heart in a left-sided diaphragmatic hernia.

Fig. 1.13 First postnatal chest radiograph of the same infant as in **Fig. 1.12** confirming the diagnosis of a left-sided congenital diaphragmatic hernia.

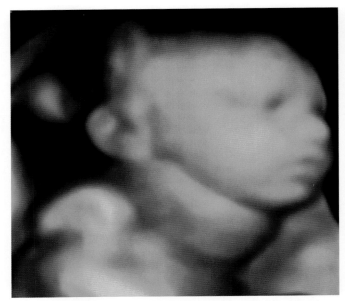

Fig. 1.14 4D ultrasound scan showing a cervical lymphatic malformation. This baby was delivered by the ex-utero intrapartum treatment (EXIT) procedure.

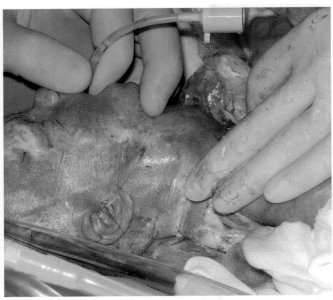

Fig. 1.15 EXIT procedure on the same infant with a cervical mass lesion.

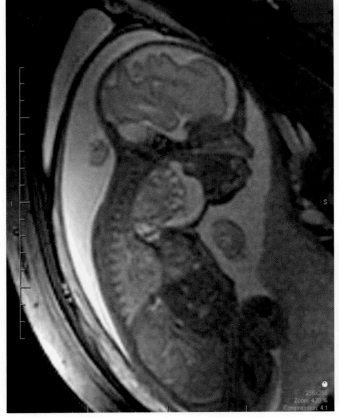

Fig. 1.16 A large cervical teratoma on antenatal MRI.

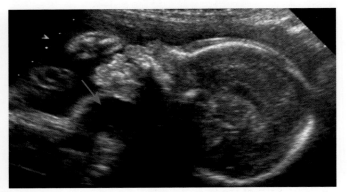

Fig. 1.17 Multicystic lymphatic malformation in the neck of a fetus (arrow) seen on ultrasound scan.

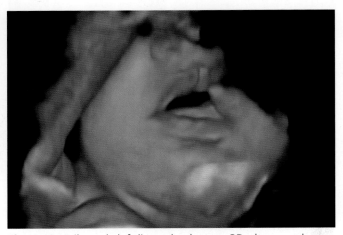

Fig. 1.18 Unilateral cleft lip and palate on 3D ultrasound scan.

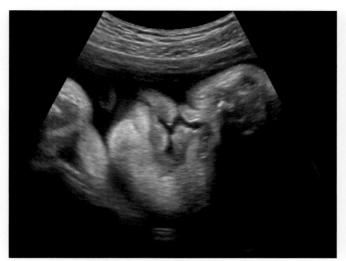

Fig. 1.19 Same fetus as in **Fig. 1.18** on 2D ultrasound scanning showing the cleft lip and palate.

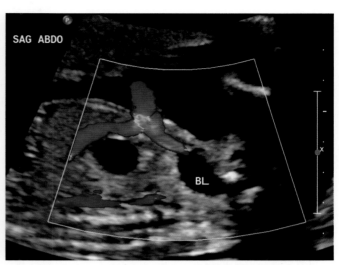

Fig. 1.20 Colour Doppler scan at 30 weeks' gestation showing an intra-abdominal fluid-filled cavity separate from the bladder, consistent with a duplication cyst.

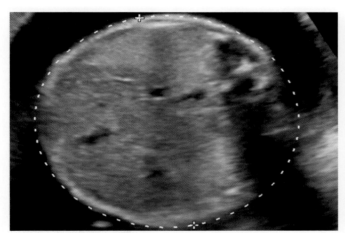

Fig. 1.21 Scan of the trunk at the level of the liver at 32 weeks' gestation, showing no stomach within the abdomen. If there is a small or absent stomach, particularly with polyhydramnios, oesophageal atresia is a possibility.

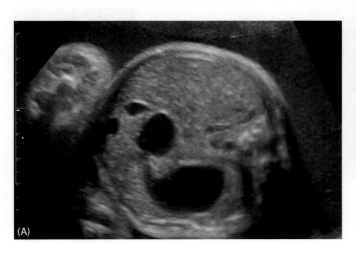

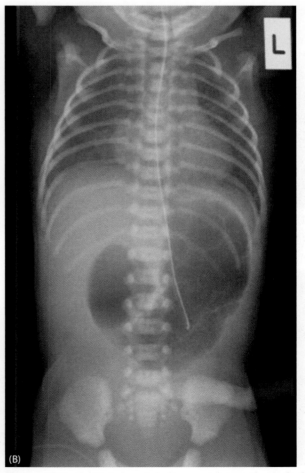

Figs. 1.22A, B (A) Antenatal ultrasound scan through the trunk showing showing two fluid-filled cavities in the upper abdomen, consistent with duodenal atresia. (B) Same baby at 3 hours after birth with classic double bubble on x-ray.

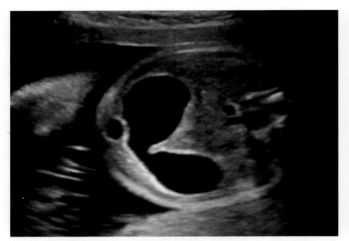

Fig. 1.23 Scan at 28 weeks' gestation showing a double-bubble sign in another fetus with duodenal atresia.

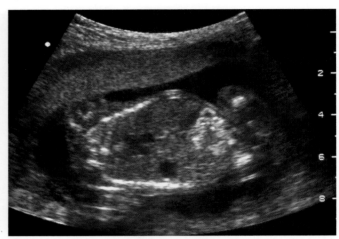

Fig. 1.24 Coronal scan of a fetus at 18 weeks showing echogenic bowel. Echogenic bowel may be seen in otherwise normal fetuses but can also be a marker for cystic fibrosis, intrauterine viral infection and aneuploidy.

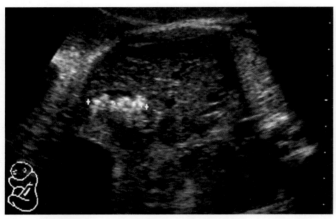

Fig. 1.25 Antenatal scan showing echogenic masses in the liver view, consistent with fetal gallstones or biliary sludge.

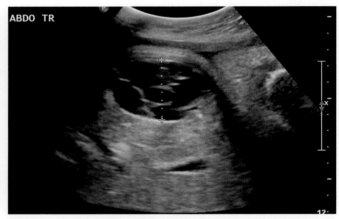

Fig. 1.26 Large multicystic ovary in a fetus at 34 weeks' gestation. Early postnatal follow-up is required.

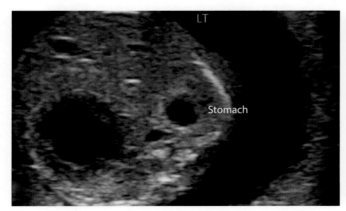

Fig. 1.27 Transverse ultrasound scan of the upper abdomen at 14 weeks' gestation showing a hepatic cyst.

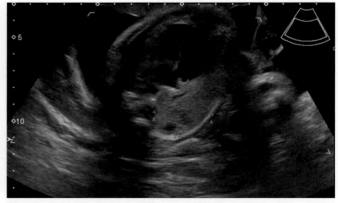

Fig. 1.28 Congenital pulmonary airway malformation (CPAM) involving the right lower lobe in a 30-week gestation fetus on transverse section.

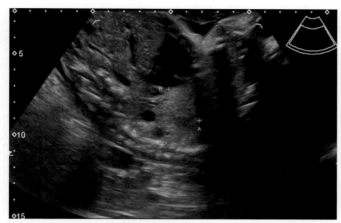

Fig. 1.29 CPAM in the right lower lobe on a longitudinal ultrasound scan of the fetus.

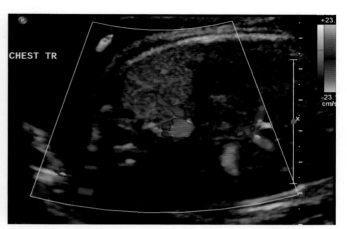

Fig. 1.30 Likely extralobar pulmonary sequestration as evident by the large vessel running directly off the aorta.

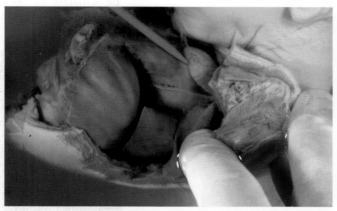

Fig. 1.31 The fetal thymus is a large structure, here exposed after removal of the left chest wall. The phrenic nerve can be seen running behind it, over the surface of the pericardium.

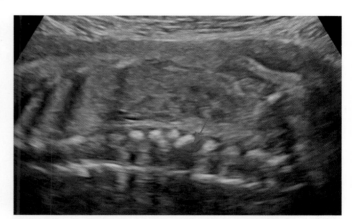

Fig. 1.32 Hemivertebrae (arrow) visible on a 28-week antenatal ultrasound scan.

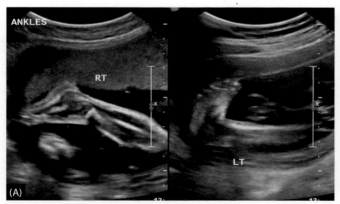

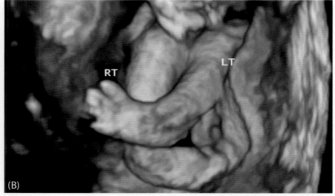

Figs. 1.33A, B (A) Ultrasound scan at 20 weeks' gestation showing both feet, with a normal right foot and club foot on the left. (B) 3D reconstruction of the same fetus at 24 weeks clearly showing bilateral talipes equinovarus.

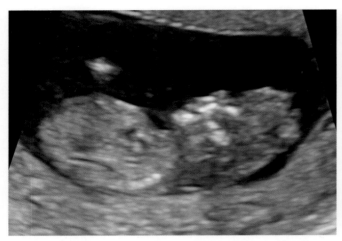

Fig. 1.34 Twelve-week' gestation ultrasound scan showing the head and face of a fetus with anencephaly.

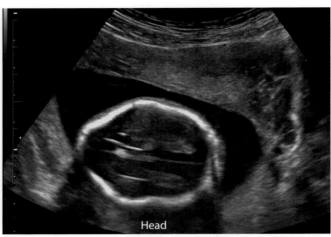

Fig. 1.35 Spina bifida was diagnosed in this fetus at 18 weeks' gestation. The lemon-shaped head is evident on ultrasonography.

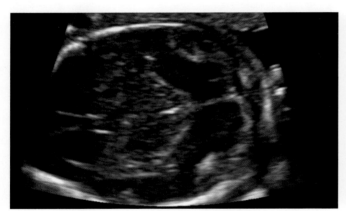

Fig. 1.36 Posterior view of the fetal skull showing dilatation of the posterior horns of the lateral ventricles in hydrocephalus.

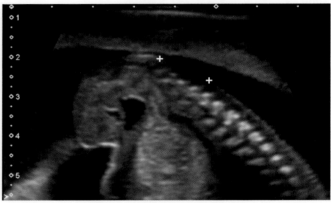

Fig. 1.37 Spina bifida of the lumbosacral spine on an antenatal scan showing an obvious gap in the dorsal arches (between the + markers).

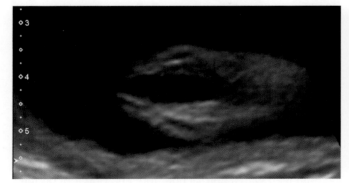

Fig. 1.38 Spina bifida showing a lumbosacral defect, which is probably myelomeningocele filled with cerebrospinal fluid (CSF).

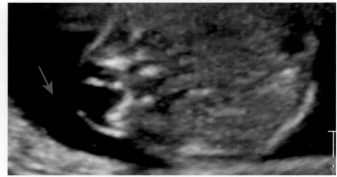

Fig. 1.39 Transverse scan of the trunk at 30 weeks' gestation showing the myelomeningocele containing CSF (arrow).

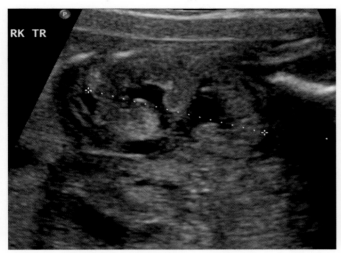

Fig. 1.40 Ultrasound scan at 28 weeks' gestation showing a duplex right kidney.

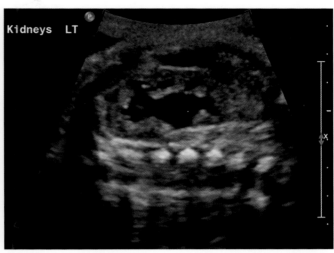

Fig. 1.41 Pelvicalyceal dilatation in the left kidney evident at 28 weeks' gestation.

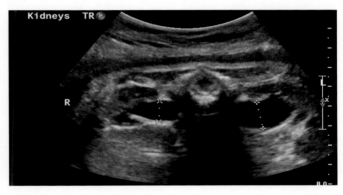

Fig. 1.42 Transverse scan of a 32-week fetus showing bilateral dilatation of the renal pelves. In this fetus posterior urethral valves must be considered and the gender, posterior urethra, thickness of the bladder wall and whether the bladder is emptying normally must also be evaluated.

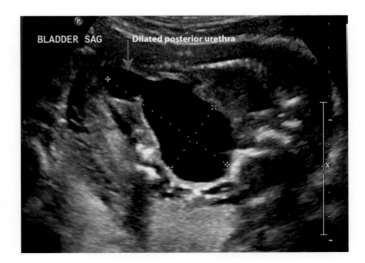

Fig. 1.43 Keyhole sign on an 18-week gestation ultrasound scan showing dilatation of both bladder and posterior urethra, consistent with a diagnosis of posterior urethral valves.

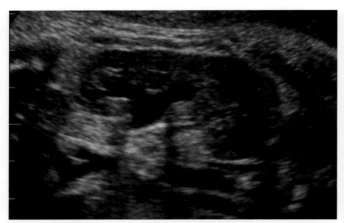

Fig. 1.44 Duplex left kidney with dilatation of the lower pole moiety.

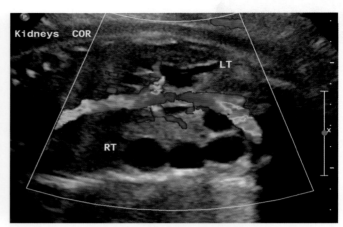

Fig. 1.45 Colour Doppler scan at 28 weeks' gestation showing both kidneys with some dilatation of the left kidney and multiple cysts in the right kidney, suggestive of a multicystic dysplastic kidney.

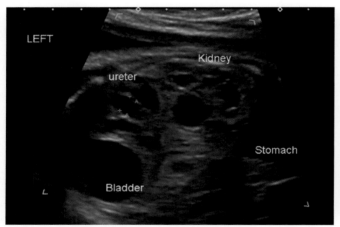

Fig. 1.46 Longitudinal view of the trunk showing hydroureteronephrosis and a full bladder in a fetus with posterior urethral valves.

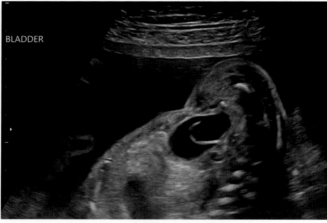

Fig. 1.47 Scan of the fetal pelvis showing a dilated bladder with a large ureterocele, which may prolapse into and block the urethra.

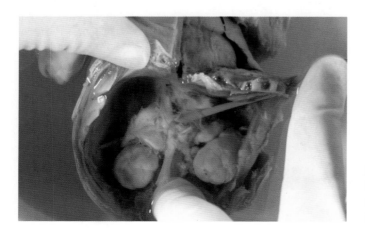

Fig. 1.48 The fetal adrenal is almost the same size as the fetal kidney. In this 16-week fetus, sectioned at the mid-abdominal level, the right adrenal dominates the right kidney on which it sits.

Most major conditions in the neonate that require surgical correction are congenital, but a few (e.g. neonatal necrotising enterocolitis and pulmonary interstitial emphysema) are acquired. They often have external manifestations and are obvious at birth (e.g. gastroschisis and imperforate anus) or cause functional disturbance, which enables them to be diagnosed within the first few days (e.g. severe respiratory insufficiency in congenital diaphragmatic hernia and bilious vomiting in duodenal atresia).

VENTRAL ABDOMINAL WALL DEFECTS

The two most common major ventral abdominal wall defects are exomphalos and gastroschisis. In exomphalos, there is a large defect at the umbilicus with protrusion of abdominal viscera into a thin membranous sac, which is formed by amniotic membrane on the outside and peritoneum on the inside. In the vast majority of infants, the sac is intact irrespective of the mode of delivery (vaginal delivery versus caesarean section). At birth the contents, usually small bowel and liver, can be seen clearly through the translucent membrane but as desiccation of the membrane occurs, it becomes opaque. The size and shape of the defect vary considerably, and in very large defects (giant exomphalos), most of the intra-abdominal viscera are within the sac, and the abdomen appears scaphoid and of small volume. The skin of the ventral abdominal wall extends up the side of the sac to a variable degree. The umbilical arteries and umbilical vein can be seen traversing within the membrane, converging at the umbilical cord. Exomphalos is associated with other major congenital abnormalities, particularly cardiac, renal and chromosomal, in about 50% of cases. In Beckwith–Wiedemann syndrome, there is hemihypertrophy, macroglossia, visceromegaly and abnormal facies. It is essential to detect and treat accompanying hypoglycaemia.

In gastroschisis, the actual defect in the ventral abdominal wall is much smaller, and nearly always lies immediately to the right of the umbilicus. The umbilical vessels are unaffected and are situated to the left of the protruding bowel. There is no covering membrane. Much of the bowel and, frequently, the stomach herniates through the defect and the bowel and mesentery may be thickened, congested and oedematous with an overlying fibrin 'peel'. Gangrene of the herniated bowel may occur if the blood supply is occluded by the narrow opening or as a result of volvulus. Where this process has occurred well before birth, the necrotic bowel is resorbed, leaving an atresia. In gastroschisis, extraintestinal abnormalities are uncommon.

EXSTROPHY

Bladder exstrophy and cloacal exstrophy are major congenital abnormalities involving failure of the lower abdominal wall to close, exposing the mucosal surface of the bladder. Other features may include exomphalos, pubic diastasis, deficient urethra, unfused genitalia and rectal prolapse.

PRUNE BELLY SYNDROME

The infant, usually a boy, is born with a flat and wrinkled-looking abdomen and undescended testes. Prune belly syndrome may be due to transient intrauterine obstruction of urinary outflow, causing gross distension of the bladder and upper urinary tract, which in turn is the cause of abdominal distension. Another theory is that the condition is due to abnormal mesodermal development.

Following spontaneous relief of obstruction, the stretched and attenuated ventral abdominal wall looks shrivelled and wrinkled ('like a prune') but the dilatation of the urinary tract persists, often for many years.

ANORECTAL MALFORMATIONS

Anorectal malformations manifest as a range of appearances. In 'low' lesions in the male, a fistula communicates with the skin via an opening in the midline anterior to the normal position of the anus, either in the perineum, scrotum or ventral midline of the penis. 'High' lesions frequently have a communication with the urinary tract, most commonly through a rectourethral fistula, but occasionally directly into the bladder neck as a rectovesical fistula. 'High' anorectal malformations may occur without any fistula; this variant is most commonly seen in Down syndrome.

In the female, the number of external orifices in the perineum will give some indication of the level of the anomaly. Where there are three openings, namely urethral, vaginal and anal, the lesion is a 'low' one; when there are two obvious openings, namely urethral and vaginal, it is a high lesion; and when there is one opening, it is known as a cloacal abnormality. The exception to this general rule is in the case of a rectovestibular fistula, which may have the same external appearance as an anovestibular fistula. The clinical distinction can be made according to the direction in which a probe runs. In the former, it will tend to run deeply parallel to the vagina, whereas in the latter, it will run first in a posterior direction in a subcutaneous plane, before it turns deeply at the level of the anus.

A fistula opening on the perineal skin is easily identified when it transmits meconium or air, but the opening can be tiny and requires a careful search with magnification and good illumination. In high lesions in males, the presence of a rectourethral or rectovesical fistula can be inferred if air or meconium is passed per urethram. The fistula is usually confirmed by subsequent contrast studies (distal loopogram and cystourethrography), which show 'beaking' of the terminal rectum where the contrast enters the urinary tract.

The use of an 'invertogram' (or shoot-through lateral radiograph of the pelvis with the baby prone) at 12–24 hours of age, once gas reaches the distal bowel, may provide additional information on the level of the abnormality. The radiograph is taken in an exact lateral projection with the baby being placed prone over a padded wedge. Gas rises to the apex of the blind-ending rectum, and the level is related to various skeletal landmarks corresponding to the levator sling. There is less reliance on plain radiographs these days to determine the level of the anorectal malformation because clinical examination with or without a perineal ultrasound scan is often sufficient.

Neonates with an anorectal malformation require investigation for associated anomalies: an ultrasound scan of the urinary tract and spine and radiographs of the chest and spine. Some also need an echocardiogram and/or karyotyping. Those with 'high' lesions usually require management with a temporary diverting stoma and are further investigated at a later date by contrast studies ± endoscopy.

AMBIGUOUS GENITALIA (DISORDERS OF SEXUAL DEVELOPMENT [DSD])

Genitalia are considered ambiguous when one or more of the following features are present:

1 The phallus is too large for a clitoris or too small for a penis.
2 The urethral opening is proximal, near the labioscrotal (genital) folds.
3 The genital folds remain unfused, giving the appearance of labia or of a cleft scrotum.
4 The testes are either not descended or impalpable.

There is variation in the degree of abnormality that may be present, making gender assignment at birth hazardous. Prompt and accurate diagnosis is imperative because of the social implications for the parents of not being able to announce the gender of the baby, and the malformation may be the outward sign of the life-threatening condition congenital adrenal hyperplasia. When congenital adrenal hyperplasia occurs in females, the appearance of the external genitalia may cover a broad spectrum, suggestive more of either male or female. In the commonest autosomal recessive variety, deficiency of the adrenocortical enzyme 21-hydroxylase causes low cortisol levels and a compensatory increase in secretion of pituitary adrenocorticotrophic hormone, resulting in adrenal hyperplasia. The excessive androgens produced in females cause virilisation of the external genitalia but the internal anatomy is normal for a female. Investigations include estimation of serum electrolytes and blood glucose (to detect hyponatraemia, hyperkalaemia and hypoglycaemia), serum 17-hydroxyprogesterone and urinary pregnanetriol. Chromosomal analysis is mandatory and screening for the known genes involved in sex development is becoming more common. A urogenital sinogram or urethroscopy will show a masculinised urethra and the presence of a vagina and cervix. A pelvic ultrasound confirms the presence of a uterus, Fallopian tubes and ovaries.

Some infants are born with normal male chromosomes and testes but with insensitivity to androgens. A genetic abnormality in the androgen receptor system prevents the normal target tissues for androgens (Wolffian ducts and external genitalia) from responding to androgen stimulation. The abnormality may be partial or complete. In the complete form (complete androgen insensitivity syndrome, CAIS), the external genitalia are completely female in appearance. The clue to the gonads being testes in a phenotypic female is their discovery in inguinal herniae. The normal secretion and response to anti-Müllerian hormone (AMH) leads to regression of the Müllerian ducts, while failure to respond to androgens prevents the development of a vas deferens.

Disorders of sex development may be produced by dysplasia of one or both testes. When both testes are dysplastic, deficiency of androgen may cause incomplete virilisation, and deficiency of AMH may allow persistence of Müllerian duct structures. Usually, both testes are undescended because they are unable to secrete enough hormones to enable testicular descent. In the asymmetrical form of dysplastic testes (mixed gonadal dysgenesis), one gonad may be a testis that has descended with preservation of the ipsilateral Wolffian duct and local regression of the Müllerian duct. The more dysplastic testis usually remains in the abdomen and has failed to cause regression of the Müllerian duct or preservation of the Wolffian duct. Infants with mixed gonadal dysgenesis may appear to be males with severe hypospadias and one palpable testis. These dysplastic testes have an increased risk of malignant degeneration.

In severe hypospadias with undescended testes the phallus may be large enough to indicate that the infant is essentially male, and usually the chromosomal karyotype is normal male (46, XY). A contrast urethrogram will demonstrate a normal male urethra without a vagina or uterus. The testes may be impalpable (in the inguinal canal or abdomen) or palpable near the pubic tubercle, on one or both sides. Severe hypospadias with undescended testes has to be distinguished from DSDs, such as severe virilising congenital adrenal hyperplasia or one of the causes of dysplastic testes.

When a newborn has ambiguous genitalia, clinical examination includes assessment of the external genitalia to determine:

1 The size of the phallus.
2 The degree of fusion of the inner genital folds to form a urethra.
3 The degree of outer genital fold fusion to form a scrotum, with its characteristically wrinkled skin.

The phallus should be lifted up to expose its ventral surface, and the genital folds spread apart to help identify the position of the urethral orifice. The skin should be carefully examined for evidence of excess pigmentation, which is common in congenital adrenal hyperplasia because of the excess melanin-stimulating hormone produced by the pituitary.

The next step is to determine the position of the gonads. Two palpable testes in the scrotum indicate that not only is the underlying sex of the child male, but also that there has been sufficient hormonal stimulation to cause testicular descent. If there are no testes palpable in the groins or labioscrotal folds, the presence of a uterus should be determined. A cervix may be palpable on rectal examination using the little finger. The presence of a uterus implies that there has been either absent or insufficient AMH.

A child with congenital adrenal hyperplasia may be vomiting, appear thin and be dehydrated, depending on the degree of salt loss and the time since birth. The nipples, skin creases and genitalia may be pigmented. Virilisation of the external genitalia is proportional to the degree of urogenital fusion. The only clue to the true sex of the child may be the absence of testes. Early and accurate diagnosis is important because:

1 Urgent medical treatment may be required if the infant has congenital adrenal hyperplasia.
2 There may be genetic implications affecting counselling.
3 The potential fertility of the infant should be established.
4 A plan for surgical management is helpful in many cases.

CONGENITAL DIAPHRAGMATIC HERNIA

Most affected children are now diagnosed from routine antenatal ultrasound scans. The defect in the diaphragm is usually left-sided and posterolateral (Bochdalek hernia). The rapidity of onset and severity of respiratory distress vary with the degree of lung hypoplasia. There is associated pulmonary hypertension from concomitant abnormal development of the pulmonary vasculature. In the most severe cases, poor peripheral perfusion and cardiovascular collapse occur within minutes of birth. A few children with a minor degree of lung hypoplasia have no symptoms for days or months and

may present later with gastrointestinal symptoms or an incidental finding on imaging.

In neonatal cases, the chest is barrel-shaped and the abdomen is scaphoid because the bowel has herniated through the diaphragmatic defect into the chest. Once air is swallowed, this sign becomes less obvious. The bowel and liver in the chest displace the mediastinum to the contralateral side. In a left-sided diaphragmatic hernia, this produces apparent dextrocardia (with the heart sounds most easily audible in the right chest) and poor breath sounds on the left side. Bowel sounds may be heard in the chest on auscultation, but this sign is not particularly reliable. The diagnosis is confirmed on a plain chest radiograph. The film should include the abdomen so that the distribution of bowel gas can be determined and an oro- or nasogastric tube should be *in situ*. The features on x-ray include:

1 Loops of bowel within the chest on the side of the defect.
2 Hemidiaphragm not visible.
3 Mediastinal shift to the contralateral side.
4 Abnormal distribution of bowel gas within the abdomen.

The radiological appearances have to be distinguished from cystic lung disease, lobar emphysema, staphylococcal pneumonia with pneumatoceles and other diaphragmatic defects.

OESOPHAGEAL ATRESIA

In oesophageal atresia, the upper oesophagus ends blindly in the upper chest and there is absence of a variable length of the mid-portion of the oesophagus. In the majority of affected patients (approximately 85%), there is a distal tracheo-oesophageal fistula. Occasionally, there may be no fistula at all, or a proximal fistula with or without a distal tracheo-oesophageal fistula. An isolated tracheo-oesophageal fistula without oesophageal atresia is often included in discussion of these abnormalities, although oesophageal continuity means that the tracheo-oesophageal fistula (H-fistula) may not be recognised until beyond the neonatal period. The infant with oesophageal atresia usually presents within hours of birth with excessive drooling (the 'mucousy' baby) from accumulation in the blind upper oesophagus of saliva that cannot be swallowed.

There may be respiratory distress, which may have a variety of causes including ineffective ventilation from escape of air down the fistula, diaphragmatic splinting from gaseous abdominal distension, aspiration pneumonia and respiratory distress syndrome of prematurity. Nearly half these babies are premature and there may be a history of maternal polyhydramnios. The diagnosis is made by passing a 10Fr feeding tube through the mouth and observing that it becomes arrested at about 10 cm from the gums. A smaller calibre tube may curl up in the blind-ending upper pouch, giving the false impression of oesophageal continuity. A plain radiograph of the chest and abdomen reveals whether there is a distal tracheo-oesophageal fistula; if present, the fistula allows gas into the stomach, which can be observed on x-ray. Associated congenital abnormalities are sought, particularly those in relation to the VACTERL association (Vertebral, Anal, Cardiac, Tracheo-Esophageal, Renal, Limb). These include imperforate anus, congenital heart disease, urinary tract abnormalities and vertebral and limb abnormalities. There is also an increased incidence of duodenal atresia. About 7% of infants born with oesophageal atresia have a significant chromosomal anomaly.

If no gas is seen below the diaphragm on x-ray, it implies there is no distal tracheo-oesophageal fistula. Most of these patients will have no fistula at all, but in 10–20% there will be a proximal tracheo-oesophageal fistula connecting the upper oesophageal pouch and the trachea. This may be identified either on tracheobronchoscopy or by performing a careful upper oesophageal contrast study, avoiding overflow of contrast into the lungs.

In isolated tracheo-oesophageal fistula, the symptoms may include respiratory distress, recurrent or repeated episodes of pneumonia, abdominal distension and choking with feeds. The fistula can be identified by a prone tube oesophageal contrast study or by tracheobronchoscopy. The fistula runs obliquely between the two structures in the lower neck, and can be divided via a cervical approach.

INTESTINAL ATRESIAS

The three cardinal symptoms of bowel obstruction in the neonate are:

1 Vomiting (particularly bilious vomiting).
2 Abdominal distension.
3 Failure to pass, or delay in the passage of, meconium.

It is important to recognise that in the neonate these symptoms represent mechanical obstruction until proved otherwise. Other causes of these symptoms include:

1 Localised or generalised sepsis.
2 Congenital heart disease.
3 Inborn errors of metabolism.

There are various causes of neonatal bowel obstruction (*Table 2.1*). Most mechanical causes present with symptoms and signs within 48 hours of birth, whereas functional obstructions (e.g. Hirschsprung disease and necrotising enterocolitis) usually present later. Bile-stained vomiting, in the absence of generalised abdominal distension, is suggestive of a high obstruction (e.g. midgut volvulus or duodenal atresia), whereas vomiting of milk, which after a period becomes bile-stained, with obvious abdominal distension, is more likely to be associated with

TABLE 2.1 Causes of neonatal bowel obstruction	
Disease	**Frequency**
Hirschsprung disease	More common
Necrotising enterocolitis	
Small bowel atresia	Less common
Malrotation with volvulus	
Duodenal atresia/stenosis	
Imperforate anus	
Meconium ileus	
Prenatal perforation (meconium peritonitis)	Uncommon

distal small bowel or colonic obstruction. Atresia of the small bowel (ileum or jejunum) is relatively common in comparison with colonic atresia, which is rare. Small bowel atresias may be multiple. Any infant who presents with green vomitus as the initial symptom should be regarded as having intestinal malrotation with volvulus until proved otherwise, because of the potentially fatal outcome of this condition.

Abdominal distension at delivery suggests distal small bowel obstruction, and is typical of meconium ileus. More distal bowel obstructions, as seen with anorectal malformations, Hirschsprung disease or necrotising enterocolitis, do not present with abdominal distension at birth. In intestinal malrotation with volvulus, abdominal distension may develop late as a result of volvulus causing obstruction of both the duodenal and colonic ends of the midgut and loss of fluid into the gut. In this situation, the abdomen may become dramatically distended and exhibit signs of peritoneal irritation. Other causes of abdominal distension/mass (e.g. massive hydronephrosis, ovarian cyst, duplication cyst, ascites or organomegaly) must be considered. Percussion of the abdomen is helpful in determining whether the distension is from dilated loops full of air or from fluid or solid structures.

Meconium is passed within 24 hours of birth in 95% of neonates born at term. One feature of Hirschsprung disease is failure to pass meconium in the first 24 hours after birth. However, in premature or very sick neonates, passage of meconium may also be delayed.

MECONIUM ILEUS

In this condition, meconium becomes excessively tenacious and sticky, causing a mechanical bowel obstruction in the ileum. The obstruction is caused by hard pellets of impacted faecal material. In most cases, meconium ileus is due to cystic fibrosis, which *in utero* causes changes to the physical properties of the meconium to make it more viscous.

The radiological appearance is variable, but classically includes air–fluid levels and a foamy pattern of air bubbles trapped around the impacted meconium. A contrast enema will demonstrate a microcolon, because the colon is unused and empty. In meconium ileus there is abdominal distension at birth, which increases subsequently. If the heavy meconium-laden ileum twists *in utero*, the infant will be born with an intestinal atresia and signs of meconium peritonitis, including intra-abdominal calcification. A localised volvulus may also occur after birth, and cause peritonitis.

The presence of ischaemic or perforated bowel must be suspected in any neonate with marked abdominal distension. Abdominal tenderness and guarding, discolouration of the thin abdominal wall, tight and shiny skin over a distended abdomen with progressive oedema and redness of the abdominal wall, and signs of sepsis and shock are all suggestive of an underlying necrotic bowel and peritonitis. On x-ray, free gas may be evident under the diaphragm or outlining the falciform ligament (football sign) or both sides of the bowel wall (Rigler sign). It is important to take a lateral decubitus or lateral 'shoot-through' radiograph, as well as a supine film, to demonstrate small amounts of free gas in the peritoneal cavity.

HIRSCHSPRUNG DISEASE

Hirschsprung disease produces a functional obstruction secondary to absence of ganglion cells in the distal large bowel. The affected segment begins at the anorectal junction and extends proximally for a variable distance – in most cases as far as the sigmoid colon. On occasions (<10%), the affected segment can extend as far as the small bowel (total colonic aganglionosis) or, very rarely, involve the entire alimentary tract, in which situation survival is unlikely. Hirschsprung disease becomes apparent clinically in the first few days of life, when it manifests as delayed passage of meconium, followed by vomiting and abdominal distension. On rectal examination, the anus and rectum may feel tight and there may be a squirt of meconium and air on extraction of the examining little finger. The plain radiological appearance is non-specific but often shows dilated bowel with absence of rectal gas. A contrast enema may demonstrate a narrow rectal lumen with a transition zone in the proximal rectum or sigmoid colon. The definitive diagnosis is made when a suction rectal biopsy shows an absence of intrinsic ganglion cells and hypertrophic extrinsic nerve fibres. In the common type of Hirschsprung disease, males outnumber females by about 4:1, and the aganglionic segment rarely extends beyond the sigmoid colon proximally. Infants with more extensive long-segment disease have an equal sex incidence; in these there is a high degree of 'penetrance' with subsequent siblings more likely to be affected.

NEONATAL NECROTISING ENTEROCOLITIS

Neonatal necrotising enterocolitis is a potentially fatal disease in which there is ischaemia of the bowel associated with inflammation and gas forming bacteria. Premature neonates are most at risk but term infants are not immune. Abnormal gut flora, formula feeds (rather than breast milk),

immature mucosal defence mechanisms, sepsis and compromised gut perfusion are all implicated in the pathogenesis of the disease. Onset is usually within 1–3 weeks of birth but is inversely related to gestational age. The infant becomes ill, lethargic and intolerant of feeds. There may be fever. Vomiting occurs early, and may become bile-stained. There is abdominal distension and the passage of loose stools containing a variable amount of blood, mucus and even necrotic tissue.

Mucosal necrosis progresses to full-thickness bowel necrosis and signs of peritonitis develop: the anterior abdominal wall becomes oedematous and red, with dilated veins. Abdominal palpation causes pain. A mass may be palpable if a localised intraperitoneal abscess has developed or if there is a persistent dilated loop of affected bowel.

The radiological features are variable. The pathognomonic finding is intramural gas ('pneumatosis intestinalis'). Gas outlining the portal vein and its branches ('portal venous gas') suggests severe disease. Free gas in the peritoneal cavity outlining the falciform ligament (football sign) or both sides of the bowel wall (Rigler sign) indicates intestinal perforation. Small amounts of free gas are best seen on a decubitus or lateral shoot-through radiograph. Other radiological features include gaseous dilatation, excessive peritoneal fluid – seen as separation of adjacent loops of bowel – and an abnormal distribution of bowel gas. At operation, the disease may be extensive and involve most or all of the bowel, or it may be localised to more discrete areas, usually within the ileum or colon.

Following medical treatment, a stricture may form, most often in the colon.

NEURAL TUBE DEFECTS

These are a group of congenital disorders in which the brain and/or spinal cord are malformed as a result of abnormal closure of the neural tube in the embryo. A range of malformations exist with variable neurological deficits. Most neural tube defects are readily detectable by antenatal screening tests including ultrasound imaging. In anencephaly, the cephalic part of the neural tube has failed not only to close, but also to develop. Deficiency of the vault of the skull exposes the brainstem and cerebellum – most of the cerebrum is missing. An encephalocele is a neural tube defect affecting the brain, and is commonest in the occipital and frontal regions.

In open spina bifida, the spinal defect is not covered by skin. There are two main variants: myelomeningocele in which neural elements are exposed (this accounts for about 90% and is associated with hydrocephalus and the Arnold Chiari malformation) and meningocele. When a baby is born with obvious open spina bifida, the vertebral level of the neural tube defect should be established as this predicts the degree of neurological deficit. Lumbosacral lesions are the most common, but fusion defects can occur at any point along the spine. The lesion may leak cerebrospinal fluid or tissue fluid from the exposed neuroepithelium. With a meningocele, a communication with the subarachnoid space can be shown when direct pressure on the lesion causes the fontanelle to bulge. Likewise, the lesion will become more tense during crying, when intracranial pressure is increased.

The level of paralysis in the neonate with myelomeningocele may be difficult to determine exactly, but observation of spontaneous movement of the hips, knees and ankles without external stimulation is revealing. The motor deficit can be estimated by observing active movement in the hips, knees and ankles. When the lesion includes nerves from or above the third lumbar segment, the legs are totally paralysed. If L3 is functional, the posture is of flexion of the hip and extension of the knee, but there is no other limb movement. When there is preservation of L4 and L5 spinal segments, there is movement of the hip and knee and the foot can actively dorsiflex, but no plantar flexion occurs. Muscular imbalance around the ankle may cause talipes. When the first two sacral segments are intact, leg movements are essentially normal, but bowel and bladder incontinence is still likely.

The sensory deficit is usually less than the corresponding motor deficit. The pattern of dermatome distribution in the neonate is the same as that in adults. The perianal skin is innervated by the third and fourth sacral segments. The sensory level is determined by commencing examination in the anaesthetic region, and proceeding towards an area of normal sensation. Rectal prolapse and absence of a natal cleft indicate paralysis of the pelvic floor muscles and adjacent bowel and bladder sphincters.

Reflex contraction of the external anal sphincter and gluteal muscles to stimulation with a blunt-ended pin will occur if the distal sacral segments are intact. Normal perineal sensation and musculature suggests that bladder function is preserved, which can be confirmed by manual compression of the lower abdomen, which should not produce incontinence of urine.

The presence and development of hydrocephalus should be sought, as well as orthopaedic deformities of the spine, hips and feet. Secondary kyphoscoliosis is common, and if there are associated hermivertebrae, may be present at birth. The lumbosacral myelomeningocele may produce imbalance of the hip muscles, causing congenital dislocation of the hip. Therefore, Ortolani's test should be performed (Chapter 9).

In closed spina bifida, the defect is covered by skin but there is a visible abnormality of the overlying or adjacent skin such as a dermal sinus, haemangioma, hairy patch, fatty lump or other cutaneous marking. These lesions are also referred to as occult spinal dysraphism and may be associated with a tethered spinal cord, which may cause neurological signs later in childhood, including dysfunctional voiding, pes cavus and clumsiness of the legs. When a sinus or dermoid cyst of the spinal canal has an external connection, meningitis may occur. A careful inspection of the dorsal midline should be conducted to identify a possible sinus opening in any patient who develops meningitis in which a skin organism is cultured. These sinuses may not be particularly obvious. They usually lie outside the coccygeal area (above the intergluteal cleft) and should be distinguished from the common sacral dimple.

Spina bifida occulta (a skin covered posterior vertebral defect with no visible external abnormalities) is a common incidental finding on x-ray of the lower spine and is rarely associated with abnormal neurology. There is a gap in the dorsal arches of the fourth and fifth lumbar vertebrae and the first sacral vertebra.

Rare variants of neural tube fusion may occur, with the spinal cord split longitudinally by a bony ridge within the vertebral canal (diastematomyelia). Some myelomeningoceles are associated with a teratoma. In the rare Currarino syndrome there is a sacral dysgenesis (typically a hemisacrum) combined with a presacral mass (e.g. an anterior sacral meningocele or teratoma) and an anorectal malformation (usually anorectal stenosis).

CONJOINED TWINS

Conjoined twins are rare, occurring in about one in 50,000–100,000 births. They are understood to be caused by early division of the inner cell mass during embryogenesis, which forms two identical, but attached, fetuses. The classification of conjoined twins relates to the site of attachment, the commonest variety being thoraco-omphalopagus, where the attachment is along the sternum and upper abdomen. Pygopagus twins, in which the pelvis of each infant is the site of connection, occur in about 20% of instances. Conjoined twins connected by the head (craniopagus) occur in only 5% of instances. Conjoined twins require detailed and careful investigation to determine the exact anatomical and functional status of each twin. Xiphopagus twins, joined around the xiphisternum and epigastrium, often share a fused liver, but this is one of the most favourable types for separation. Surgery is best deferred until detailed imaging has been performed and an opportunity to observe function of the various organs. The ultimate aim of surgery is to separate the twins to produce two live, separate infants. Sometimes, unequal distribution of organs does not allow equal separation. In addition, in some instances of conjoined twinning, the development of each twin is not symmetrical, so that one twin is much larger than the other. In its more extreme form, this may present at birth with the appearance of a parasitic, dysmorphic twin attached to the external surface of the otherwise normal twin.

SACROCOCCYGEAL TERATOMA

This is a rare congenital germ cell tumour occurring at the caudal end of the developing vertebral column (notochord). The tumour is usually attached to the coccyx. It may be a large (exophytic) tumour obvious at birth, or may be concealed (endophytic) growing anteriorly from the coccyx into the pelvis behind the rectum. Large external tumours diagnosed at birth are excised promptly. Endophytic tumours may not be diagnosed until later and are more likely to have become malignant. Many sacrococcygeal tumours are now detected by prenatal ultrasound scan and affected fetuses require monitoring *in utero* because of the potential of the tumour to recruit a high blood flow and cause fetal hydrops. All sacrococcygeal teratomas, irrespective of their external appearance, need prompt excision after birth because of the high risk of malignant degeneration in the first few months of life.

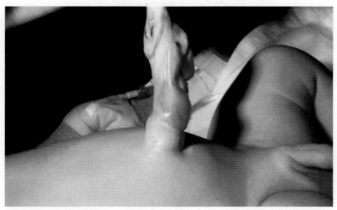

Fig. 2.1 This is the most minor form of exomphalos, essentially a hernia into the umbilical cord. Care must be taken when clamping the cord to avoid inadvertent injury to the bowel within the defect.

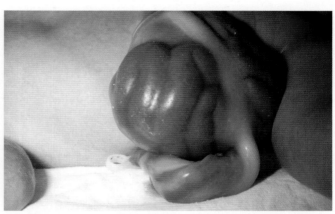

Fig. 2.2 A typical intermediate-sized exomphalos, with loops of small bowel visible through the translucent sac. The sac consists of apposed layers of amnion and peritoneum. As the sac dries it becomes opaque, such that the sac contents become more difficult to see.

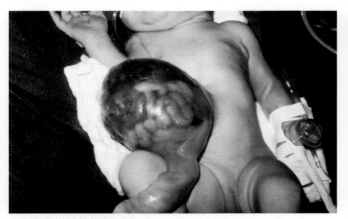

Fig. 2.3 A large exomphalos into which have herniated loops of bowel and the liver. The relatively small size of the abdominal cavity may make an exomphalos of this size difficult to close at birth with primary surgery.

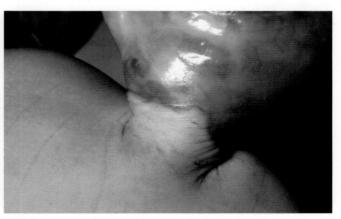

Fig. 2.4 In this moderate-sized exomphalos, the neck is relatively narrow and the skin of the abdominal wall can be seen encroaching on the sac.

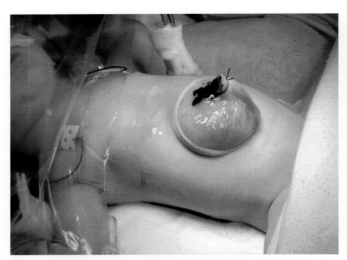

Fig. 2.5 Exomphalos major with a wide defect in the abdominal wall.

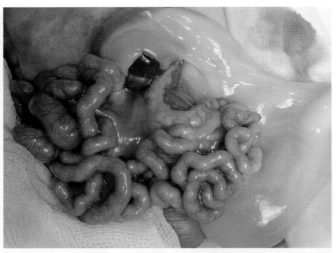

Fig. 2.6 Exomphalos with early rupture of the sac.

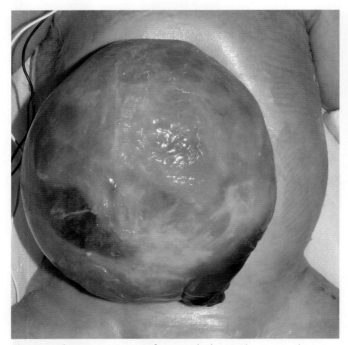

Fig. 2.7 The appearance of exomphalos major, sometimes known as 'giant exomphalos, several days after birth.

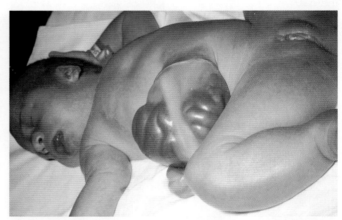

Fig. 2.8 This large baby presented with exomphalos and visceromegaly, features suggestive of Beckwith–Weidemann syndrome. The enlarged viscera may be the result of excess insulin production by the fetal pancreas. The babies are at risk of profound postnatal hypoglycaemia, which might be severe enough to cause cerebral injury. The hypoglycaemia and excess insulin production usually resolve spontaneously within a week or two of birth.

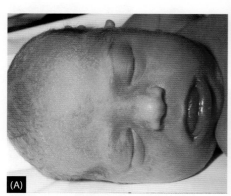
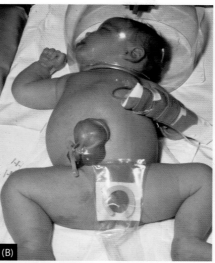
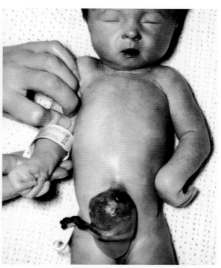

Figs. 2.9A, B (A) An infant born with Beckwith–Weidemann syndrome and exomphalos usually will have an abnormal facial appearance, with an enlarged tongue (seen here) and abnormal grooves in the earlobes. Later in life the child is predisposed to some solid tumours, including Wilms tumour, adrenal tumours and hepatoblastoma. (B) An infant with Beckwith–Weidemann syndrome with obvious macrosomia and exomphalos minor. Note the macroglossia.

Fig. 2.10 A baby with exomphalos who has trisomy 18.

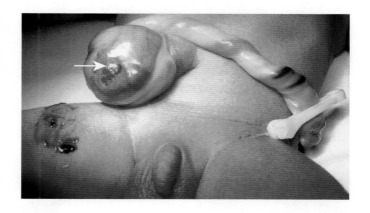

Fig. 2.11 Perforation of the sac in exomphalos, caused by pressure during transfer to the tertiary centre. The leakage of meconium can be seen as a stain on the right thigh (perforation arrowed).

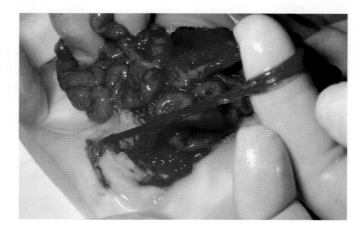

Fig. 2.12 A Meckel band from the ileum to the under surface of the fundus of the exomphalos sac, demonstrated at operation.

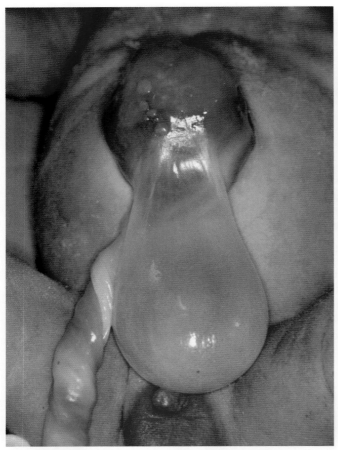

Fig. 2.13 A common finding is peritoneal fluid collecting in a sacculus related to the exomphalos. It has no particular significance.

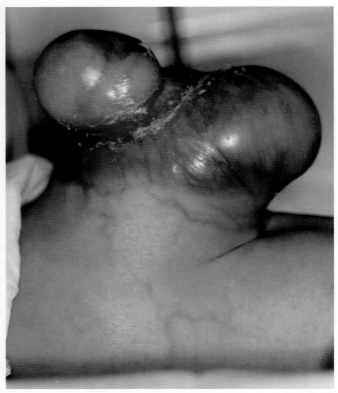

Fig. 2.14 The late appearance of a large exomphalos treated non-operatively by topical application of antiseptic at birth. In this infant, at 6 months of age, the skin has largely covered the defect, giving the appearance of a somewhat irregular incisional hernia. These are difficult to repair.

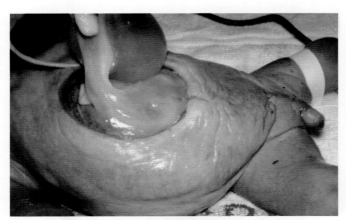

Fig. 2.15 Exomphalos in association with prune belly syndrome.

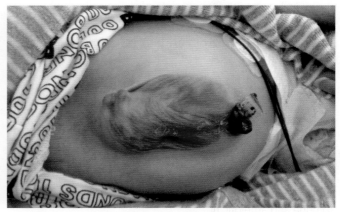

Fig. 2.16 Pentalogy of Cantrell, showing the abdominal wall defect extending up to include the xiphisternum, making the possibility of defects in the diaphragm, pericardium and heart very likely.

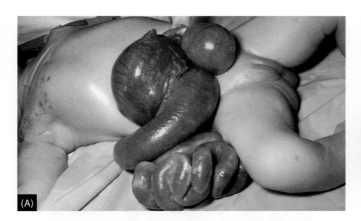

(A)

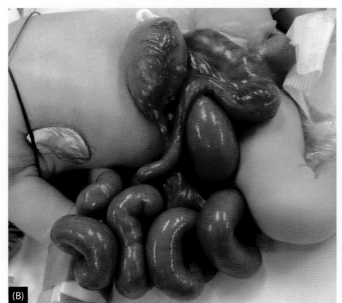

(B)

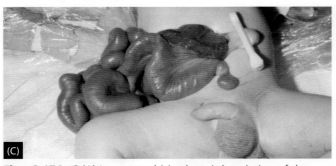

(C)

Figs. 2.17A–C (A) In gastroschisis, there is herniation of the abdominal contents, sometimes including bladder, through a defect adjacent to the umbilicus. The bowel is covered with a fibrinous exudate (or 'peel'), believed to be caused by exposure to urine and amniotic fluid *in utero*. (B) Gastroschisis in which herniation of the stomach, small bowel and colon has occurred. The calibre change from dilated proximal bowel to narrow ileum should alert the surgeon to possible atresia of the small bowel. (C) A baby with gastroschisis, where the testis has prolapsed out of the defect in the abdominal wall.

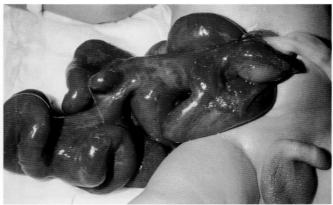

Fig. 2.18 A close-up view of the oedema and foreshortening of the thickened bowel, adjacent loops of which are matted together. The defect is almost always to the right of the umbilicus. In this infant, the umbilicus can be seen to the left of the protruding bowel.

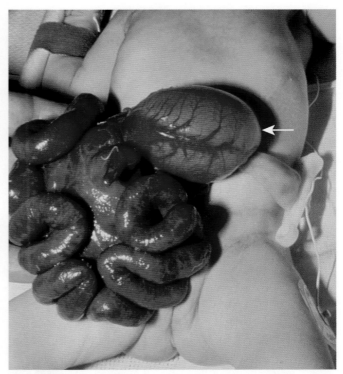

Fig. 2.19 The oedema and exudate is confined to the small bowel, which has been exposed to the amniotic fluid *in utero*. Postnatally, after the infant swallowed air, the stomach (arrow) also protruded through the defect, but is not oedematous and is not covered with exudate.

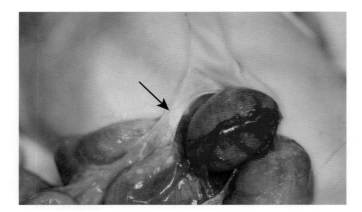

Fig. 2.20 An amniotic band (arrow) with secondary attachment to the mesentery of the herniated bowel, consistent with it being a ruptured umbilical cord prior to birth. The general features were those of gastroschisis rather than exomphalos.

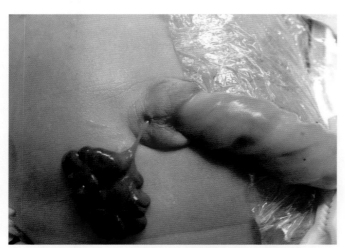

Fig. 2.21 Infarction of the herniated gut in gastroschisis ('vanishing gastroschisis') secondary to vascular compression of the gut mesentery by a very narrow abdominal wall defect.

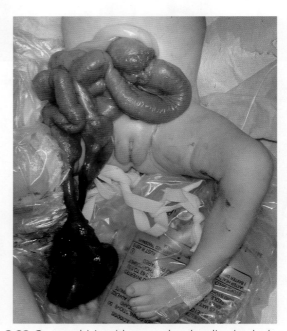

Fig. 2.22 Gastroschisis with secondary localised volvulus and necrosis of the gut.

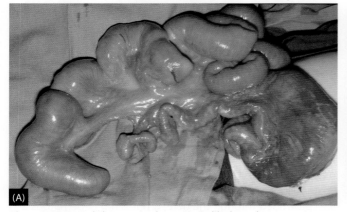

(A)

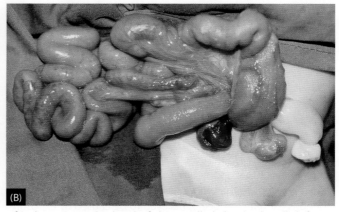

(B)

Figs. 2.23A, B (A) Intestinal atresia is likely to be a consequence of ischaemia at the level of the small abdominal wall defect or to volvulus of the herniated bowel, both of which cut off the supply of blood to the bowel and result in its atrophy and resorption *in utero*. (B) Gastroschisis with both testes extruded along with multiple loops of bowel.

Fig. 2.24 Prolapse of a vitello-intestinal duct associated with an ileal atresia. Superficially, this looks similar to a gastroschisis, but on careful inspection the surface of the bowel is mucosal, rather than serosal, suggesting that it has intussuscepted through the wide vitello-intestinal duct.

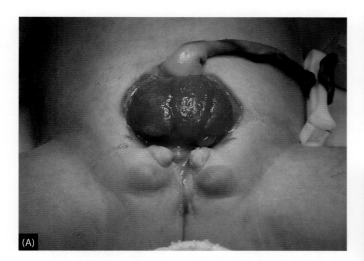

(A)

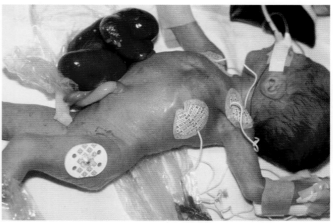

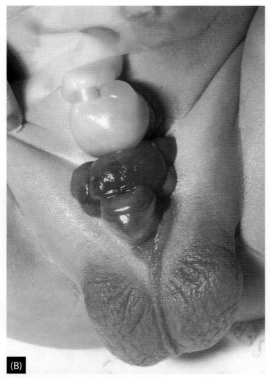

(B)

Figs. 2.25A, B (A) The usual appearance of bladder exstrophy in a girl. The clitoris is in two parts and the labia majora are displaced laterally. (B) The usual appearance of bladder exstrophy in a boy. There is foreshortening of the lower abdominal wall with the umbilical cord lower than normal and the ectopic prepubic skin is displaced caudally to lie between the penis and the scrotum.

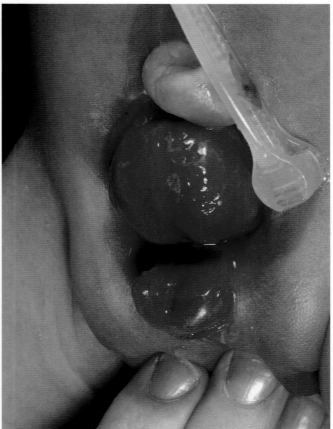

Fig. 2.26 Exposed bladder mucosa rapidly becomes oedematous. It then ulcerates and bleeds. The penis is short and the urethral plate is exposed as it runs from the penis to the base of the bladder. Urine leaks continuously from the ureteric orifices.

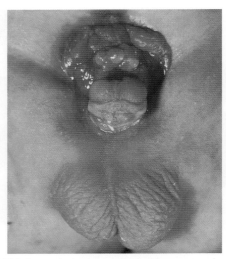

Fig. 2.27 This is a relatively small bladder exstrophy. The penis is moderately well developed. Note the blistering and oedema of the bladder mucosa.

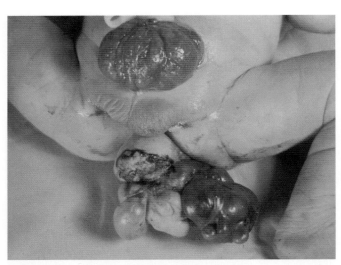

Fig. 2.28 This boy with bladder exstrophy has an associated sacrococcygeal teratoma.

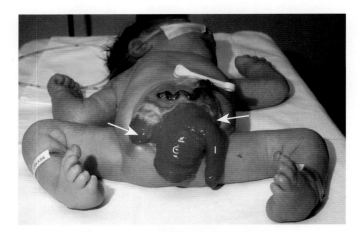

Fig. 2.29 Cloacal exstrophy. This is a gross defect of the lower abdominal wall extending into the perineum. There is an exomphalos in continuity with bladder on either side of a cloacal defect, into which the terminal ileum has intussuscepted. The bladder on either side is marked (arrows). The ileum (I) and colon (C) are seen in the centre.

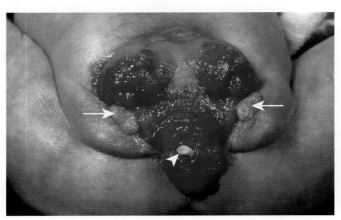

Fig. 2.30 A female infant with cloacal exstrophy. The bladder mucosa can be seen on either side with central colonic mucosa with faeces (arrowhead) coming from it. The two halves of the clitoris can be seen on the edge of the defect (arrows).

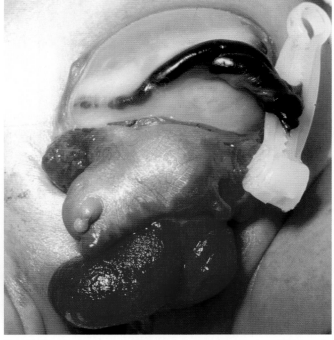

Fig. 2.31 Cloacal exstrophy with exomphalos superiorly and prolapsing bowel inferiorly. Exposed bladder mucosa can be seen on either side.

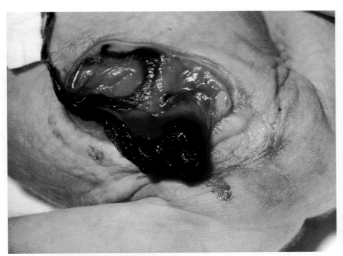

Fig. 2.32 Cloacal exstrophy with an imperforate anus and prolapse of the hindgut through the defect.

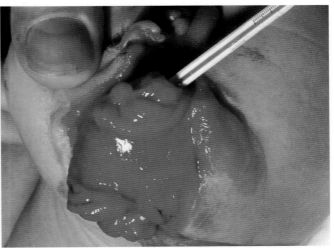

Fig. 2.33 Cloacal exstrophy should be distinguished from other rare abnormalities of the region. This infant has a split notochord syndrome with myelomeningocele, with an anterior and posterior spina bifida. There is a sacral defect and an absent anal canal with the rectum opening directly to the surface posteriorly adjacent to a diastematomyelic spur. In the neonatal period, the infant also developed hydrocephalus, hypercalcaemia and purulent sialadenitis.

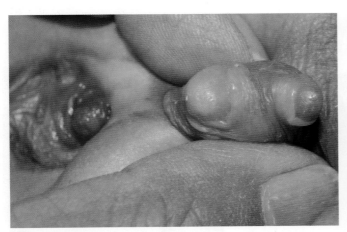

Fig. 2.34 Exstrophy of the bladder associated with duplication of the glans penis.

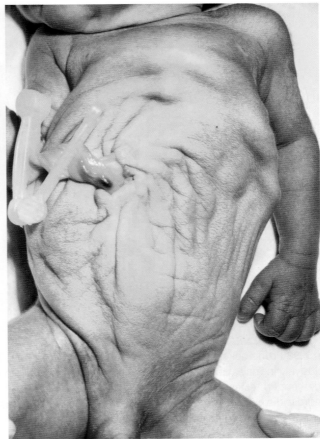

Fig. 2.35 In prune belly syndrome, the abdomen is flat and wrinkled because of deficient muscular development. This condition was previously known as 'the triad syndrome', on account of the three main features: prune belly, urinary tract distension and undescended testes. It may be caused by severe, distal urinary tract obstruction, which resolves spontaneously before birth.

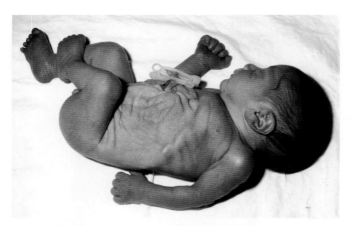

Fig. 2.36 The gross distension of the bladder and upper urinary tract *in utero* results in flaring of the costal margins, in addition to the stretching of the abdominal wall musculature. Following relief of this obstruction, the abdominal wall appears redundant (hence wrinkled) but flaring of the costal margin may persist after birth.

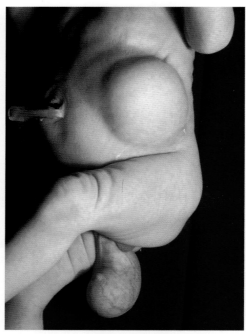

Fig. 2.37 A variant of prune belly syndrome showing localised attenuation of the ventral abdominal wall musculature. In many cases of prune belly syndrome, it is believed that obstruction occurs in the distal urethra at the junction of the penile and glandular urethra. This often results in megalourethra as seen here.

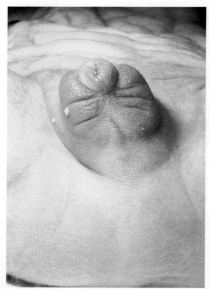

Fig. 2.38 Prune belly syndrome occurs almost exclusively in males and is associated with undescended testes. The empty scrotum is because the gross distension of the bladder antenatally prevents the testes gaining access to the internal inguinal ring, such that they cannot descend.

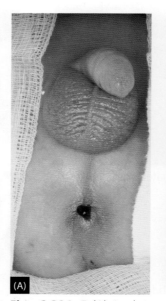
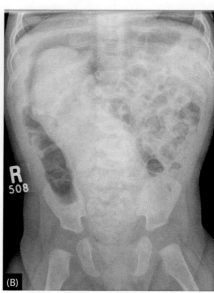

Figs. 2.39A, B (A) Anal stenosis, showing a bead of meconium on the perineum. (B) Massive faecaloma in an infant with anal stenosis. The sacrum is obscured. Currarino syndrome needs to be excluded in this case.

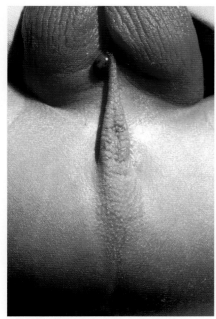

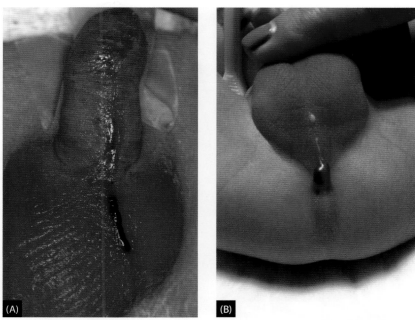

Fig. 2.40 Imperforate anus in the male, with a perineal fistula opening at the base of the scrotum. Meconium is discharging from the opening. This is a low anorectal malformation that can be treated by neonatal anoplasty.

Figs. 2.41A, B (A) A cutaneous fistula extending along the median raphé anteriorly, as far as the ventral shaft of the penis. (B) Cutaneous fistula in a boy containing meconium and sebaceous material in the median raphé. This fistula extends posteriorly to connect with the anorectum.

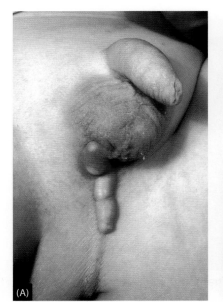

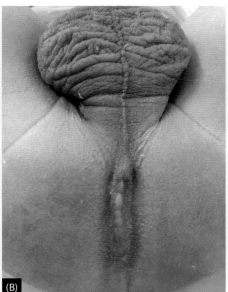

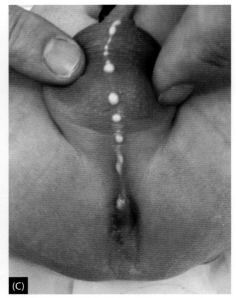

Figs. 2.42A–C (A) An anocutaneous fistula that has become filled with desquamated debris (white meconium). (B) Anorectal malformation with a cutaneous fistula containing non-pigmented meconium. (C) Another infant with a cutaneous fistula containing white debris.

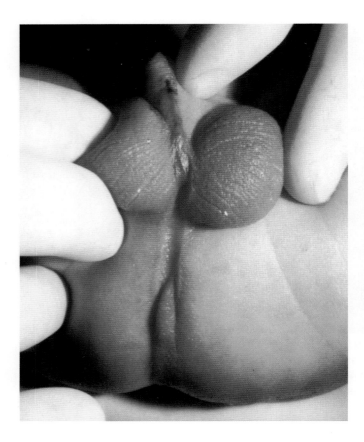

Fig. 2.43 In this infant with a cutaneous fistula opening on the penis, there is a completely bifid scrotum.

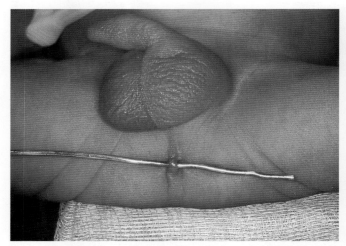

Fig. 2.44 Bucket-handle deformity in a boy with a cutaneous fistula.

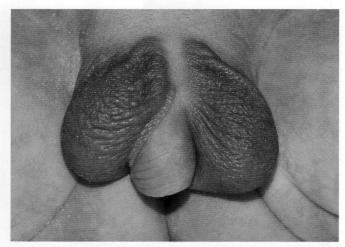

Fig. 2.45 Penoscrotal transposition in a male with a rectourethral fistula.

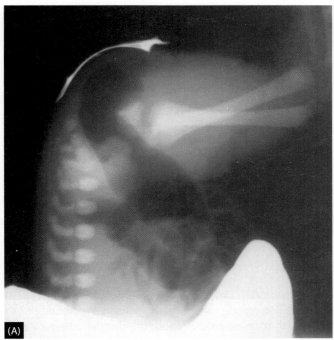

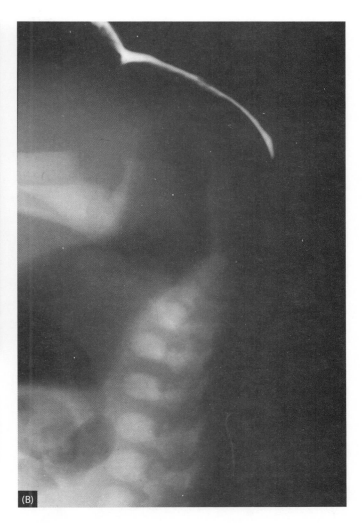

Figs. 2.46A, B In some cases it may be difficult to determine the exact level of the anorectal malformation from clinical examination alone. For this reason, an 'invertogram' is sometimes employed. The infant is radiographed prone with head down or inverted, allowing gas in the rectum to ascend. If the buttock crease is marked with contrast, the distance between the skin and the anorectum can be determined. The termination of the rectum is related to known anatomical bony landmarks. Both these infants have low lesions (and a normal looking sacrum).

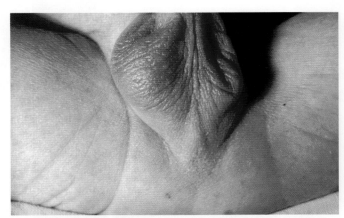

Fig. 2.47 The featureless perineum of a high imperforate anus in the male. There is no evidence of meconium under the skin. It is likely that there is a rectourethral fistula, which may be identified on urethrography.

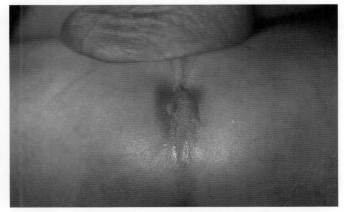

Fig. 2.48 Rectoprostatic fistula with a relatively flat perineum; the position of the anus is suggested by a skin tag.

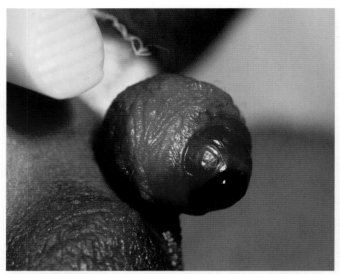

Fig. 2.49 When there is a rectourethral fistula, meconium may be observed to be passed per urethram.

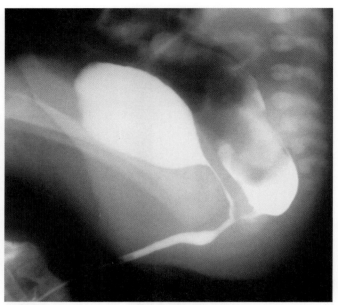

Fig. 2.50 Retrograde urethrogram showing a rectobulbar fistula with contrast entering both the bladder anteriorly and the rectum posteriorly.

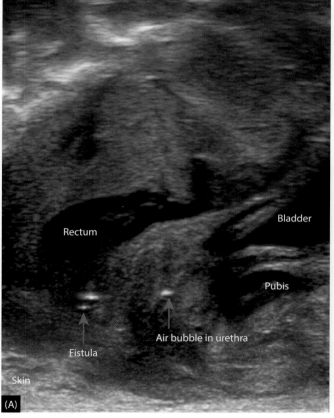

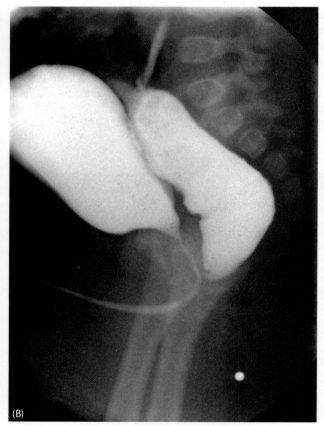

Figs. 2.51A, B (A) Perineal ultrasound scan in an infant with a rectourethral fistula showing the bright echoes from air bubbles in the fistula and in the urethra. The fistula is 1.3 cm from the perineal skin. (B) Distal loopogram demonstrating the rectourethral fistula. The opaque dot marks the skin at the site of the imperforate anus.

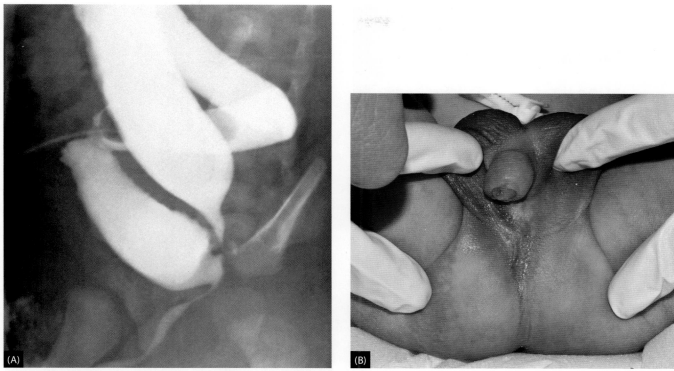

Figs. 2.52A, B (A) Distal colostogram demonstrating a rectovesical fistula. (B) Same patient showing the absent anal opening. The sacrum is deficient.

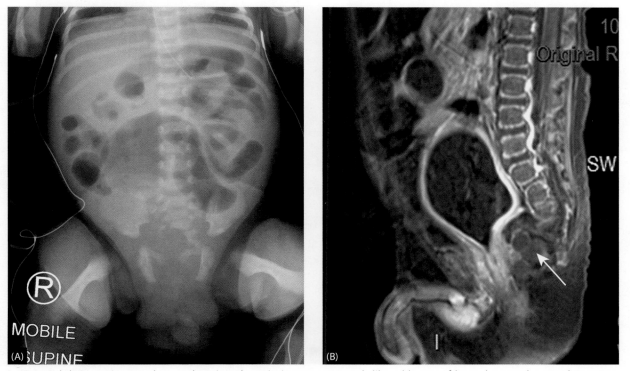

Figs. 2.53A, B (A) Currarino syndrome showing the scimitar sacrum and dilated loops of bowel secondary to the anorectal stenosis. (B) Sagittal MRI of Currarino syndrome showing an anterior neural tube defect associated with a teratoma (arrow) and deficient sacrum. Note the severe constipation caused by the extrinsic compression of the rectum and anorectal stenosis.

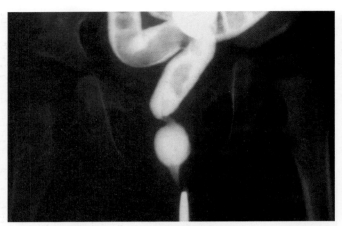

Fig. 2.54 Rectal stenosis. The stenosis is at an intermediate level in relation to the levator musculature. Rectal stenosis is a rare type of anorectal malformation and may be associated with a presacral mass (but not necessarily the Currarino syndrome).

Fig. 2.55 The number of external orifices in the perineum will indicate the level of the abnormality in female infants. In this girl, there are three orifices, and the anus is situated anterior to its usual position. There is a skin tag at the normal site of the anus.

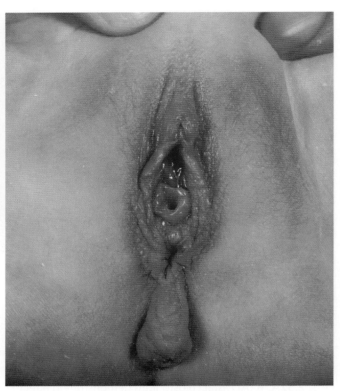

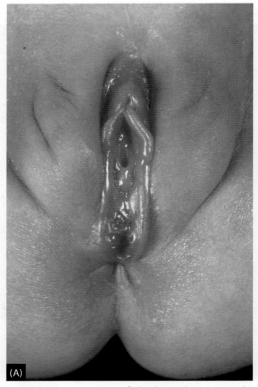

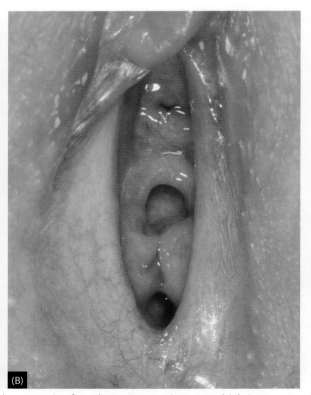

Figs. 2.56A, B (A) The opening of the bowel is situated in the posterior fourchette in a moist area which is an extension of the introitus. There are three orifices. (B) Rectovestibular fistula evident as the most posterior of the three openings at the introitus. There is a common wall between the lower part of the posterior wall of the vagina and anterior wall of the rectum.

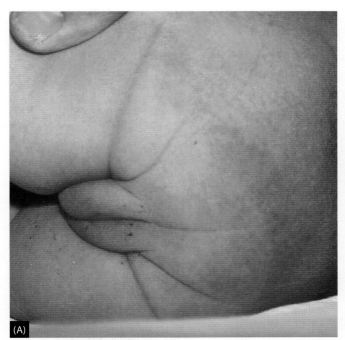
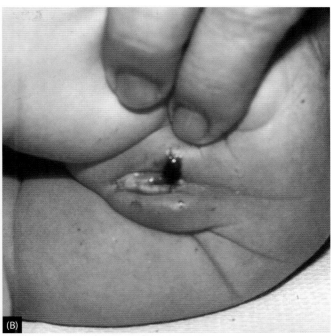

Figs. 2.57A, B (A) The site of the fistula opening in the perineum may not be evident unless the labia are parted. (B) In this girl, meconium is seen issuing from the anovestibular fistula.

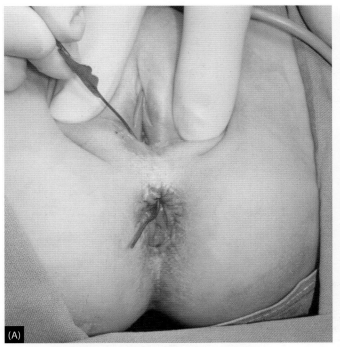
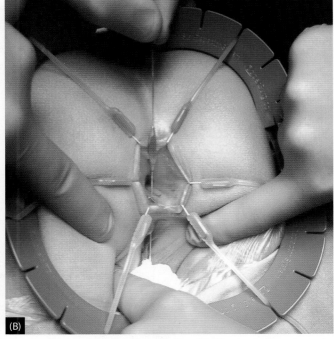

Figs. 2.58A, B (A) An H-type fistula between the anal canal and the vestibule, shown with a probe. (B) Fistula demonstrated during surgery by a probe passing from the anterior wall of the anal canal to the vestibule. These are rare anorectal malformations in the West but more common in Asians. They may present with vulval sepsis.

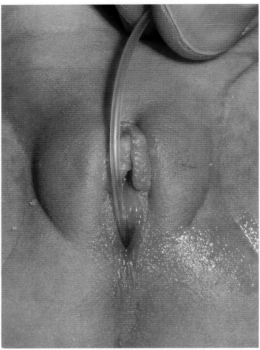

Fig. 2.59 An anovestibular fistula has an opening which, from the outside, looks the same as that of a rectovestibular fistula. The distinction can be made clinically by the direction in which a probe can be passed. In an anovestibular fistula, the probe passes first posteriorly in the subcutaneous plane before turning upwards.

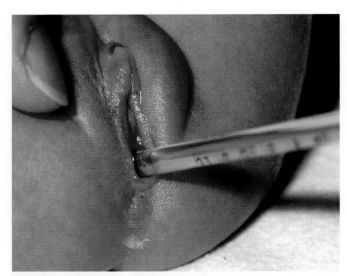

Fig. 2.60 In the rectovestibular fistula, the probe can only be passed upwards, parallel to the posterior wall of the vagina. This distinguishes it from an anovestibular fistula. At surgery it will be found that the rectum and posterior wall of the vagina share a common wall for a variable distance.

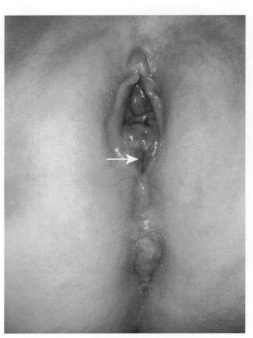

Fig. 2.61 In this infant with a vestibular fistula, the opening of the bowel can be seen in the vestibule (arrow) and there is a skin tag at the site of a normal anus.

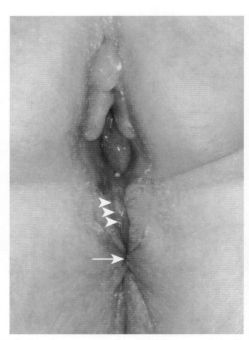

Fig. 2.62 Perineal groove. In this child the anus is in the normal place (arrow), anterior to which there is a moist mucosal-lined groove connecting with the vestibule (arrowheads). The father of this child was incorrectly accused of sexual abuse.

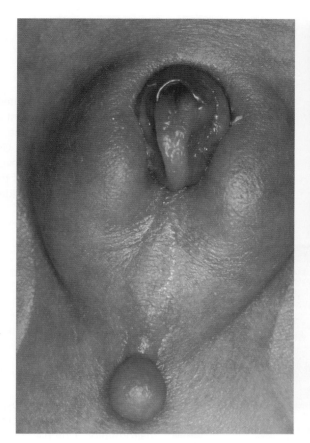

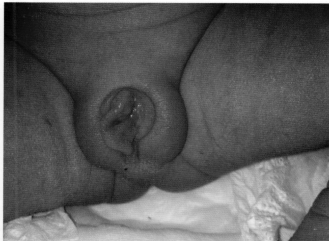

Fig. 2.64 Cloacal anomaly, showing redundant foreskin of the clitoris. Urine flow was obstructed by the pinhole cloacal opening.

Fig. 2.63 A cloacal anomaly. There is only one opening for the urogenital system and rectum. This is hidden behind the foreskin of the clitoris, which may be enlarged. The labia majora are largely fused and there is a skin tag at the normal site of the anus. The vagina was rudimentary.

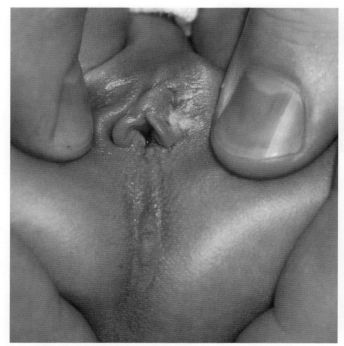

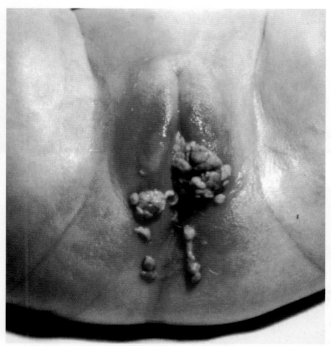

Fig. 2.65 There is a tiny bead of meconium appearing at the cloaca, the common opening for the urethra, vagina and rectum.

Fig. 2.66 Faeces are appearing through the common cloacal channel.

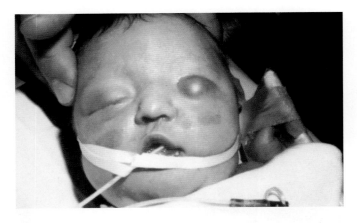

Fig. 2.67 Anorectal anomalies are frequently associated with other major congenital abnormalities. This infant girl with a rectovestibular fistula has CHARGE (Coloboma, Heart defects, Atresia choanae, growth Retardation, Genital abnormalities, Ear abnormalities) association. Whenever a child presents with an anorectal anomaly, patency of the oesophagus must be established to exclude oesophageal atresia.

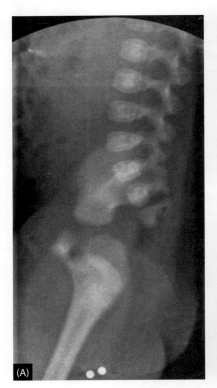

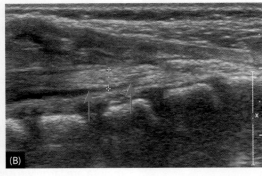

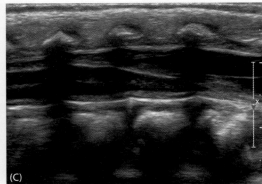

Figs. 2.68A–C (A) Lateral radiograph of the spine demonstrating sacral agenesis in an infant with an anorectal malformation. Completeness of the sacrum is one of the main determinants of subsequent continence. There are radiopaque markers on the perineum where the anus should be. (B) Spinal ultrasound scan showing a low-lying conus (arrows) in the sacral area and a fatty filum terminale (between cursors). (C) Spinal ultrasound scan showing a normal conus medullaris.

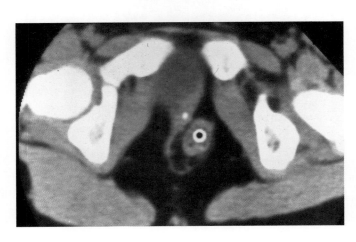

Fig. 2.69 CT scan (or more usually MRI) may be useful to identify the location of the bowel in relation to the sphincters and levator ani muscles. In this patient, the bowel can be seen to be eccentrically placed, perhaps contributing to the poor faecal continence that occurred postoperatively.

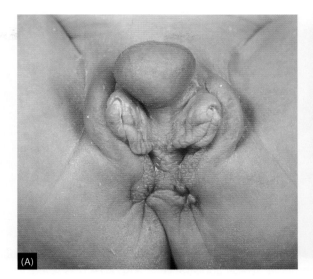

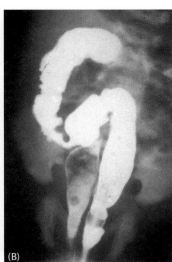

Figs. 2.70A, B (A) Duplication of the hindgut. This girl, in addition to duplication of her clitoris and introitus, has a duplicated anorectum, as demonstrated on the contrast study. (B) The contrast study of the same girl shows the distal duplication of the hindgut.

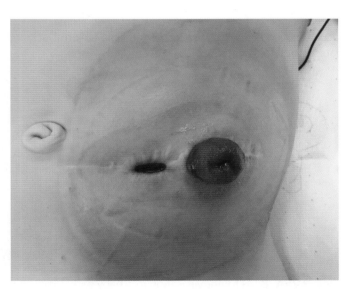

Fig. 2.71 Divided colostomy in proximal sigmoid colon in an infant with a high anorectal malformation. The mucous fistula lies medially.

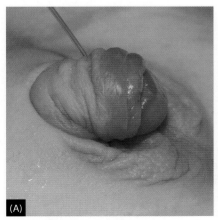

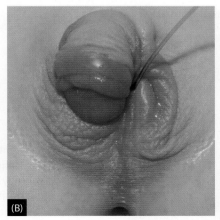

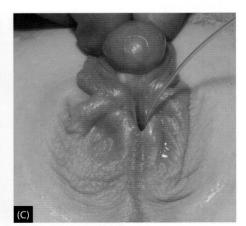

Figs. 2.72A–C (A) Ambiguous genitalia with a probe in the urogenital sinus in a baby with obvious virilisation but no visible testes bilaterally. Congenital adrenal hyperplasia is likely here. The feeding tube is in the urogenital sinus. (B) Same patient with Prader 3 virilisation. (C) View from below of the same patient with the feeding tube demonstrating the opening of the urogenital sinus.

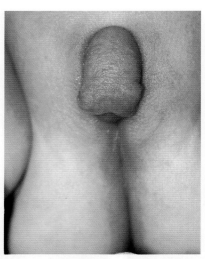

Fig. 2.73 Congenital adrenal hyperplasia. Typical appearance of ambiguous genitalia where there is moderate to severe deficiency of 21-hydroxylase. Clitoral enlargement is accompanied by masculinisation of the labia to form labioscrotal folds (Prader3).

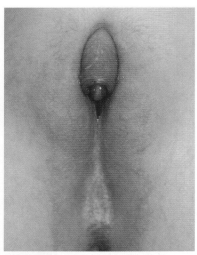

Fig. 2.74 Less severe variant of congenital adrenal hyperplasia without pigmentation or wrinkling of the labia majora, minimal fusion of the labia minora and some clitoral enlargement (Prader 2).

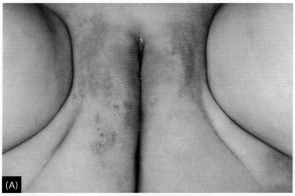

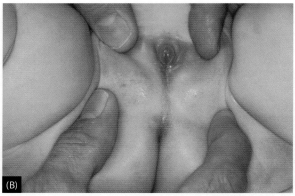

Figs. 2.75A, B (A) Minor virilisation in a baby with congenital adrenal hyperplasia in which the clitoral enlargement is not visible externally (Prader 2). (B) When the labia are parted the enlarged clitoris and labial fusion become apparent. Any degree of clitoral enlargement should be regarded as abnormal.

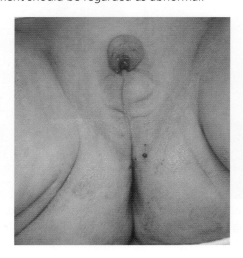

Fig. 2.76 A baby with severe congenital adrenal hyperplasia (21-hydroxylase deficiency) who received dexamethasone suppression therapy during pregnancy. There is marked masculinisation of the labia and urethral fusion, but the clitoris is not as large as would be expected. This is because the treatment failed to prevent virilisation initially because of an inadequate dose, but later in gestation it did prevent phallic growth.

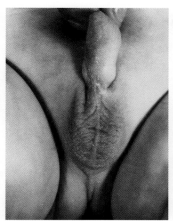

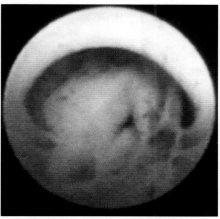

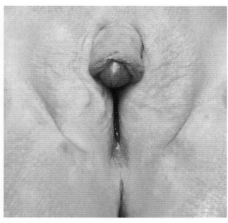

Fig. 2.77 Congenital adrenal hyperplasia in a completely masculinised baby displaying a 'penis' and empty 'scrotum' (Prader 5). The child had a rare variant of congenital adrenal hyperplasia that caused extreme virilisation so that the external genitalia appear the same as in a boy. Note that there are no visible gonads, since this baby has normal intra-abdominal ovaries.

Fig. 2.78 On urethroscopy, the opening into the vagina can be identified in the posterior wall of the urethra.

Fig. 2.79 Exposure to exogenous androgens. This girl received exogenous androgens (extract of bull testis) contained in homeopathic medicines ingested by her mother during pregnancy. Note that there is no labial fusion (fusion occurs between 8 and 12 weeks) but that the clitoris is enlarged (phallic growth occurs from 10–40 weeks).

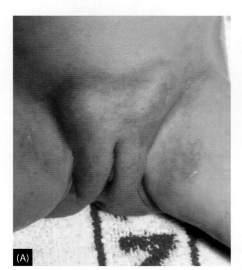

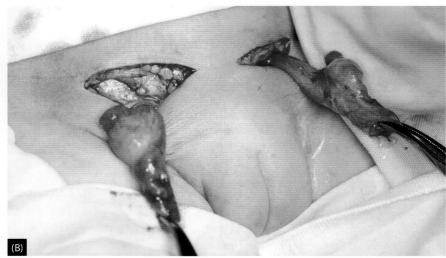

Figs. 2.80A, B (A) Complete androgen insensitivity (CAIS). Despite XY chromosomes and normal testicular development (the testes are visible inside inguinal herniae), the external genitalia have not responded to androgens, resulting in a normal female phenotype. The defect is a mutation, which renders the androgen-receptor totally inactive. These children have no uterus or tubes, because the testis makes normal amounts of anti-Müllerian hormone (AMH). The vagina is present, but is shorter than in normal females, since the lower vagina forms from the urogenital sinus. The upper third of the vagina has regressed because it is derived from the Müllerian ducts. The testes themselves are larger than in a normal male because of loss of the negative feedback on the hypothalamus. (B) In the same patient, normal testes are exposed in inguinal herniae prior to their neonatal excision.

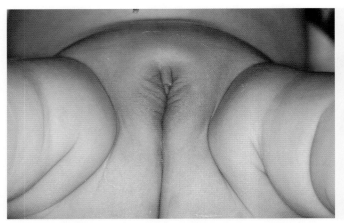

Fig. 2.81 Partial androgen insensitivity in an XY male with a severe androgen-receptor defect, such that the external genitalia are significantly feminised.

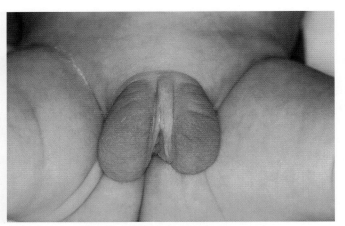

Fig. 2.82 Partial androgen insensitivity has permitted good masculinisation of the hemiscrota, but the phallus has not been stimulated sufficiently to produce a normal penis.

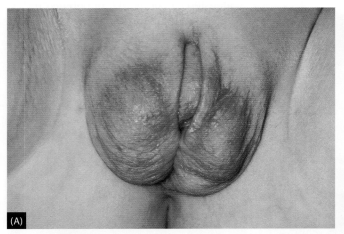

(A)

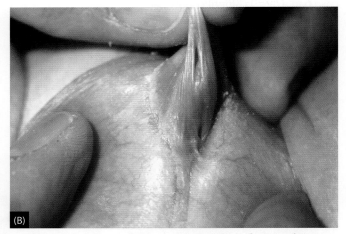

(B)

Figs. 2.83A, B XY/XX mosaicism. (A) Phenotypic male with inadequate development of the phallus and little fusion of the genital folds, leaving a perineal opening and hemiscrota. (B) The phallus with its dorsal hood is lifted up, while the fingers of the other hand stretch the labioscrotal skin folds to expose the opening of the urogenital sinus.

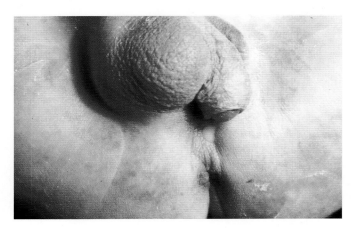

Fig. 2.84 In mixed gonadal dysgenesis, the gonadal mosaicism leads to asymmetrical development. On the right side, the gonad is more testicular (and undergoes greater descent) while on the opposite side, there is a dysplastic streak gonad (which is undescended) and an empty hemiscrotum. The subsequent genital asymmetry may be striking, as in this baby. The hypospadiac phallus is of moderate size. A vaginal cavity is present within the urogenital opening, as can be predicted by the presence of vaginal mucus appearing below the phallus. Mucus production is caused by maternal hormones stimulating the vagina. This child was reared as a boy, with the gonads left *in situ*. He re-presented in adolescence with a seminoma in the intra-abdominal gonad.

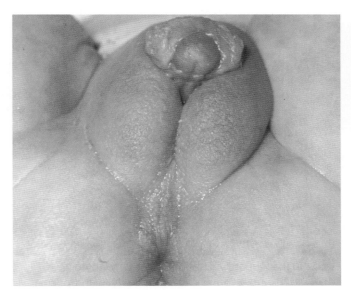

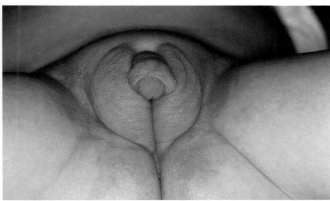

Fig. 2.86 Mixed gonadal dysgenesis involving a baby with severe dysplasia of both gonads. Consequently, there has been less virilisation of the external genitalia. Note the moderate-sized hypospadias phallus and 'shawl' labioscrotal folds. These children are usually reared as females, with early genital reconstruction, because of the risk of malignancy in the dysplastic gonads. When the intra-abdominal gonads were excised at 2–3 months of age, the right gonad contained a gonadoblastoma.

Fig. 2.85 Mixed gonadal dysgenesis. Obviously ambiguous external genitalia with impalpable gonads. The asymmetry of gonadal development and descent is not apparent here because neither gonad has descended below the inguinal canal.

Fig. 2.87 Some patients with 46,XY DSD have Drash syndrome, where the kidneys have diffuse mesangial sclerosis and develop Wilms tumours. This child had ambiguous genitalia with dysplastic testes at birth, and underwent gonadal excision and genital reconstruction as a female. She died suddenly at 9 months of age, with unrecognised renal failure. At postmortem, the kidneys showed mesangial proliferation, global glomerulosclerosis, chronic interstitial inflammation and tubular ectasia, all of which are seen here.

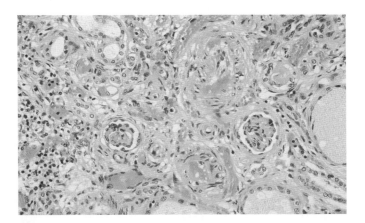

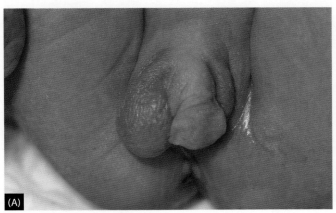

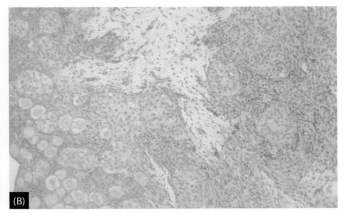

Figs. 2.88A, B (A) Ovotesticular DSD in a baby with asymmetrical ambiguous genitalia similar to that seen in mixed gonadal dysgenesis. The gender of rearing selected was female, and at gonadal excision, the left gonad was found to be an ovotestis, while the right gonad was a testis. (B) The histology in the same patient shows normal seminiferous tubules adjacent to ovarian stroma.

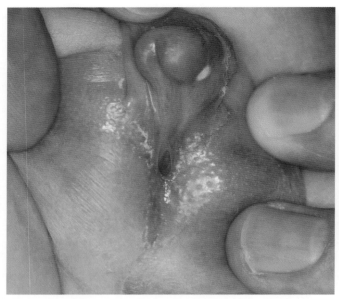

Fig. 2.89 Examination of the external urogenital opening in an infant with ovotesticular DSD to determine the degree of masculinisation of the urethra. This is proportional to the amount of androgen present in the 8–12-week gestation fetus, and correlates closely with the degree of testicular development.

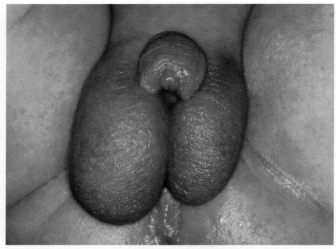

Fig. 2.90 Inadequate virilisation in a baby with 46,XY DSD who had no recognisable abnormality in androgenic function, despite inadequate virilisation. This has led to severe hypospadias and a bifid scrotum. This child represents the overlap in presentation between DSD and 'hypospadias'. Any baby with hypospadias where the scrotum is bifid (as seen here), or where one or both testes are impalpable, should be referred immediately after birth for exclusion of causes of DSD and to allow correct gender assignment.

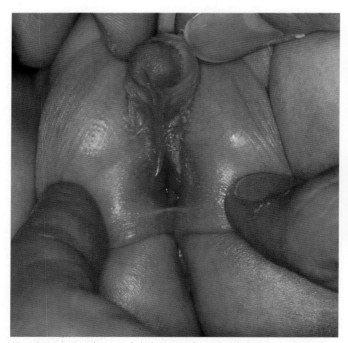

Fig. 2.91 Mixed gonadal dysgenesis. Careful separation of the labioscrotal folds is essential to examine the urogenital sinus opening. In this baby with mixed gonadal dysgenesis, the opening of the vagina is identified by the purplish hymen, which is easily distinguished from the darker red of the urethral mucosa.

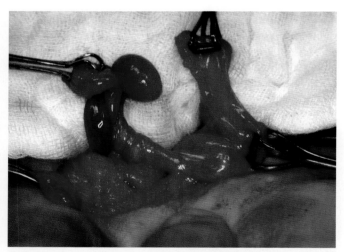

Fig. 2.92 Operative photograph of the intra-abdominal gonads in a 46,XX baby with mixed gonadal dysgenesis. The Babcock forceps hold each Fallopian tube. Seen on the left is the testicular gonad (with an intragonadal gonadoblastoma), while on the right the gonad is streak.

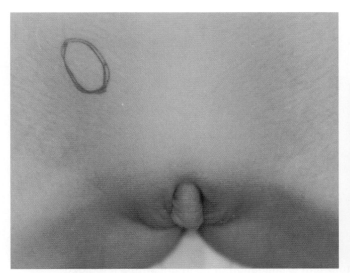

Fig. 2.93 Androgen secretion deficiency in a baby with 46,XY DSD with an enzyme defect in androgen production (17-beta-hydroxysteroid dehydrogenase-3 deficiency) leading to ambiguous genitalia and female phenotype. The inguinal testis and enlarged phallus are shown.

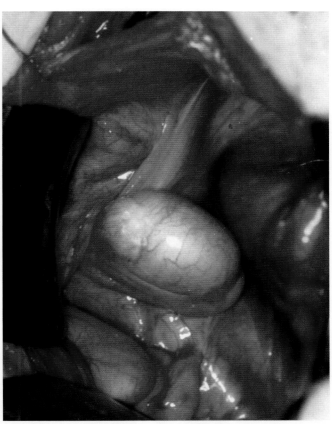

Fig. 2.94 Laparotomy on the patient in **Fig. 2.93** reveals an enlarged testis, which has been pulled back out of the right inguinal canal. Note the lack of normal epididymis because of Wolffian duct degeneration.

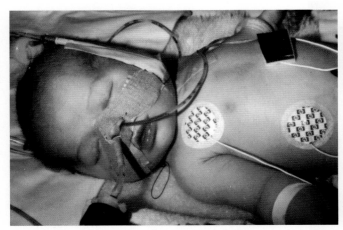

Fig. 2.95 In severe cases of congenital diaphragmatic hernia, poor peripheral perfusion and cardiovascular collapse occur within minutes of birth. This infant remained cyanosed despite intensive ventilatory assistance and died several hours after birth.

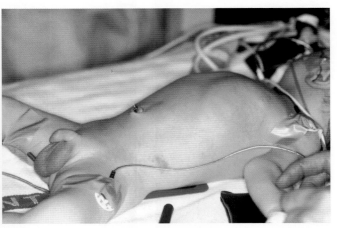

Fig. 2.96 The infant with a diaphragmatic hernia will have a barrel-shaped chest and a scaphoid abdomen. This is because most of the contents of the abdomen have moved up into the left hemithorax through the defect in the left hemidiaphragm. The presence of bowel and liver in the chest displaces the mediastinum to the right. This produces apparent dextrocardia with the heart sounds most easily audible in the right chest, and poor breath sounds in the left chest.

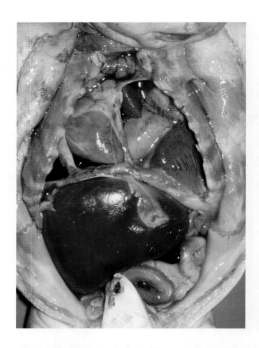

Fig. 2.97 A postmortem examination of an infant with a left-sided diaphragmatic hernia, who died of respiratory distress shortly after birth. The prolapsed liver can be seen compressing the intrathoracic structures and pushing the heart to the right. There is little room for the lungs.

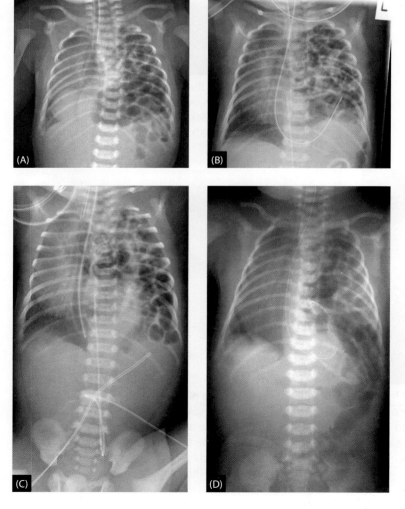

Figs. 2.98A–D (A) Chest radiograph showing bilateral congenital diaphragmatic hernias. Note the absence of a nasogastric tube. (B) Diaphragmatic hernia showing nasogastric tube displaced into the chest. (C) Same patient at 2 hours of age and before correct placement of a nasogastric tube. At the time the radiograph was taken the tube was in the lower oesophagus. (D) Diaphragmatic hernia on x-ray with nasogastric tube position confirming that the stomach is in the left chest.

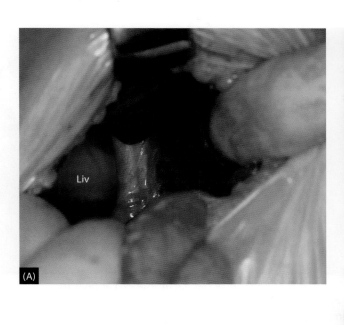

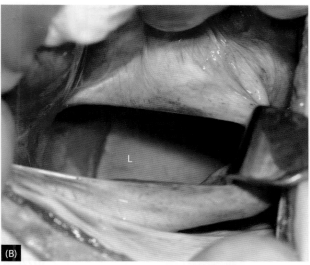

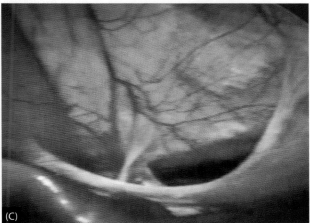

Figs. 2.99A–C (A) Operative appearance of a right diaphragmatic hernia. The liver (Liv) has been returned to the abdomen, revealing the rim of the defect in the right hemidiaphragm. In this view, the small hypoplastic right lung cannot be seen in the right hemithorax.
(B) Operative picture of a left congenital diaphragmatic defect in a child with delayed presentation. Note the reasonably good sized lung (L) in this case.
(C) Laparoscopic view of a Morgagni hernia.

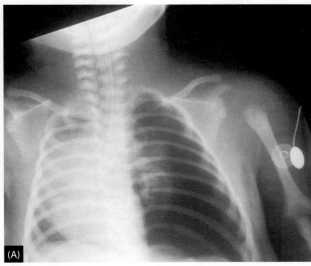

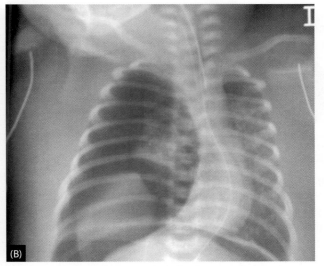

Figs. 2.100A, B (A) Chest radiograph showing hypoplastic lung after repair of a left congenital diaphragmatic hernia.
(B) Tension pneumothorax on the right in a patient with a congenital diaphragmatic hernia.

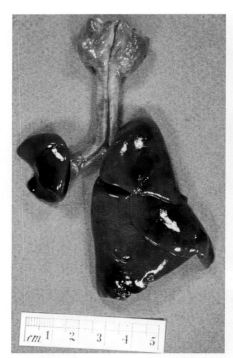

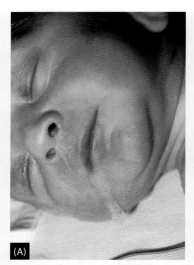

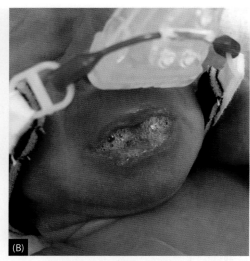

Figs. 2.102A, B (A) An infant with oesophageal atresia will appear to drool excessively ('mucousy baby') because saliva accumulates in the upper oesophageal segment and cannot be swallowed. (B) Mucousy baby with frothy saliva that cannot be swallowed in oesophageal atresia.

Fig. 2.101 As viewed from behind, in severe cases of congenital diaphragmatic hernia, there is marked pulmonary hypoplasia, with the lung on the side of the hernia being the more severely affected. This is a postmortem specimen of a child with a left diaphragmatic hernia who died as the result of severe lung hypoplasia. Note the small size of both lungs, particularly the left.

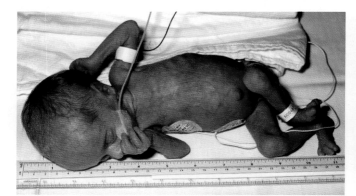

Fig. 2.103 A 27-week gestation 594 g infant with oesophageal atresia and mild abdominal distension from air passing down the distal tracheo-oesophageal fistula. The combination of prematurity and maternal polyhydramnios is suggestive of oesophageal atresia. The anomaly was repaired on day 1.

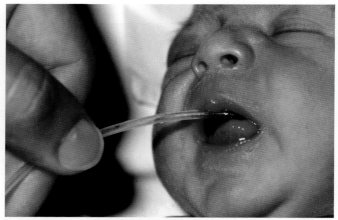

Fig. 2.104 The diagnosis of oesophageal atresia is made when a stiff No.10 gauge nasogastric tube passed through the mouth becomes arrested at about 10 cm from the gums.

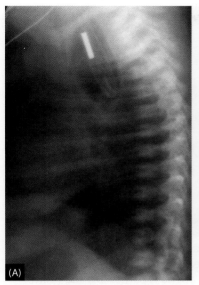
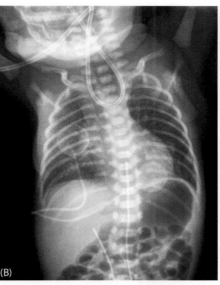

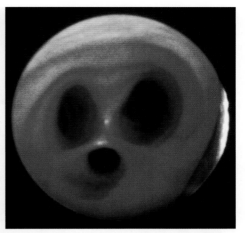

Fig. 2.106 The bronchoscopic appearance of a distal tracheo-oesophageal fistula in oesophageal atresia. This tracheo-oesophageal fistula arises at the level of the carina and runs behind both main bronchi to communicate with the distal oesophageal segment.

Figs. 2.105A, B (A) If a tube of small calibre is used to diagnose oesophageal atresia, it may curl up in the blind-ending upper pouch (as seen here) giving the false impression of oesophageal continuity. For this reason, a larger, stiffer catheter should be used. (B) Neonatal radiograph showing gas-filled upper oesophagus and a nasogastric tube, which is too small to identify the atresia. The tube has ended up in the nasopharynx!

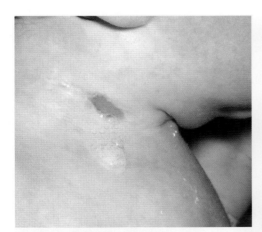
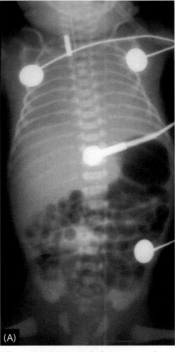
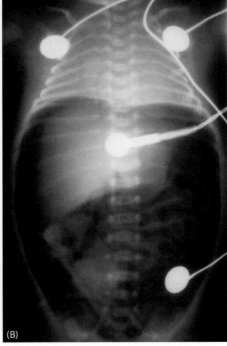

Fig. 2.107 Cervical oesophagostomy, which is occasionally needed in the management of complicated oesophageal atresia. The stoma (end of the upper pouch of the oesophagus) is seen opening onto the right side of the neck, with saliva dribbling out of it.

Figs. 2.108A, B (A) In oesophageal atresia the baby is at risk of aspiration of saliva, and there is often prematurity, so the lungs are at risk. (B) If the respiratory resuscitation is too vigorous, the baby may develop a gastric perforation caused by too much air passing down to the stomach through the tracheo-oesophageal fistula.

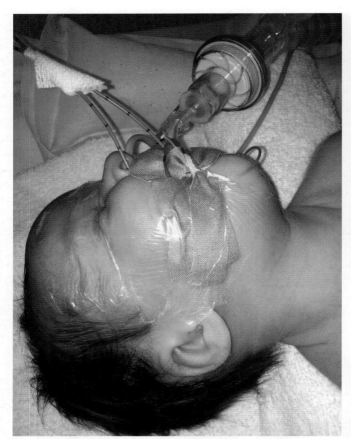

Fig. 2.109 Long-gap oesophageal atresia with proximal fistula. A ureteric catheter has been passed through the nose and into the trachea via the bronchoscope and retrieved from the oesophagus.

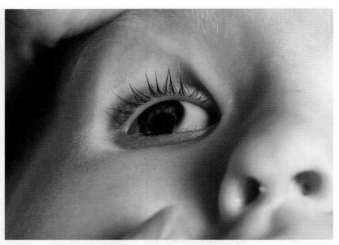

Fig. 2.110 The CHARGE association is seen in about 1–2% of babies with oesophageal atresia. The combination of colobomata and choanal atresia is particularly suggestive. This child has a coloboma of the right eye, involving deficiency of the iris.

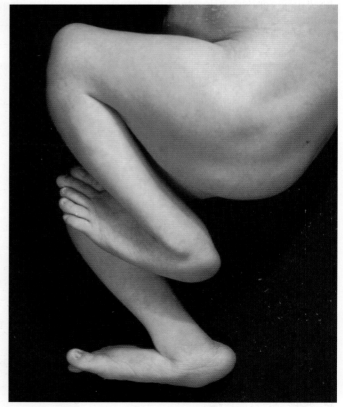

Fig. 2.111 Dysmorphic features and 'rocker-bottom feet' are suggestive of trisomy 18, which has a known association with oesophageal atresia. It may be appropriate to await chromosomal analysis before proceeding with surgical repair of the oesophageal atresia if suspicion is high, because the outlook in trisomy 18 is very poor.

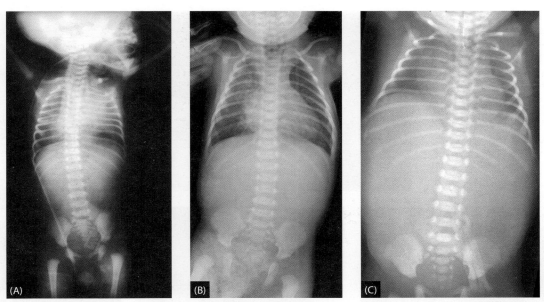

Figs. 2.112A–C (A) Oesophageal atresia with no fistula, producing a gasless abdomen on x-ray. Note that there are 13 pairs of ribs. (B) Long-gap oesophageal atresia with gasless abdomen. (C) The gasless abdomen in oesophageal atresia suggests that there is no distal fistula. Most of these infants will have no fistula at all, while about 20–25% will have a proximal tracheo-oesophageal fistula and about 10% will have an occluded distal tracheo-oesophageal fistula.

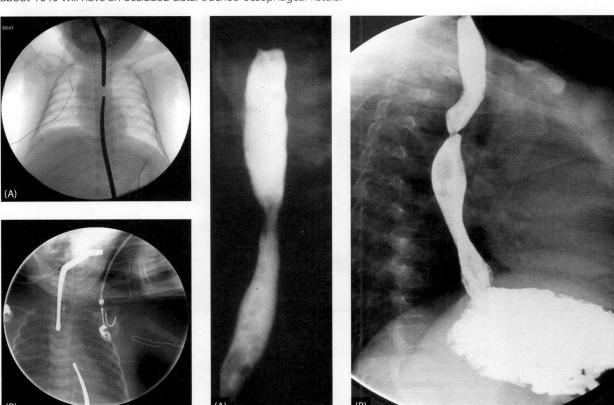

Figs. 2.113A, B (A) Determining the gap between the two ends of the oesophagus with metal sounds passed through the mouth and gastrostomy. (B) Gap study in long-gap oesophageal atresia.

Figs. 2.114A, B (A) Following repair of oesophageal atresia, there is often a persistent slight narrowing at the site of the anastomosis. (B) Contrast swallow showing an anastomotic stricture after oesophageal atresia repair.

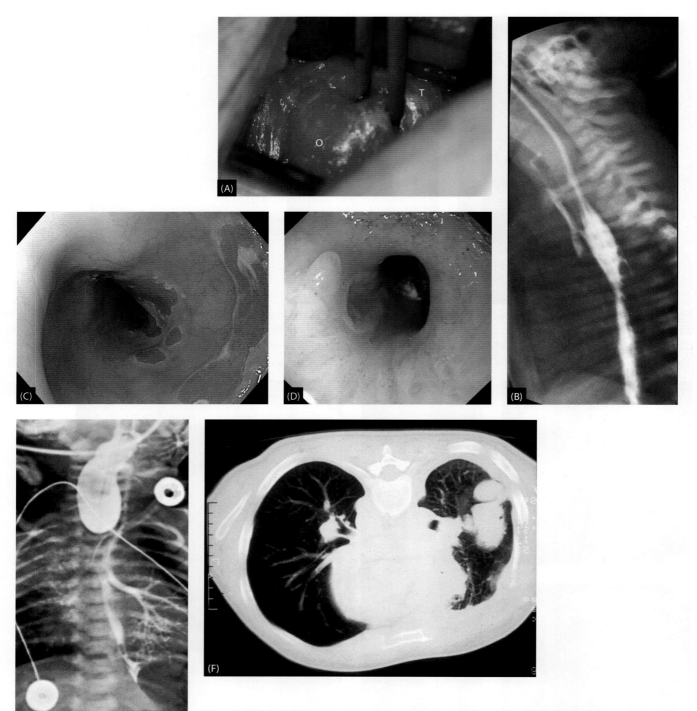

Figs. 2.115A–F (A) Isolated tracheo-oesophageal fistula (H-fistula). The blue vascular sling is around the fistula which runs from the oesophagus (O) to the trachea (T). Care must be taken to avoid damage to the recurrent laryngeal nerves. (B) H-type tracheo-oesophageal fistula demonstrated on prone tube oesophagogram. (C) Heterotopic gastric mucosa in oesophagus in a child with a repaired oesophageal atresia. (D) Endoscopic view of anastomotic stricture and ulcer after oesophageal atresia repair. (E) Inappropriate contrast study in a baby with oesophageal atresia causing soiling of the airways and accidental identification of the lower pouch fistula. (F) Aspiration pneumonia demonstrated on chest CT in an infant with oesophageal atresia.

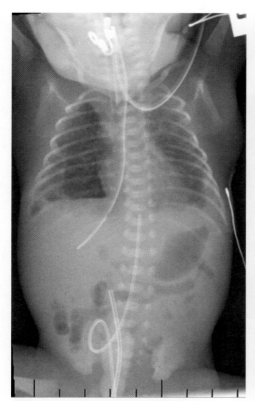

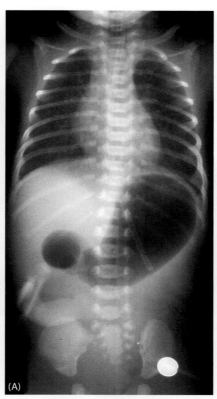

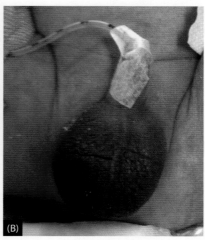

Fig. 2.116 Chest and abdominal radiograph showing a perforated oesophagus with extraluminal nasogastric tube.

Figs. 2.117 A, B (A) Duodenal atresia. Plain radiograph of the abdomen shows a 'double bubble', with gas in the stomach and proximal duodenum. There is no gas beyond the atresia, which is at the level of the ampulla of Vater, the junction of the foregut and midgut. (B) Intestinal perforation in neonates may allow bowel contents to reach the scrotum through the patent processus vaginalis. In this patient with a complex duodenal atresia and secondary perforation, bile has reached the tunica vaginalis bilaterally.

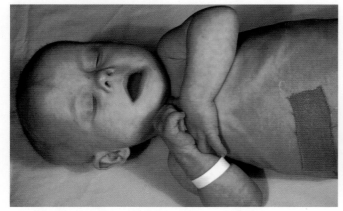

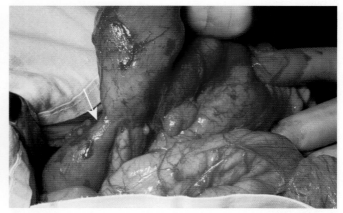

Fig. 2.118 Down syndrome is present in 30% of infants born with duodenal atresia. An infant with undiagnosed duodenal atresia usually presents with bile-stained vomiting shortly after birth. Apart from epigastric fullness from the distended stomach, the abdomen is scaphoid, because the bowel beyond the atresia contains no air and is collapsed.

Fig. 2.119 Duodenal stenosis may present with symptoms similar to duodenal atresia, but on plain radiographs air is present in the small bowel. It is less common than duodenal atresia. The narrow segment of duodenum is arrowed. At operation, a small pinhole opening was found at this point. The child also had Down syndrome and was diagnosed after a long history of recurrent vomiting.

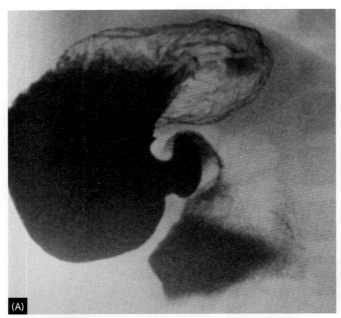

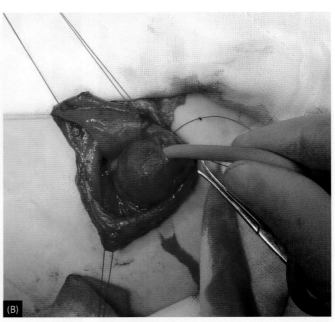

Figs. 2.120A, B (A) Contrast swallow showing a dilated stomach and duodenal obstruction caused by a web. (B) Operative view in the same patient showing the web has developed into a 'windsock', with a small central aperture shown by the tube. The duodenum has been opened.

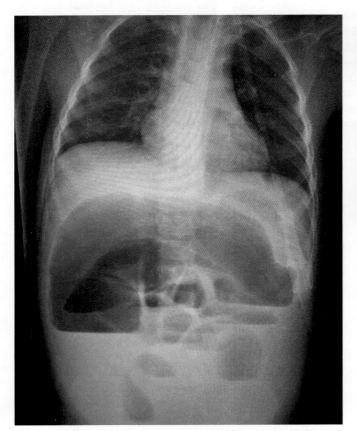

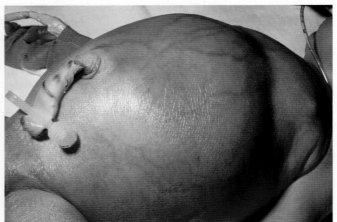

Fig. 2.122 Ileal atresia with gross distension of the abdomen. No meconium was passed. The clinical appearance may be indistinguishable from meconium ileus and some cases of Hirschsprung disease.

Fig. 2.121 Erect abdominal radiograph showing very dilated bowel loops in a distal intestinal atresia.

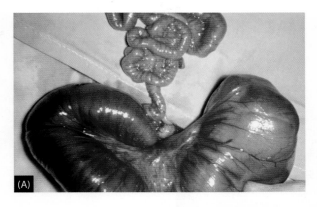

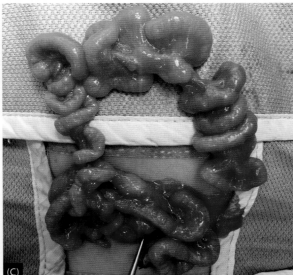

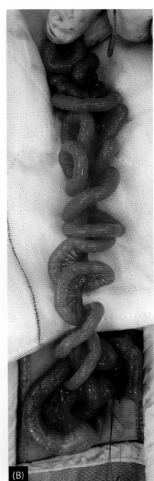

Figs. 2.123A–C (A) Operative appearance of jejunal atresia with gross distension of the jejunum proximal to the obstruction with small collapsed bowel distal to it. One of the operative difficulties is anastomosing the distended proximal bowel to the collapsed distal bowel. (B, C) Apple-peel atresia with distal small bowel surviving on the marginal artery.

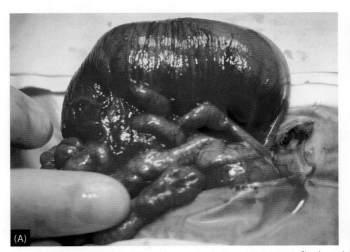

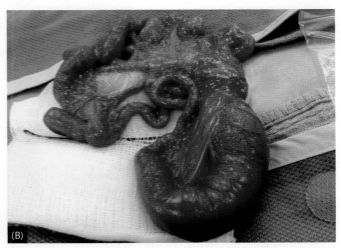

Figs. 2.124A, B (A) In jejunal atresia, it is common to find multiple atretic segments. The grossly distended proximal jejunum ends abruptly at the first atresia, after which there are multiple short segments of collapsed bowel of varying length, which sometimes have an appearance of 'a string of sausages'. It is important to recognize this possibility at surgery. (B) Jejunal atresia at surgery showing dilated proximal jejunum and collapsed distal bowel.

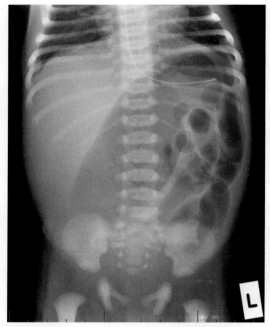

Fig. 2.125 In colonic atresia there is massive distension of the proximal colon above the level of the atresia, which may be confused with massive ileal dilatation in meconium ileus.

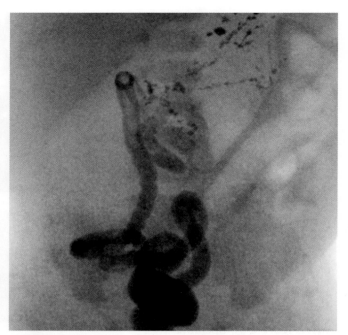

Fig. 2.126 Contrast enema in colonic atresia showing the distal microcolon.

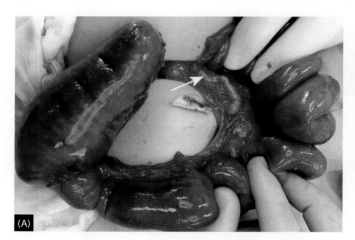

(A)

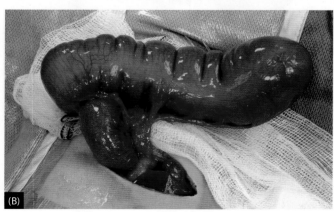

(B)

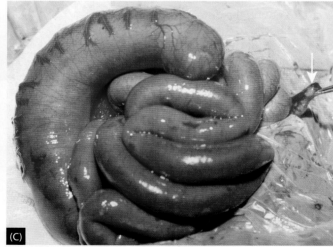

(C)

Figs. 2.127A–C (A) Colonic atresia at operation: dilated ileum and proximal colon. The distal microcolon is visible near the edge of the mesenteric defect (arrow). (B) Operative photo showing dilated ascending colon in colonic atresia. (C) Colonic atresia at neonatal laparotomy. The distal microcolon is visible laterally (arrow).

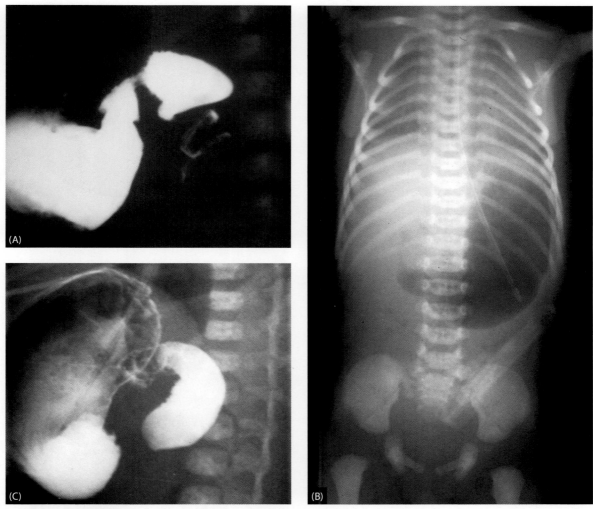

Figs. 2.128A–C (A) Any child who presents with strongly bile-stained vomiting as the initial symptom should be regarded as having malrotation with volvulus until proved otherwise. A contrast meal, even in the absence of complete duodenal obstruction, may reveal a 'spiral' of the duodenum, with failure of it to cross the midline and re-ascend to the level of the pylorus. This feature is diagnostic. (B) Abdominal radiograph in a baby with malrotation and volvulus, showing acute dilatation of the stomach but no chronic dilatation of the duodenum, as would be seen in duodenal atresia. Note the paucity of gas in the midgut. (C) Malrotation with midgut volvulus on contrast study, with slight dilatation of the proximal duodenum and complete obstruction in the second part of the duodenum.

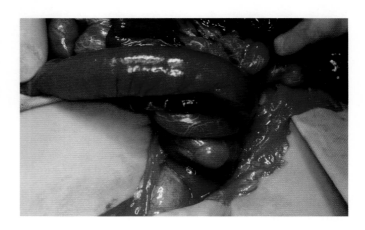

Fig. 2.129 An operative photograph of the base of the small bowel mesentery in malrotation complicated by volvulus, showing a 720-degree clockwise twist. The root of the mesentery is extremely narrow and predisposes to volvulus. Note the gross distension of the superior mesenteric vein and the lymphatic obstruction.

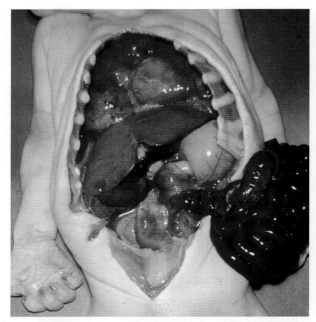

Fig. 2.130 Postmortem photograph of a child who died of unrecognised neonatal midgut volvulus, showing the narrow small bowel mesentery, which has allowed the entire midgut to twist on its axis and cut off its blood supply. The infarction was the cause of the child's demise.

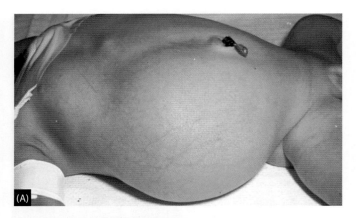

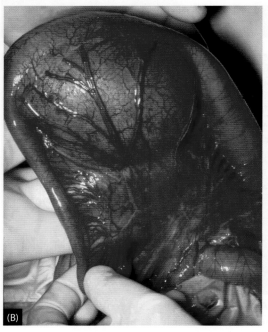

Figs. 2.131A, B Jejunal duplication. (A) This neonate presented with a bowel obstruction in association with a large cystic mass palpable in the abdomen. (B) Jejunal duplication cyst in the same patient causing bowel obstruction. The cyst lying in the mesentery of the jejunum has compressed and attenuated the normal jejunum adjacent to it.

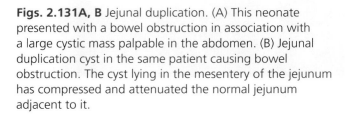

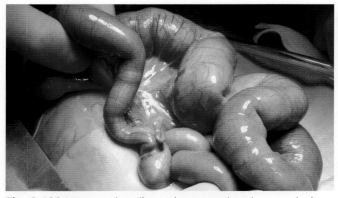

Fig. 2.132 In meconium ileus, the meconium is excessively tenacious and sticky, causing a mechanical bowel obstruction in the ileum. Beyond the distended mid-ileum, the terminal ileum is small and collapsed and contains multiple hard pellets. Meconium ileus is caused by cystic fibrosis in at least 90% of cases.

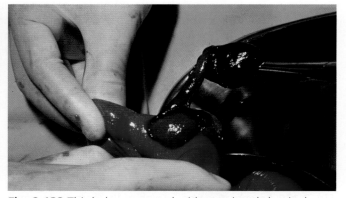

Fig. 2.133 This baby presented with massive abdominal distension at birth. At laparotomy the bowel has been opened and the sticky meconium is so tenacious it may be winched out of the bowel like a piece of rope. This extreme viscosity of the meconium and mucus is the reason for one of the original names for cystic fibrosis: 'mucoviscidosis'.

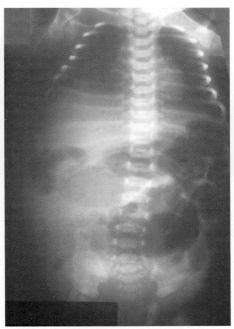

Fig. 2.134 Abdominal radiograph in meconium ileus with dilated loops in the left upper quadrant and ground-glass appearance in the right lower quadrant.

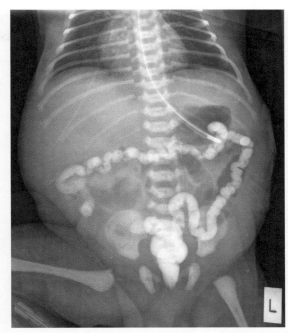

Fig. 2.135 Contrast enema showing microcolon in meconium ileus.

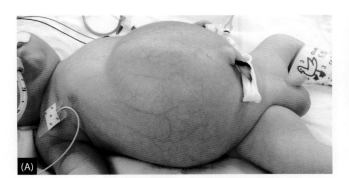

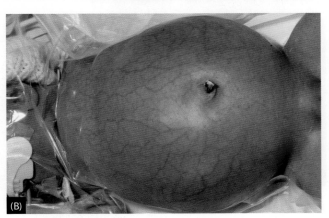

Figs. 2.136A, B (A) If the meconium-laden ileum twists *in utero*, the infant will be born with signs of meconium peritonitis, where the abdomen is red, oedematous and tender. (B) Meconium peritonitis showing gross distension and early vascular changes in the skin.

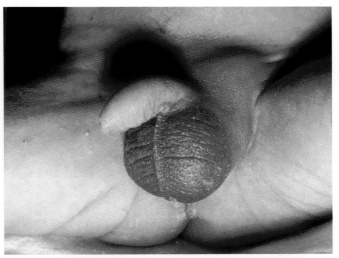

Fig. 2.137 Volvulus of the meconium-laden ileum has occurred well before birth in this infant and the meconium released has tracked down through the tunica vaginalis to collect in the scrotum, giving it a dark appearance.

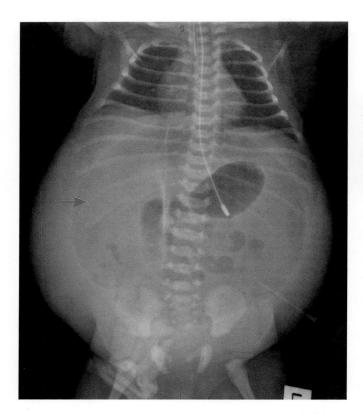

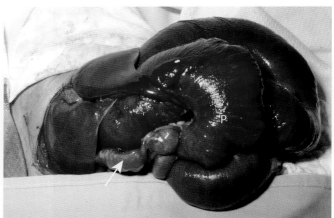

Fig. 2.139 The operative appearance of an infant with meconium peritonitis secondary to localised volvulus of the ileum and adjacent ileal atresia (the legacy of *in-utero* volvulus). Note the dilated proximal ileum (P), which is in contrast to the collapsed distal ileum (arrow).

Fig. 2.138 Meconium peritonitis with free air and ascites, and a subtle line of calcification over the surface of the liver (arrow).

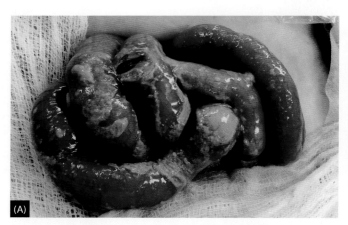

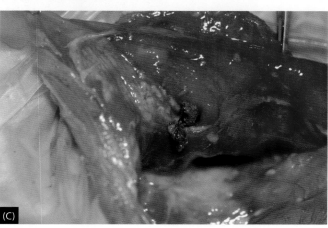

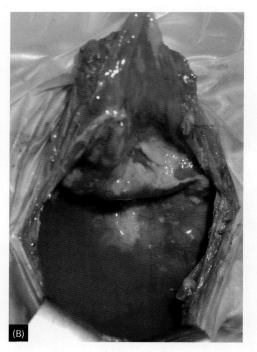

Figs. 2.140A–C (A) Severe soiling of the peritoneal cavity following ileal perforation in meconium ileus complicated by localised volvulus and necrosis. (B) Meconium peritonitis showing extravasation of bowel contents at laparotomy. (C) Same patient showing the peritoneal soiling and the site of intestinal perforation.

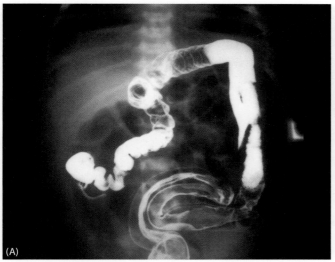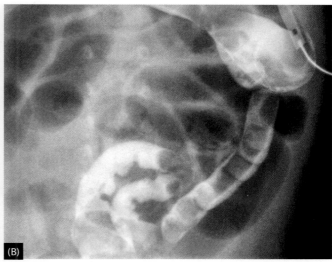

Figs. 2.141A, B (A) In meconium plug syndrome, a cast of thick inspissated meconium obstructs the colon, producing the appearance of a distal bowel obstruction. A contrast enema will outline the cast within the colon and demonstrate normal patency above this level. A meconium plug is usually passed spontaneously. It may affect sick neonates. Most affected infants have no underlying disease but Hirschsprung disease and cystic fibrosis are potential causes. (B) Contrast enema in a baby with small left colon syndrome, showing meconium pellets in the descending colon and an abrupt calibre change at the splenic flexure. This causes a transient functional bowel obstruction. There is an association with maternal diabetes.

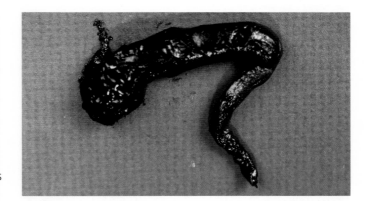

Fig. 2.142 The appearance of a meconium plug following its spontaneous passage.

Figs. 2.143A, B (A) Intraluminal radiopaque crystals may be difficult to distinguish radiologically from the extraluminal calcification of meconium peritonitis. It is a rare finding for which there is sometimes no obvious cause, but in some patients may be related to the presence of urine in the gastrointestinal tract (e.g. in patients with imperforate anus and a rectovesical fistula). It can be distinguished from meconium peritonitis by the absence of abdominal signs, and the fact that the position of the calcification alters on a plain radiograph as it moves through the colon. The crystals usually contain magnesium ammonium phosphate. (B) A radiograph of meconium passed by an infant with intraluminal radiopaque crystals confirms that it is the meconium itself that contains the radiopaque material.

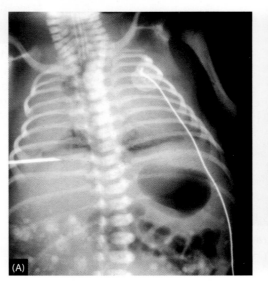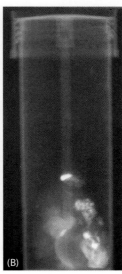

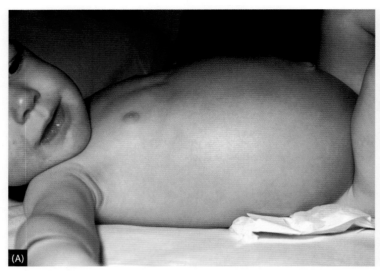

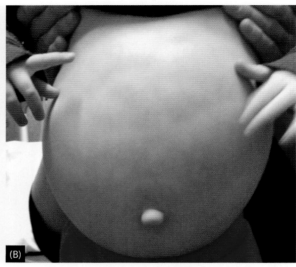

Figs. 2.144A, B (A) An infant with Hirschsprung disease will usually appear normal at birth, but over the first 3 or 4 days of life develops increasing abdominal distension and vomiting, and there is delay in the passage of meconium. Meconium is passed within the first 24 hours in 95% of normal, term infants, but in Hirschsprung disease, may not be passed for 2 or 3 days. (B) Chronically distended abdomen in a child who had a previous pull-through for Hirschsprung disease, but where the transition zone was pulled down, and the child still has functional obstruction.

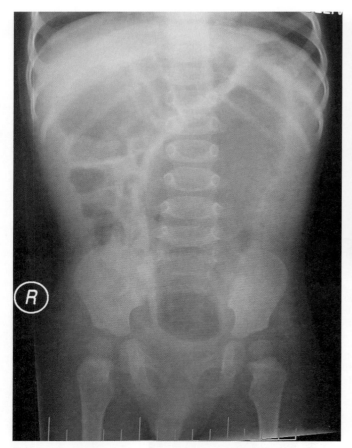

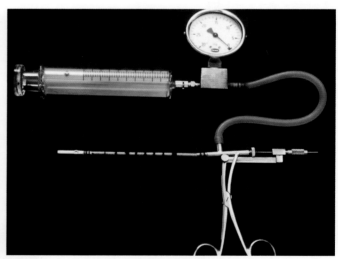

Fig. 2.146 The diagnosis of Hirschsprung disease is confirmed on rectal suction biopsy. The original suction rectal biopsy device (described by Helen Noblett) attached to a syringe via a pressure manometer.

Fig. 2.145 Abdominal radiograph showing dilated distal bowel in a patient with Hirschsprung disease.

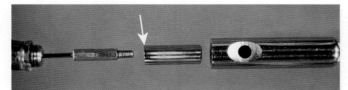

Fig. 2.147 Disassembled, the cutting edge of the inner cylinder of the rectal suction biopsy device is arrowed. This is screwed on to the stem of the instrument, over which an outer sheath is screwed. The outer sheath contains a small side-hole through which a portion of the rectal mucosa is sucked. The cylindrical knife then cuts off a piece of mucosa.

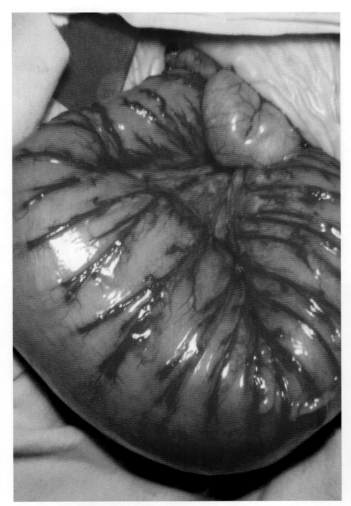

Fig. 2.148 The operative appearance of Hirschsprung disease showing grossly dilated colon above the aganglionic segment. It has prominent surface vessels and increased thickness of the muscle wall. Seromuscular biopsies can be taken for frozen section to locate the exact level of the transition zone. If a temporary colostomy is used to overcome the obstruction, it is sited a few centimetres proximal to the transition zone.

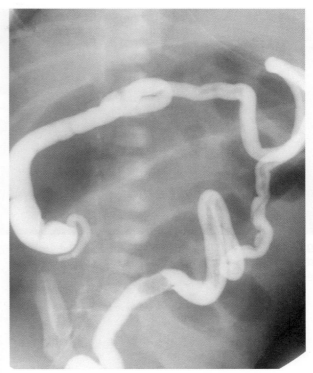

Fig. 2.149 Contrast enema showing a microcolon in a baby with total colonic Hirschsprung disease.

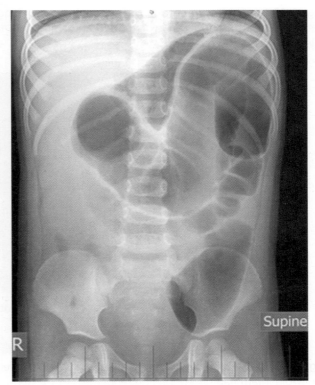

Fig. 2.150 Acute dilatation of the distal bowel in an infant with Hirschsprung-associated enterocolitis.

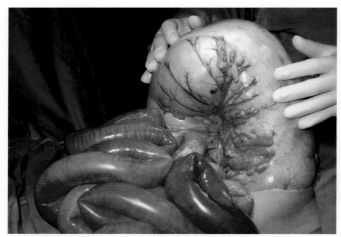

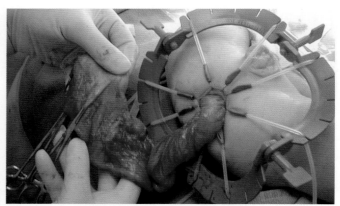

Fig. 2.152 Dilated colon in Hirschsprung disease at an endorectal pull-through operation.

Fig. 2.151 Toxic megacolon and enterocolitis in a 14-year-old girl with Hirschsprung disease. The grossly distended megacolon is obvious.

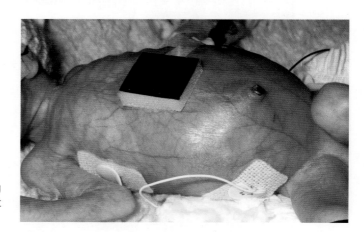

Fig. 2.153 A premature infant with neonatal necrotising enterocolitis. The abdomen is distended and shiny, but at this stage is not discoloured.

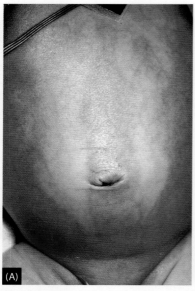

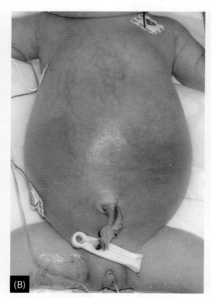

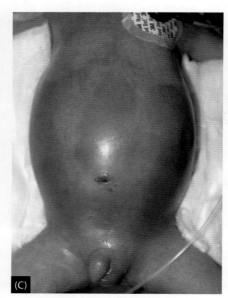

Figs. 2.154A–C (A) The appearance of the abdomen in severe necrotising enterocolitis (NEC) in the premature infant. This 4-day-old infant had distension and tenderness of the abdomen with erythematous discoloration reflecting underlying peritonitis. At operation, there was total infarction of the right colon and distal ileum. (B) Erythematous, distended abdomen in a baby with NEC. (C) The erythematous abdominal wall in a premature infant with NEC totalis (affecting the whole small and large bowel), showing how the thickness of the rectus muscles affects the pattern of redness.

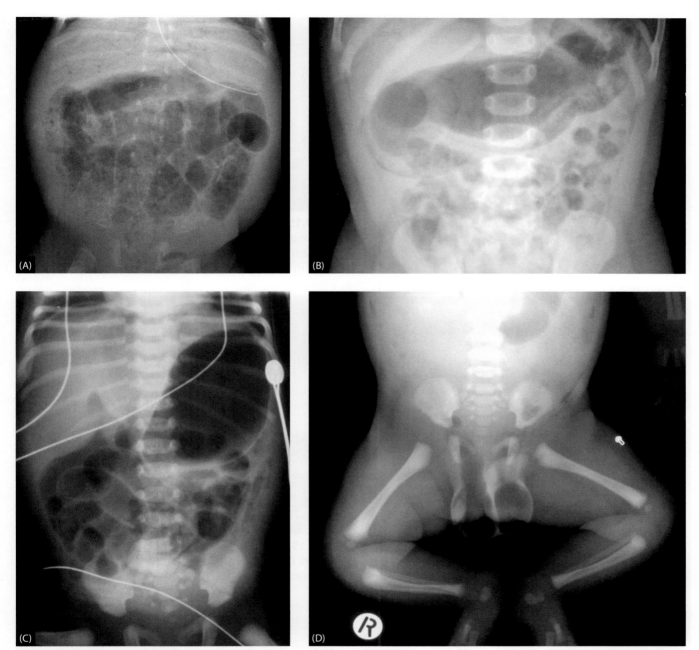

Figs. 2.155A–D (A) A plain radiograph of the abdomen in NEC will show pneumatosis or intramural gas of the affected bowel. This needs to be distinguished from meconium and faeces. The bowel wall often looks thickened and there may be free peritoneal fluid between the affected loops. This baby also has visible portal venous gas. (B) Gross pneumatosis of the stomach and duodenum in an infant with necrotising enterocolitis. (C) Abdominal radiograph of necrotising enterocolitis with perforation. Note the Rigler sign and free air alongside the falciform ligament and under the right hemidiaphragm. (D) Baby with necrotising enterocolitis and secondary perforation where the gas has tracked down into the scrotum (scrotal pneumatocele).

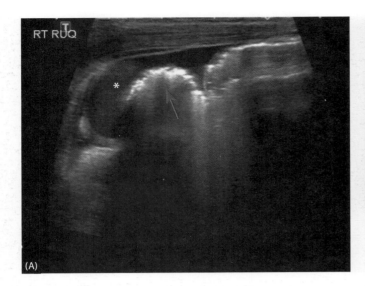

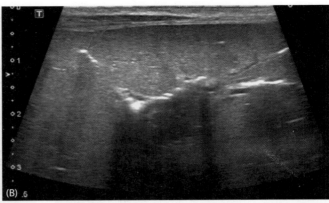

Figs. 2.156A, B Abdominal ultrasound scan showing (A) pneumotosis within the bowel (arrow) and complex free fluid with debris (*). (B) Homogeneous echotexture of the liver with presence of portal venous gas (arrow).

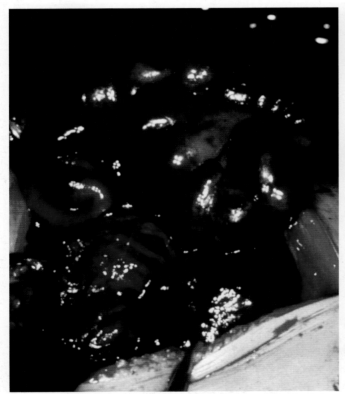

Fig. 2.157 Severe necrotising enterocolitis causing necrosis of virtually the entire small and large bowel (NEC totalis). This infant did not survive.

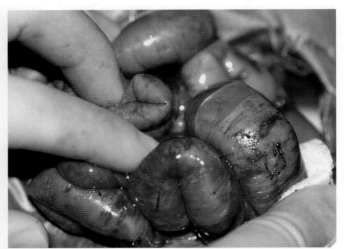

Fig. 2.158 Moderately severe involvement of several loops of small bowel with full-thickness bowel necrosis and intramural gas.

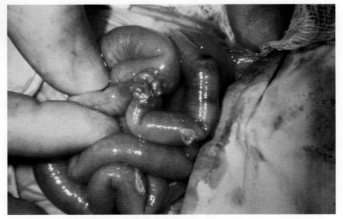

Fig. 2.159 Localised necrotising enterocolitis showing patchy involvement of the small bowel: in places there is full-thickness gangrene; other areas are ischaemic but viable.

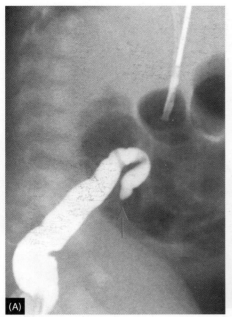
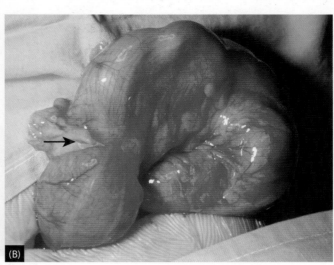

Figs. 2.160A, B (A) Lower gastrointestinal enema with water-soluble contrast (Omnipaque™) introduced into the patient's rectum by gentle hand injection. There is satisfactory distension of the rectum and the distal part of the sigmoid colon with an abrupt cut-off with tapering at the mid-sigmoid level (arrow). This is suggestive of a severe stricture. (B) Bowel affected by necrotising enterocolitis can produce a fibrotic stricture. This usually occurs in the colon (arrow) but has been reported in the small bowel as well.

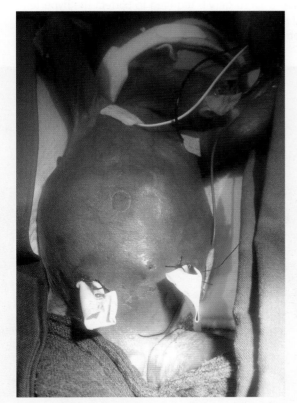

Fig. 2.161 Extremely premature baby (23 weeks) with necrotising enterocolitis and peritonitis treated by abdominal Penrose drains inserted under local anaesthesia.

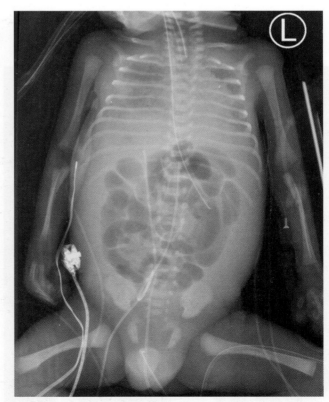

Fig. 2.162 Abdominal radiograph showing neonatal ascites secondary to a misplaced umbilical vein catheter and leakage of total parenteral nutrition fluid into the peritoneal cavity.

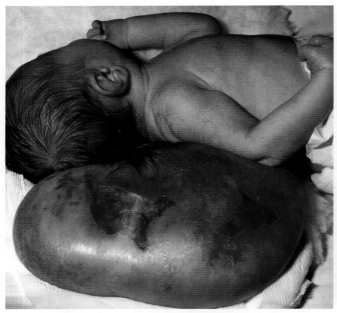

Fig. 2.163 Encephalocele. This enormous occipital meningoencephalocele is best left untreated because of the inevitable hydrocephalus, mental retardation and brain dysfunction. Most such anomalies are now diagnosed on antenatal scan and treated by termination of pregnancy after parental counselling and consent.

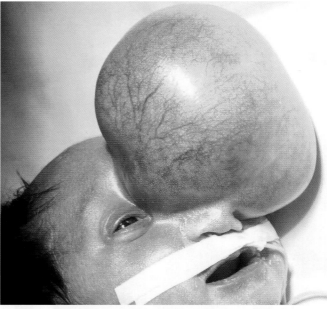

Fig. 2.164 Fronto-nasal encephalocele. The region of the glabella represents the most cranial portion of the neural tube. A neural tube defect at this site produces a nasal or frontal encephalocele. This usually contains meninges, frontal cortex and one (or more) anterior horn(s) of the lateral ventricles. If treatment is offered, then secondary craniofacial surgery is required to correct the hypertelorism and reconstruct the nose once the encephalocele has been excised.

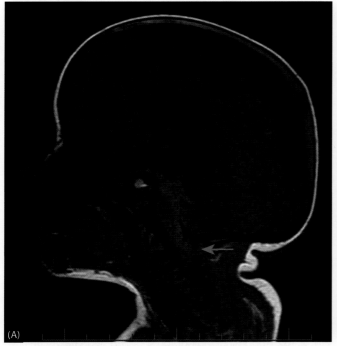

(A)

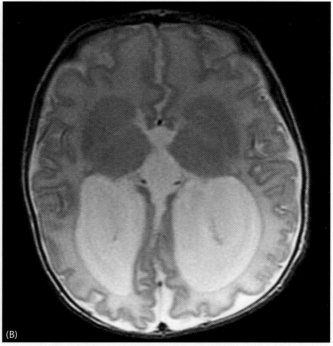

(B)

Figs. 2.165A, B (A) Chiari malformation; part of the cerebellum (arrow) extends below the foramen magnum into the upper spinal canal. There is associated hydrocephalus. (B) Hydrocephalus showing dilated lateral ventricles and third ventricle.

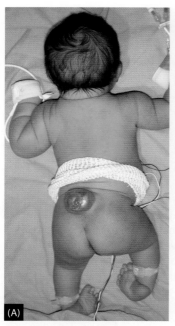 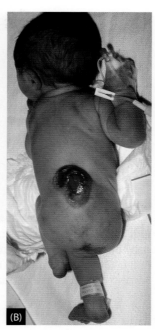

Figs. 2.166A, B (A) Lumbar myelomeningocele. This baby has wasting of the buttocks and a patulous anus caused by paralysis of the gluteal muscles and pelvic floor. Note the bilateral talipes equinovarus caused by paralysis of the muscles in the lower limbs. (B) A lumbar myelomeningocele showing more severe buttock wasting and a patulous anus.

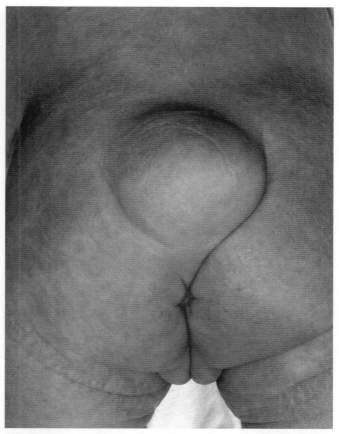

Fig. 2.167 A lumbosacral meningocele covered by skin. This lesion transilluminates brilliantly, and contains no neural tissue. It freely communicates with CSF pathways. If excised carefully, there should be no neurological dysfunction.

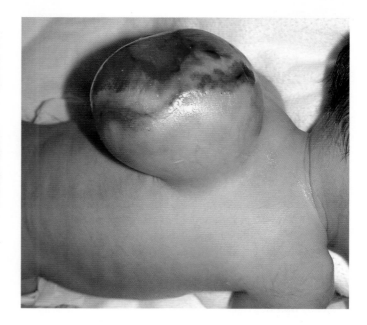

Fig. 2.168 This newborn baby has a rare cervicothoracic myelomeningocele. This is an uncommon site for a live-born infant with spina bifida, since most fetuses with a defect of this size would die before delivery. Note the dysplastic skin over the apex of the lesion.

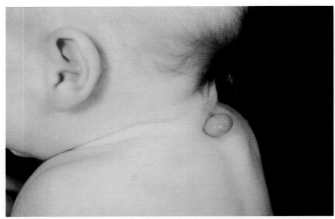

Fig. 2.169 Thoracic meningocele. A rare high thoracic neural tube defect showing protrusion of skin-covered meninges but no neurological deficit.

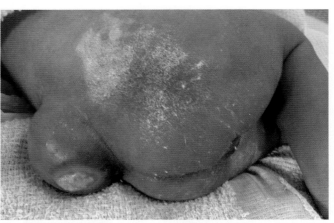

Fig. 2.170 Lumbar lipomyelomeningocele. This newborn baby has an ulcerated skin-covered neural tube defect in the lumbar region, which contains a large amount of hamartomatous fat in association with the myelomeningocele.

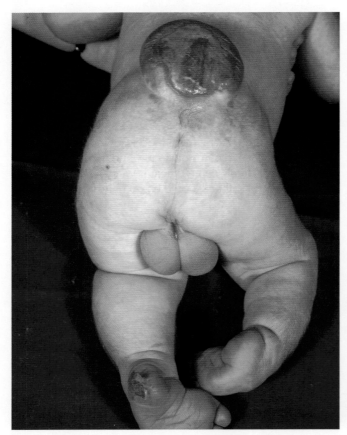

Fig. 2.171 Physical examination. Examination of the motor system should include inspection of spontaneous movements and any deformities secondary to paralysis or paresis. This baby with a high lumbar myelomeningocele has a flat perineum indicative of perineal and levator ani paralysis, as well as bilateral talipes equinovarus. This suggests that the child had paralysis of the legs prenatally, which led to the secondary deformity of the feet.

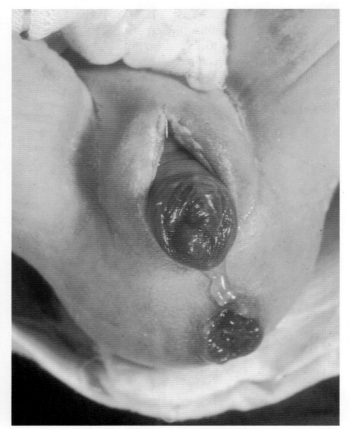

Fig. 2.172 Vaginal and rectal prolapse with continuous leakage of urine. This is secondary to total paralysis of the pelvic floor.

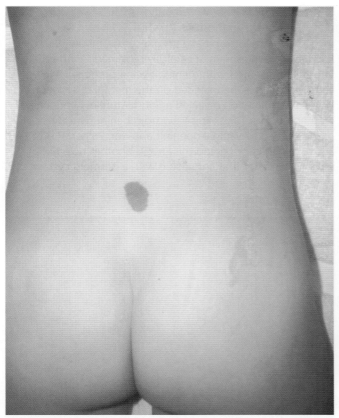

Fig. 2.173 Occult spinal dysraphism. Underlying spinal dysraphism is indicated by the pigmented patch in the midline in this child. The ectodermal dysplasia is secondary to the underlying neural tube defect. Such children need careful investigation to exclude tethering of the spinal cord.

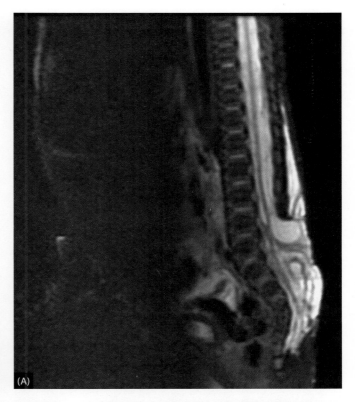

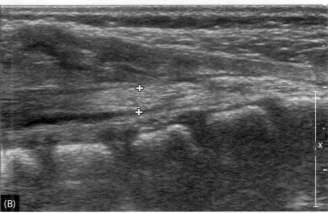

Figs. 2.174A, B (A) Spinal dysraphism on sagittal MRI. (B) Spinal ultrasound scan showing a fatty filum (between cursors) in an infant with an anorectal malformation.

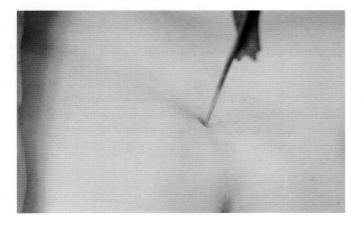

Fig. 2.175 Occult spinal dysraphism with dorsal dermal sinus. This child had failure of neural tube fusion but did not present in the neonatal period. Later in childhood the diagnosis became apparent because of recurrent gram-negative meningitis. Physical examination revealed a small sinus in the midline over the lumbosacral region. At operation, a lacrimal probe was inserted into the sinus, which communicated directly with the vertebral canal. Excision of the sinus prevents further meningitis.

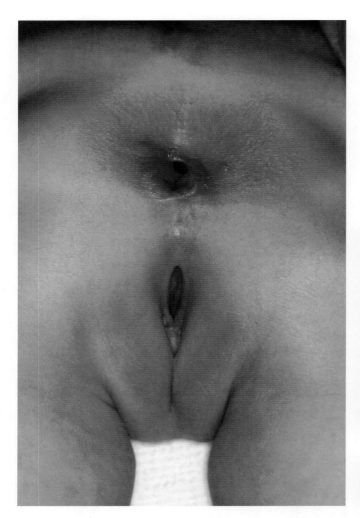

Fig. 2.176 Intravertebral dermoid cyst. This 2-year-old had a defect of chromosome 7, which is known to be associated with intraspinal dermoid cysts. The perineum had never been examined carefully by a medical attendant. The child presented with meningitis and progressive lower limb weakness, superimposed on the mental retardation. Physical examination revealed a flat, featureless perineum with no buttock folds. This view from behind with the child prone shows the vaginal opening anterior. Posterior is the anus. Immediately behind the anus is another hole about 1 cm in diameter that connected with a dermoid cyst within the vertebral canal.

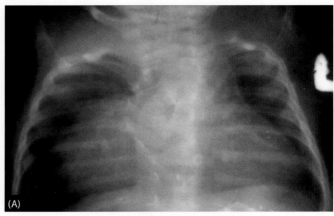

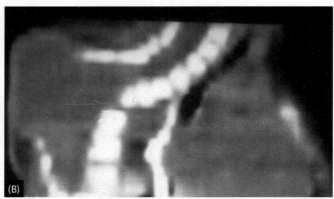

Figs. 2.178A, B (A) Split notochord syndrome in a 2-day-old male infant. The child presented with a lesion on the upper back and abdominal distension. The plain chest radiograph shows the defect in the upper thoracic vertebrae and a mediastinal mass on the right. At laparotomy, a long tubular duplication of the ileum was discovered. (B) In the same patient, a CT scan showed the vertebral defect (arrow) and the cystic skin-covered lesion in the back. The communication between the mediastinal lesion and the dorsal lesion is evident.

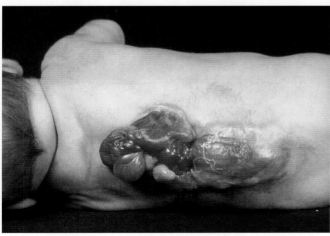

Fig. 2.177 A thoracolumbar myelomeningocele associated with development of a teratoma.

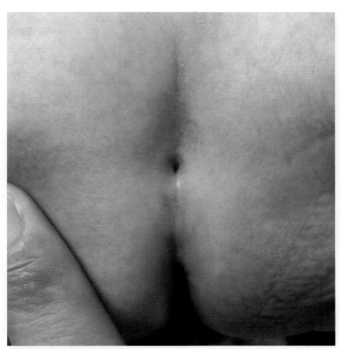

Fig. 2.179 A sacral dimple or pit posterior to the anus. The skin should be stretched over the coccyx to expose the base of the dimple. These are common and benign. The differential diagnosis is a dorsal dermal sinus (see Fig. 2.175), which is usually more than 2.5 cm cranial to the anus and may be associated with hair, naevus, a discharge or a swelling. Unlike a sacral pit, a dorsal dermal sinus may communicate with the spinal canal.

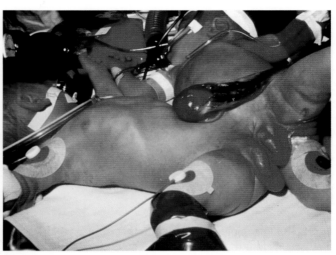

Fig. 2.180 These conjoined twins are connected from the umbilicus to the perineum. There is a common umbilical cord with a small exomphalos, but otherwise the twins are well formed. The surgical problems in separation of conjoined twins depend on the individual anatomical variants. Some organs are duplicated (one for each baby) whereas others are single and shared. Ischiopagus twins may have three limbs (tripus) or four limbs (tetrapus).

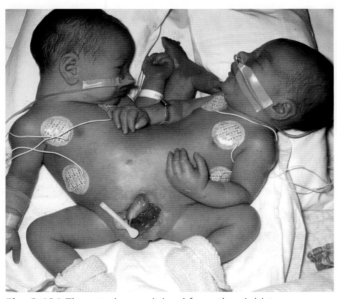

Fig. 2.181 These twins are joined from the xiphisternum to the perineum and share a liver and bowel from the duodenum to caecum. The aim of surgery is to separate the twins equally, to produce two live infants.

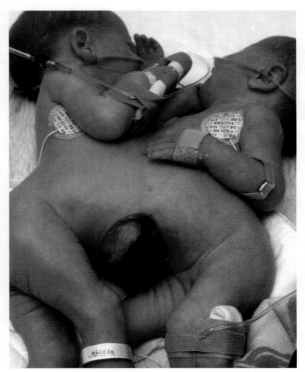

Fig. 2.182 Thoracopagus, where the twins are attached from the sternum to the umbilical region, is the most common variety of conjoined twins, and accounts for about two-thirds of reported cases undergoing separation. Some degree of pericardial fusion is usual.

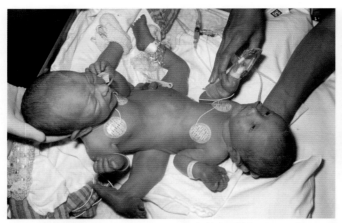

Fig. 2.183 In conjoined twins, a number of bizarre variants may occur. Note the fused common limb in the foreground.

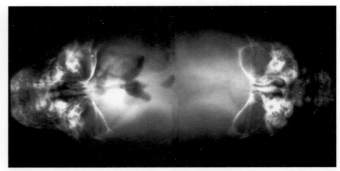

Fig. 2.184 Craniopagus is the rarest form of conjoined twins. This plain radiograph shows the skull separation. Separation can be achieved if there is a superior sagittal sinus for each brain.

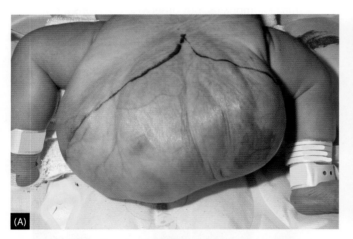

(A)

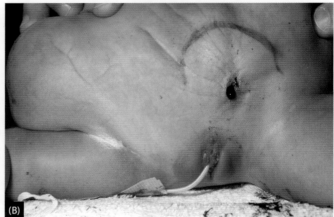

(B)

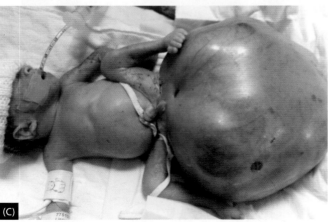

(C)

Figs. 2.185A–C (A) Sacrococcygeal teratoma causing gross distortion of the perineum and some abnormal blood vessels in the overlying skin. (B) Sacrococcygeal teratoma with secondary compression of the anal canal. (C) Sacrococcygeal teratoma is one of the few tumours that can be larger than the infant. Note the ventral displacement of the anus.

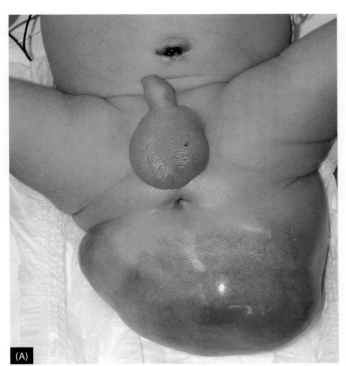
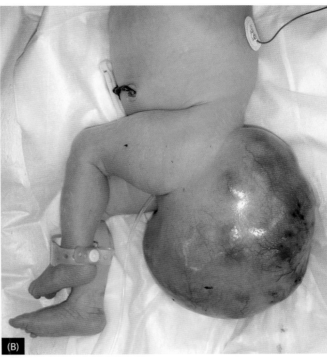

Figs. 2.186A, B (A) A large sacrococcygeal teratoma, which was excised completely in the neonatal period. The coccyx was removed with the tumour to reduce the likelihood of recurrence and malignant degeneration. (B) Lateral view of the same tumour.

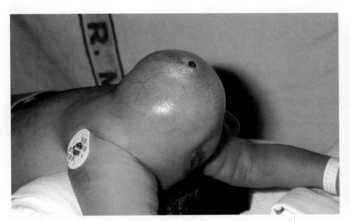

Fig. 2.187 A smaller cystic exophytic sacrococcygeal teratoma. These lesions are readily excised. Note the small area of skin necrosis on the surface of the lesion.

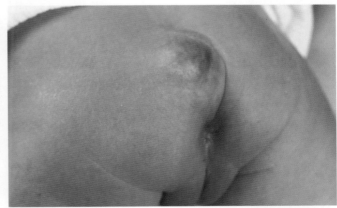

Fig. 2.188 A partially concealed sacrococcygeal teratoma that was initially and erroneously thought to be a vascular anomaly. Most of this tumour was growing anterior to the sacrum and coccyx in the pelvis behind the rectum.

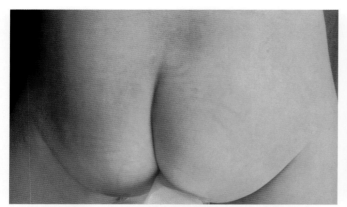

Fig. 2.189 A completely concealed sacrococcygeal teratoma in an infant (Altman type 4). On rectal examination, a presacral mass could be felt. These are potentially the most dangerous because there is often delay in diagnosis and a consequent greater likelihood of malignant degeneration.

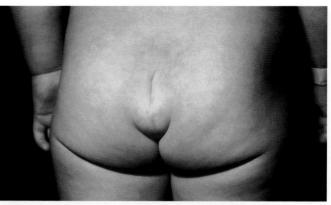

Fig. 2.190 Sacrococcygeal teratoma may present with a benign-looking coccygeal mass later in childhood.

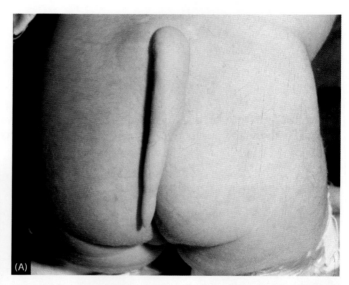

(A)

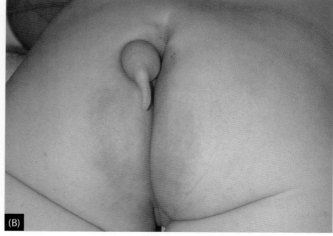

(B)

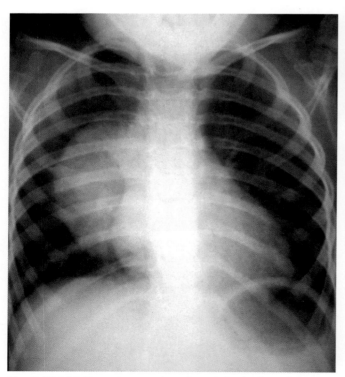

Fig. 2.191 Malignant secondary deposit in the lung from an incompletely excised sacrococcygeal teratoma. This child highlights the importance of complete excision of the tumour at birth, before malignant degeneration occurs.

Figs. 2.192A, B (A) Human tail in a newborn baby. The lesion was attached to the sacral region. There was no neurological deficit, although the tail was sensitive to touch and pain. There was no spinal defect. (B) Another baby with a tail.

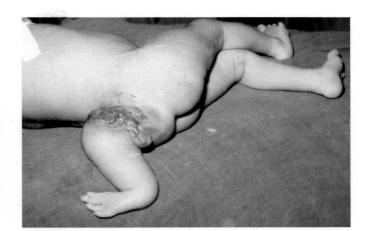

Fig. 2.193 Well-formed accessory limb attached to the lumbosacral region, which is likely to be the result of loss of a conjoined twin. The spine had no abnormality. The limb had sensation but no motor function.

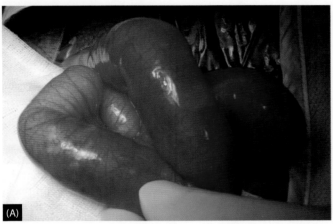

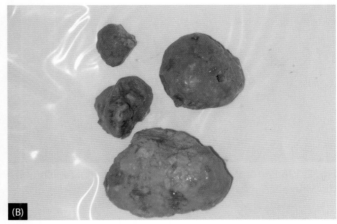

Figs. 2.194A, B (A) Neonatal faecoliths in the bowel. (B) Neonatal faecoliths after removal.

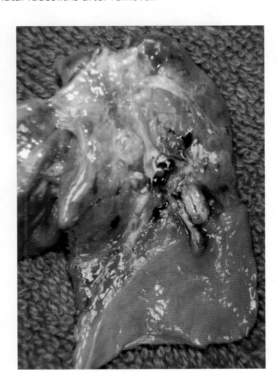

Fig. 2.195 Meconium aspiration can cause respiratory failure in the newborn. Most cases respond to intensive care. In this postmortem specimen of the lungs, the bronchi filled with meconium.

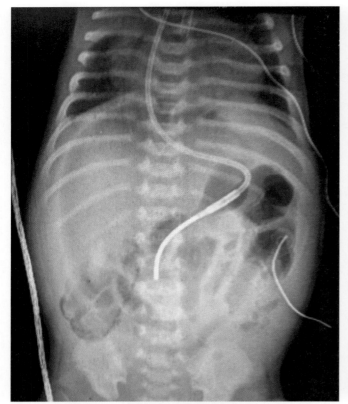

Fig. 2.196 Perforated stomach on an abdominal radiograph, showing a large gas bubble over the liver.

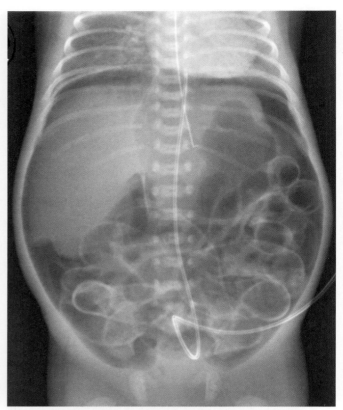

Fig. 2.197 Spontaneous perforation in a 24-week premature baby showing Rigler sign on x-ray, with air outlining both sides of the bowel wall and an obvious falciform ligament.

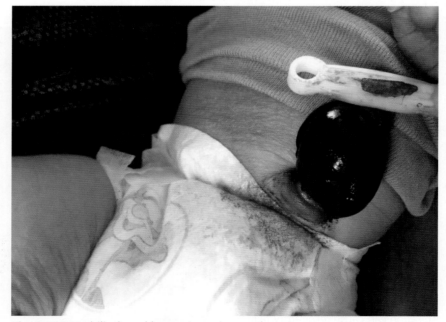

Fig. 2.198 Umbilical cord haematoma in an otherwise normal neonate with no bleeding diathesis.

Head and neck | CHAPTER 3

THE SKULL

The size and shape of the vault of the skull are determined by growth of the brain. The commonest abnormality of the cranium is hydrocephalus, which is caused by congenital abnormalities of the CSF pathway or by acquired obstruction of the CSF flow from haemorrhage, infection or tumour. Spina bifida with Arnold-Chiari malformation was once the commonest cause of hydrocephalus, but now intracranial haemorrhage in very premature babies is seen more frequently. Other disorders causing abnormalities of the skull vault include: plagiocephaly, a positional head deformity caused by pre- or postnatal external pressure on the developing skull that may be associated with intrauterine compression, prematurity or congenital torticollis; microcephaly, as a primary abnormality or secondary to brain injury; encephalocele, which is a severe neural tube fusion defect; and craniosynostosis, where there is premature closure of suture lines.

Hydrocephalus

Hydrocephalus is confirmed by observing an enlarged head circumference relative to that expected on a standard growth chart. Clinical signs of hydrocephalus include frontal bossing, a bulging fontanelle, wide sutures, dilated scalp veins and a small face. Also there may be 'setting-sun eyes', where the iris is partly concealed by the lower lid; this is thought to be caused by compression of periaqueductal structures from raised intracranial pressure resulting in an upward gaze paresis. Severe hydrocephalus in infants can be demonstrable by transillumination of the skull (a bright light and a dark room are required), although an ultrasound scan is a more appropriate and accurate investigation.

Congenital or chronic acquired hydrocephalus is usually treated by insertion of a ventriculoperitoneal shunt to drain the excess CSF into the peritoneal cavity where it is reabsorbed into the circulation. This relieves the raised intracranial pressure and allows skull growth and mental development.

Craniosynostosis

Abnormal or premature closure of the sutures causes distortion of the shape of the vault. As the brain continues to enlarge, skull expansion is produced by increased growth at alternative suture lines, leading to distortion of the head shape. The degree of abnormality varies enormously from minor flattening of one area of the head to severe cranial deformities.

When appropriate, craniosynostosis is now treated by early interventional surgery by craniofacial surgeons. Sutures are opened surgically and the skull and facial skeleton are repositioned to overcome the bony deformity.

Encephalocele

Failure of neural tube fusion in the region of the developing forebrain produces an encephalocele. This commonly involves the occipital region and, less frequently, the glabella. There is a skin-covered cystic swelling containing dysplastic brain and an extension of the CSF pathway. Occipital encephaloceles are often associated with secondary hydrocephalus, blindness and ataxia, because of the non-function of the herniated neural tissue. Encephaloceles are readily identified on antenatal ultrasound (see Chapter 1).

External angular dermoid

This common abnormality is caused by a nest of skin cells becoming separated from the surface during development of the face. The external angle of the eye is along the line of fusion between the frontonasal and maxillary processes, and is therefore a frequent site of a congenital inclusion cyst. Rarely, dermoid cysts may be present over the vault of the skull, behind the ear, or at the internal angle of the eye. The cyst contains desquamated epithelium and skin secretions. It is frequently located below the periosteum, giving it a firmer consistency than would normally be expected of a cyst. It is treated by elective excision in early childhood before it becomes too large. Other lumps on the vault of the skull in childhood are quite rare, although haemangiomas and an occasional primary or secondary tumour may be seen. The commonest neoplasms are Langerhans cell histiocytosis and neuroblastoma metastases.

THE EAR

Common abnormalities affecting the external ear are protruding (bat) ears, preauricular skin tags and preauricular sinuses. Failure of formation of the antihelical fold in the pinna produces protruding ears, and this is corrected with surgery should the cosmetic defect be severe. Preauricular skin tags are really partial duplications of the pinna and often contain a cartilaginous core, which needs to be removed to correct the abnormality. Preauricular skin tags are found anterior to the tragus.

Preauricular sinuses occur on the anterior edge of the upper helix. The sinus runs anteriorly and downwards, and may branch; it may also contain a cartilagenous element. Infection at the blind end of a preauricular sinus produces an abscess anterior to the helix of the ear. Only those infants with a preauricular skin tag or sinus associated with other congenital malformations need to be investigated for potential renal abnormalities.

In more complicated deformities, particularly those related to certain syndromes, there may be severe deficiency or complete agenesis of the external ear. Hearing tests need to be performed to determine whether a middle and inner ear are present. A low position of the pinna in relation to the line of the eye ('low-set ears') may be seen in some malformation syndromes.

SUPERFICIAL INFECTION

Periorbital cellulitis occurs with lower lid oedema and erythema, proptosis and chemosis. The affected eyelids are sometimes closed. Children with periorbital cellulitis tend to be systemically ill, unlike those with preseptal cellulitis. Proptosis with painful limitation of eye movement is the classical sign. Orbital cellulitis is a sight-threatening and occasionally life-threatening infection. It usually arises from the contiguous paranasal sinuses and vision is threatened by compression of the optic nerve and compromise of intraocular circulation. Urgent CT scanning of the orbits and adjacent sinuses, followed by drainage of involved sinuses, is indicated. True orbital abscesses are relatively uncommon.

PAROTID REGION

Overall, the commonest cause of a parotid swelling in children is mumps. The main surgical cause is non-tuberulous mycobacterium (*Mycobacterium avium intracellulare scrofulaceum* [MAIS], previously known as atypical mycobacterium) infection involving parotid nodes. Haemangiomas may also occur in the parotid region. Infection of the parotid gland may damage the duct system, producing sialectasis and recurrent bacterial infection presenting as a recurring painful unilateral parotid swelling. Recurrent parotid sialectasis in children is not necessarily related to infection and the sialectasis in these cases will ultimately resolve without the need for surgery.

THE LIP

Cleft lip is caused by failure of fusion of the maxillary process with the globular process of the premaxilla. It may be unilateral or bilateral, and is associated with distortion of the upper lip and nose, with or without a defect in the alveolar margin and the palate. It is a conspicuous abnormality at birth, and therefore surgery is recommended in the first few months to overcome the cosmetic defect as well as allow normal development of the alveolar margin and dentition. Infants with isolated cleft lip can breast-feed successfully.

Cleft palate is caused by failure of fusion of the palatal shelves, and may affect just the soft palate or both the soft and hard palates. This produces a less severe cosmetic defect, but breast-feeding is impossible because of lack of oral suction. It requires repair before the end of the first year so that normal speech can be acquired. Isolated cleft palate occurs in some instances as part of the Pierre-Robin sequence, where it is due to inability of the tongue to sink into the floor of the mouth because of the abnormally small mandible. The tongue then prevents palatal fusion and leads to a large rectangular cleft. Cleft lip and palate are often inherited together, and are commonly associated with multiple malformation syndromes. They may not only cause feeding difficulties but can also affect speech, dentition and hearing and so are best managed by a multidisciplinary team.

Palatal clefts may involve the soft palate only, hard and soft palate, or are submucosal (consisting of a bifid uvula, notched hard palate and a midline mucosal lucency representing palatal muscle diastasis).

The mucus retention cyst is a minor but common lesion of the lip, usually found on the inside of the lower lip.

THE TONGUE

Tongue-tie (ankyloglossia) is where a tight, short frenulum prevents normal mobility of the tongue. This may interfere with normal latching and breastfeeding and, in more severe cases, with speech. Protrusion of the tongue enables the degree of tongue-tie to be assessed: where the child can protrude the tongue beyond the incisor teeth, release of the frenulum is required rarely.

Enlargement of the tongue may be congenital, as in Beckwith–Wiedemann syndrome, hypothyroidism (cretinism) or Down syndrome, or may be acquired, due to a space-occupying lesion such as a haemangioma or lymphangioma. Displacement of the tongue producing apparent enlargement is present in Pierre-Robin syndrome. Overgrowth of the tongue with Beckwith–Wiedmann syndrome may require surgical reduction, while lymphangioma, although producing an enlarged tongue, may be more difficult to treat surgically. A mass in the midline of the tongue posteriorly may be a lingual thyroid, caused by failure of the normal descent of the thyroid from the region of the foramen caecum; it may be the only functioning thyroid tissue present.

MOUTH, GUMS AND PHARYNX

A ranula is a large cystic lesion in the floor of the mouth pushing up into the oral cavity and distorting the position of the tongue. It is treated by marsupialisation of the overlying mucosa to prevent reaccumulation of mucus. It needs to be differentiated clinically from a lymphangioma, which is more likely to be an infiltrating cystic lesion spreading through the floor of the mouth from the neck.

When a stone is present in the duct of the submandibular salivary gland, it produces intermittent pain and swelling of the gland and obstruction to salivary flow. The calculus is visible through the overlying mucosa inside the mouth just proximal to the duct orifice. If the stone does not pass spontaneously, it can be removed by surgical incision into the duct.

Two abnormalities affecting the gums are an alveolar abscess from a deep-seated infection around a permanent tooth, and a dentigerous cyst, which is a cystic swelling around an unerupted tooth. The latter produces a mass on the external side of the alveolus, which is painless and uninflamed.

Inflammation of the tonsils – tonsillitis – is common in early childhood. The child complains of a sore throat and pain on swallowing; the child is febrile and the tonsils appear enlarged, inflamed and covered with exudate. With increasing age, recurrent infection becomes less common. Severe tonsillitis may lead to a retropharyngeal or peritonsillar abscess ('quinsy'), both of which are severe and potentially life-threatening conditions. They cause severe toxicity, loss of pharyngeal movement (so the child has difficulty in swallowing saliva) and occasionally upper airway obstruction. Such abscesses need incision and drainage in a specialised centre where the airway can be maintained adequately until resolution of the inflammation.

Large adenoids may obstruct the nasopharynx in 4–7-year-old children but treatment is usually unnecessary unless there is severe airway obstruction during sleep (sleep apnoea) or recurrent middle ear infections. Adenoidal tumours are seen occasionally.

CHOANAL ATRESIA

Choanal atresia is unilateral or bilateral bony or membranous occlusion of the posterior choanae. About 50% of affected infants have other congenital anomalies (e.g. the CHARGE association). Bilateral choanal atresia presents immediately after birth with cyanosis and/or respiratory distress relieved by crying because neonates are obligatory nose breathers. These infants require urgent insertion of an oral airway until more definitive investigation and treatment is possible.

LARYNX AND TRACHEA

Abnormalities in the upper airway are rare, except in oesophageal atresia, where tracheomalacia and other airway anomalies are common. Congenital malformations, including stenosis, cysts or webs, may present as respiratory obstruction stridor or aspiration. The exact abnormality is usually determined by fibreoptic transnasal laryngoscopy.

MIDLINE CERVICAL SWELLING

There are four main causes of a midline cervical swelling in childhood, of which thyroglossal cyst is the most frequent. The other causes are infected submental lymph nodes, dermoid cyst and the rare ectopic thyroid. The site of the lump, the degree of movement on swallowing and protrusion of the tongue, and whether the lump is transilluminable usually enable the diagnosis to be made on clinical grounds. Examination includes inspection of the inside of the mouth: the cause of submental nodal infection is usually severe untreated dental caries. A dermoid cyst is mobile in the subcutaneous plane and may have a creamy hue through the skin. Thyroglossal cysts and dermoid cysts are best excised; the thyroglossal cyst and its tract should be removed in their entirety, which involves excision of the middle third of the hyoid bone and a suprahyoid core of tongue muscles. If an ectopic thyroid is suspected, the location of all functioning thyroid tissue can be demonstrated on a radionucleide scan of the neck.

LATERAL NECK LUMPS

Reactive hyperplasia of the lateral cervical lymph nodes is by far the most frequent cause of a lump in the side of the neck. In infants and young children, acute lymphadenitis may lead to secondary abscess formation, an acute cervical abscess. Other lateral cervical masses include lymphatic malformations (previously termed 'cystic hygromas'), haemangioma or a non-tuberculous mycobacterium (MAIS) lymphadenitis. In a child over 6 years of age with painless enlargement of cervical nodes, with or without fever and night sweats, malignant lymphadenopathy from lymphoma must be considered. Other tumours occur occasionally. A branchial cyst may be seen in late childhood: the swelling is deep to sternocleidomastoid and may be associated with signs of inflammation if secondary infection has occurred.

Acute lymphadenitis may progress to abscess formation in a few days. The presence of a fluctuant swelling suggests abscess formation, but when the cavity is beneath the investing cervical fascia, even a large abscess may be tense and not obviously fluctuant. Non-tuberculous mycobacterial lymphadenitis has a longer history with low-grade inflammatory signs, and after about 4–6 weeks produces a purple discoloration of the skin as the subcutaneous portion of the collar-stud abscess points. Untreated, a chronic discharging sinus will develop. Lymphatic malformations involving the neck or side of the face may present as non-tender swellings at birth. In the absence of haemorrhage into the cysts, they transilluminate. They may enlarge rapidly from both infection and haemorrhage. Surgery at birth is not necessary unless the lesion is enormous and causes obstruction of the airway, in which situation urgent provision of an airway may be required. Lymphatic malformations are often treated by interventional radiology.

Haemangiomas can be distinguished from lymphatic malformations by the fact that they contain spongy blood-filled tissue. There may be overlying dysplastic vessels in the skin and, if blood flow is rapid, they may produce a bruit on auscultation. Haemangiomas can be emptied by compression and may be associated with systemic features such as cardiac failure caused by excessive blood flow through the lesion or thrombocytopaenia from trapping of platelets, leading to secondary haemorrhage (Kassabach–Merritt syndrome). When haemangiomas occur in a limb or appendage, local tissue overgrowth may be dramatic (Klippel-Trenaunay syndrome).

A sternomastoid tumour is a fibrous swelling of the sternocleidomastoid muscle, the cause of which is unknown but may be related to abnormal intrauterine positioning and/or an ischaemic muscle injury. It presents a few weeks after birth with shortening of the sternomastoid muscle and rotation of the head to the opposite side. In infants this may produce secondary plagiocephaly because of the effect of gravity on one side of the head. The sternomastoid tumour resolves spontaneously within several months, but in some children there is residual fibrosis and shortening of the muscle, often with concomitant unilateral facial hypoplasia. This produces the classic torticollis or wry neck of later childhood, where the head is held level but one shoulder is elevated in compensation. The head is flexed towards and rotated away from the side with the short sternomastoid. The differential diagnosis of torticollis includes ocular imbalance, congenital cervical hemivertebrae, atlantooccipital subluxation and occasionally a posterior fossa tumour causing brain stem compression. In none of these is there shortening of the sternocleidomastoid muscle.

Malignant disease in lymph nodes presents with rapidly growing, non-tender nodes that feel rubbery and have no features of inflammation. In pre-school children, leukaemia or secondary neuroblastoma is the most likely cause. In older children, lymphoma and leukaemia are more common causes of malignant nodal enlargement. If a diagnosis cannot be made on a blood film or bone marrow aspiration, lymph node biopsy is performed.

Branchial cysts are rare congenital remnants of the second or third branchial clefts. A single cyst is usually present beneath the middle third of the sternocleidomastoid muscle. Persistence of the cartilaginous remnants of the branchial arches may present as skin-covered, cartilaginous lesions in the same area. Persistence of the second branchial cleft will present with a sinus opening at the anterior border of the lower third of the sternomastoid muscle. Mucus, saliva or pus may exude from the opening. The sinus may communicate with the tonsillar fossa as a fistula.

THE EYE

Physical examination of the eye is important in infancy because the patient is unable to give a clear history. The eye should be clear and the pupil black, and the pupillary reflexes should be normal.

Nystagmus

Nystagmus is abnormal at any age, and the baby should be able to fix on a point of light by the age of 6 weeks. By 2–3 months of age, the infant should be able to follow a moving object, demonstrating that normal macular function is established. The ability to identify and pick up small objects and coloured beads is a way of testing visual acuity in toddlers. Visual acuity in children more than 3 years of age is tested with the E-chart or the Sheridan-Gardiner tests. In the latter, the child identifies the correct one of several letters held by the examiner, by pointing to the same letter on cards held by the child.

Strabismus

Strabismus, or squint, is a common abnormality where there is failure of coordination of the eyes. After 2–3 months, when normal macular vision should be established, persisting strabismus is abnormal and needs immediate investigation. If untreated, the brain will suppress the double image caused by the deviated eye. This may be permanent. Blindness or oculomotor nerve injuries need to be excluded, but the common problem is a refractive error. While shining a light on the eyes and observing the corneal reflection, the non-squinting eye is covered to see if the deviated eye can take up macular fixation. This occurs as long as there is no severe defect in the visual pathway. Head tilt may be an adaptation to a vertical squint.

Obstruction of the nasolacrimal duct at birth is due to epithelial debris or an occluding membrane in the duct. It tends to resolve spontaneously within the first 6 months, and usually requires no treatment apart from measures to avoid or treat infection. If photophobia is present with watering, this suggests more serious abnormalities, such as corneal irritation caused by congenital glaucoma, corneal abrasion or foreign body keratitis.

The white pupil (leukocoria)

The black pupil has a red reflex when reflecting incident light from the surface of the retina. A white reflex is a serious physical sign suggesting:

1 space-occupying lesion in the eye, such as retinoblastoma.
2 An inflammatory mass due to toxoplasmosis or *Toxocara* infestation.
3 Retinal detachment, seen in retinopathy of prematurity.
4 A congenital or acquired cataract.

Retinoblastoma, although rare, is an important abnormality, since early recognition improves the prognosis. The tumour spreads directly along the optic nerve to the central nervous system, or via the bloodstream. In some families it is hereditary. It produces either a white reflex or a convergent squint, since the resulting decrease in vision is not recognised.

Ptosis

Ptosis is seen in a variety of conditions in childhood, but may be quite subtle in its presentation. Severe ptosis, which results in occlusion of the pupil, will cause amblyopia if not corrected promptly – the same applies to other lesions that occlude the visual pathway.

SPECIFIC SYNDROMES

A number of specific syndromes are associated with recognisable deformities or peculiarities of the head, face and neck.

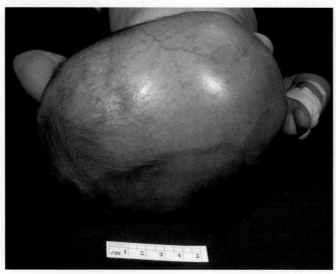

Fig. 3.1 Hydrocephalus. This baby has a large head with a bulging fontanelle and dilated veins on the scalp.

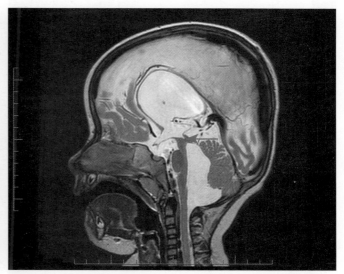

Fig. 3.2 MRI of skull showing aqueduct stenosis (arrow).

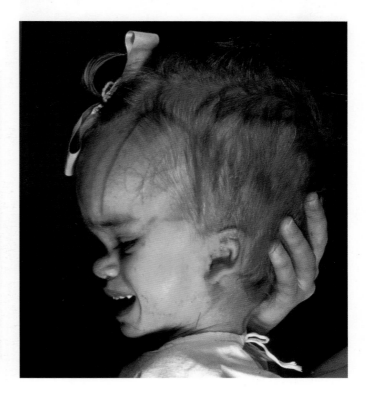

Fig. 3.3 This infant with gross hydrocephalus has an enlarged head circumference, bulging fontanelle, overhanging forehead, distended scalp veins and separation of the sutures. The face looks small in comparison to the size of the head.

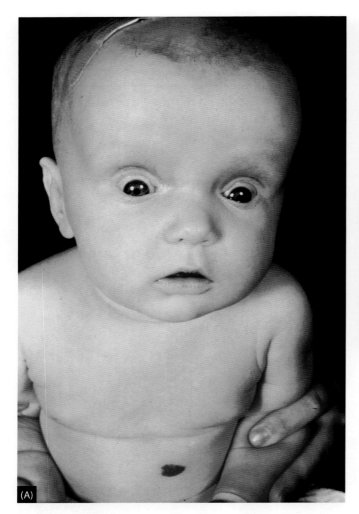

(A)

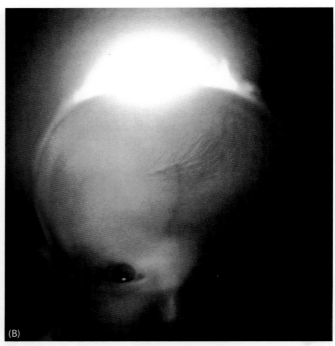

(B)

Figs. 3.4A, B (A) Dandy–Walker syndrome with hydrocephalus. The wide-open anterior fontanelle is visible. (The small dressing at the lateral angle of the fontanelle is where CSF has been aspirated). The large head circumference, frontal bossing and 'setting-sun' eyes are evident. In addition, the child has a small infantile haemangioma on the anterior chest wall. (B) Transillumination of the head of the same child with gross hydrocephalus as in A. Much of the cavity of the vault contains fluid, which in this age group can be transilluminated by a bright light (same patient as in A).

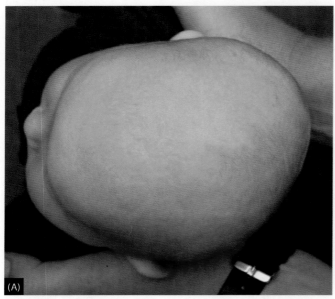

(A)

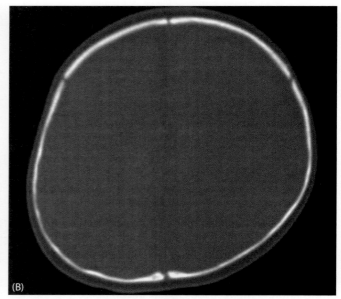

(B)

Figs. 3.5A, B (A) Deformational plagiocephaly. (B) Skull CT showing patent sutures in plagiocephaly.

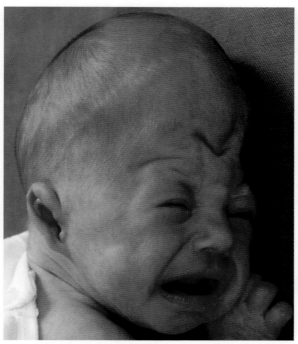

Fig. 3.6 Turricephaly. This baby has vault synostosis producing a small deformed head, which is elongating upwards to form a turret.

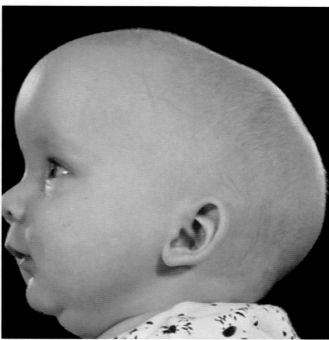

Fig. 3.7 Scaphocephaly. Premature fusion of the sagittal suture produces scaphocephaly, with a long, narrow boat-shaped head. This baby is 3 months of age.

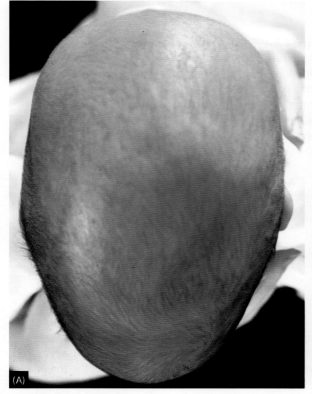

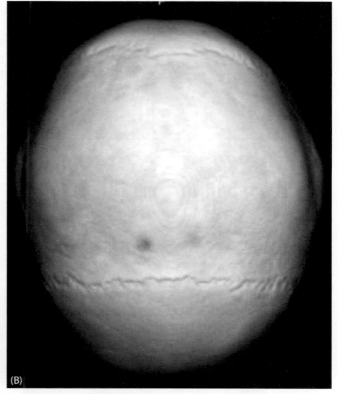

Figs. 3.8A, B (A) View from above showing the narrow skull in scaphocephaly. (B) CT reconstruction in scaphocephaly showing the coronal and parietal sutures open but the sagittal suture closed.

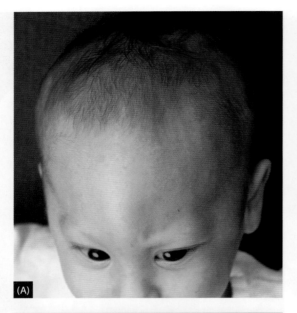

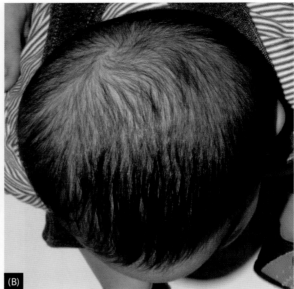

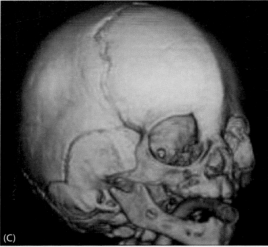

Figs. 3.9A–C (A) Craniosynostosis in a child who has premature closure of the metopic suture, causing a trigonocephalic skull deformity. There is a prominent ridge passing from the anterior fontanelle to the bridge of the nose and the narrow forehead. (B) Trigonocephaly caused by premature closure of the metopic suture. (C) CT reconstruction of skull in trigonocephaly.

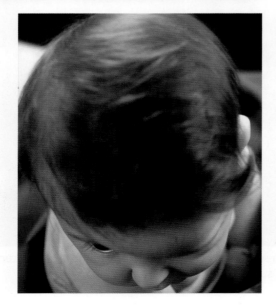

Fig. 3.10 Coronal synostosis in an infant with frontal plagiocephaly caused by premature closure of the right coronal suture. There is recession of the right side of the forehead, best seen from above, as in this picture. In addition to the deformity of the forehead, it shows the typical curvature of the facial skeleton that occurs in this condition, with convexity of the cheek greatest on the side of the forehead deformity.

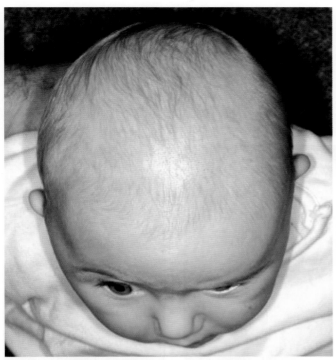

Fig. 3.11 Unicoronal synostosis showing the asymmetry of the orbits.

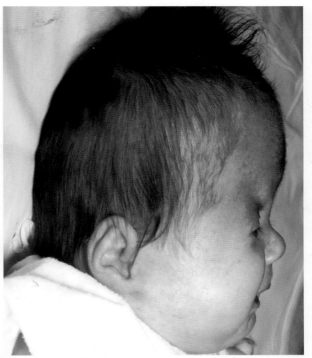

Fig. 3.12 Brachycephaly. This 1-month-old infant has bilateral coronal synostosis producing a narrow head from front to back.

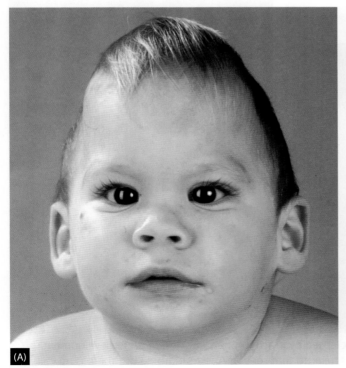

(A)

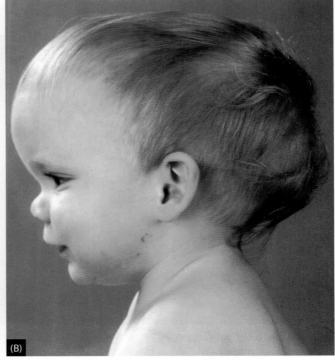

(B)

Figs. 3.13A, B Scaphocephaly affecting an older child with sagittal suture closure showing the progressive deformity that occurs in scaphocephaly, as seen from the front in (A) and from the side in (B).

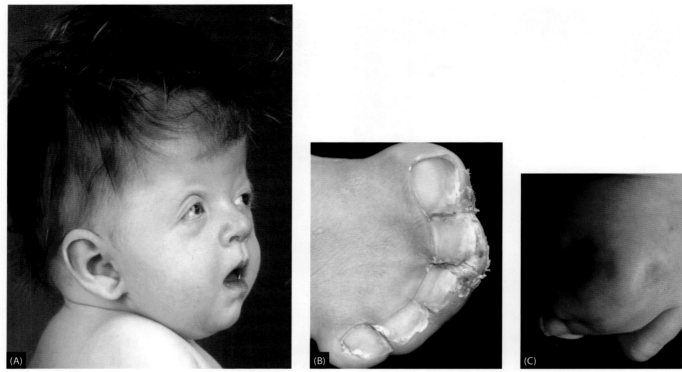

Figs. 3.14A–C Craniosynostosis in Apert syndrome. (A) In this inherited deformity there is brachycephaly associated with underdevelopment of the middle third of the face. There is also syndactyly which can affect the foot (B) or the hand (C).

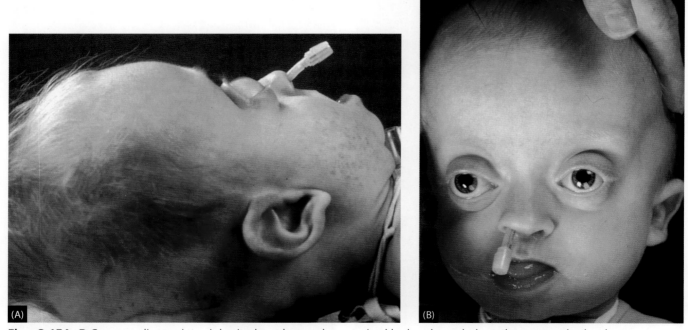

Figs. 3.15A, B Crouzon disease is an inherited syndrome characterised by brachycephaly and severe underdevelopment of the middle third of the face. It produces a facial appearance similar to that seen in Apert syndrome but there is no syndactyly. This child also has hydrocephalus and choanal atresia, which necessitated insertion of a nasal airway. Note that a tracheostomy was required in early infancy to establish an adequate airway. (A) Lateral view; (B) frontal view.

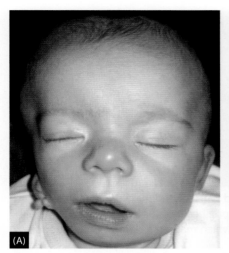
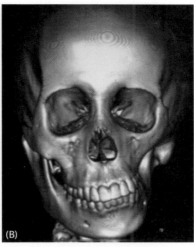
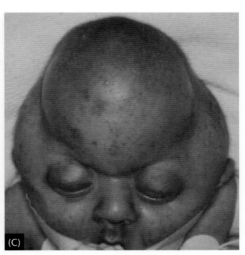

Figs. 3.16A–C (A) Hemifacial microsomia and microtia in Goldenhar syndrome. (B) CT reconstruction of hemifacial microsomia. (C) Complex cranioisynostosis with Kleeblattschädel anomaly (cloverleaf deformity).

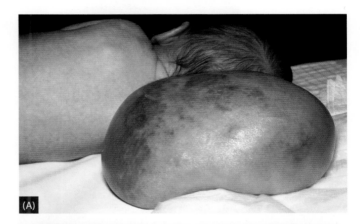

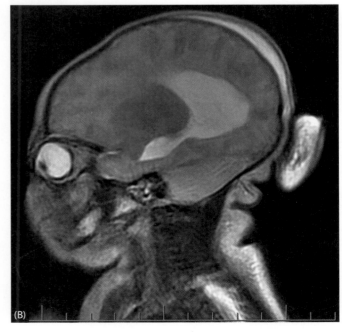

Figs. 3.17A, B (A) Massive occipital encephalocele containing predominantly fluid (CSF), but also some brain tissue, which has herniated through the defect in the skull. Many of these children are now diagnosed antenatally (see Chapter 1) and the pregnancy terminated. (B) MRI of occipital encephalocele.

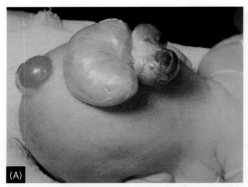
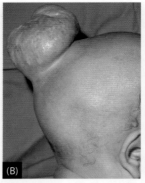
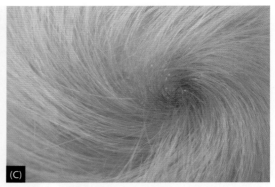

Figs. 3.18A–C (A) Multiple encephaloceles in the occipital region. This was associated with secondary hydrocephalus, blindness and ataxia because of non-function of the herniated neural tissue. (B) Encephalocele of the cranial vault. (C) A neural tube defect presenting as a tuft of different-coloured hair on the scalp, which marked a dermal sinus extending down to the dura.

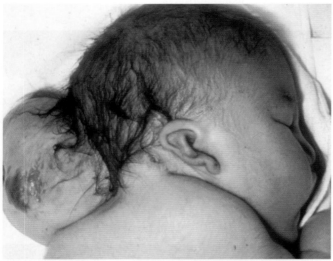

Fig. 3.19 Meckel syndrome is a rare genetic disorder characterised by an encephalocele, polydactyly and multicystic kidneys. It is usually fatal as a result of renal failure, oligohydramnios and pulmonary hypoplasia. The flabby skin conceals a sac that contains brain, meninges and CSF, and in this child is associated with secondary microcephaly and significant distortion of the CSF pathways. Should the defect be excised, hydrocephalus is an almost inevitable consequence. This child would be severely retarded and blind if it survived. A concomitant major abnormality of the cervical spine has caused the shoulder girdle to ride high to the extent of distorting the lobe of the right ear. The infant dies from renal failure shortly after birth.

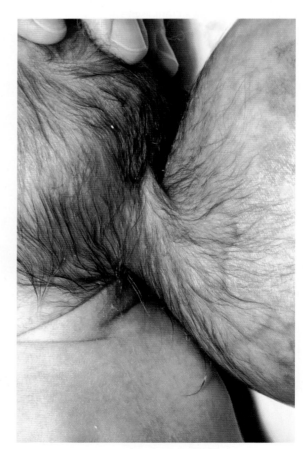

Fig. 3.20 Large occipital encephalocele with a small, narrow, pedunculated attachment to the head.

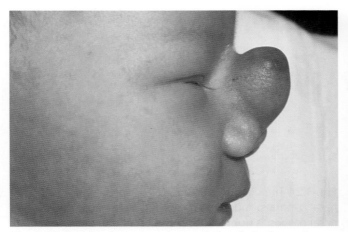

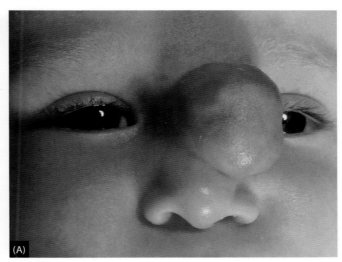

(A)

Fig. 3.21 An anterior or nasal encephalocele in the region of the glabella. It is present at birth and may produce orbital hypertelorism and nasal deformity. It is soft and compressible and enlarges on crying.

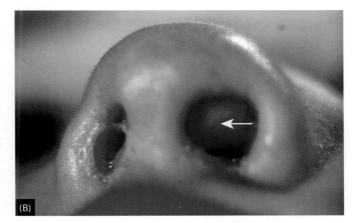

(B)

Figs. 3.22A, B (A) A nasal encephalocele may look similar to a nasal glioma, the difference being that an encephalocele has maintained a communication with the brain and is within the dural sac, whereas the neural tissue within a nasal glioma has become walled off from the brain and meninges. (B) The lower margin of a nasal glioma may be seen bulging into the anterior nares (arrow).

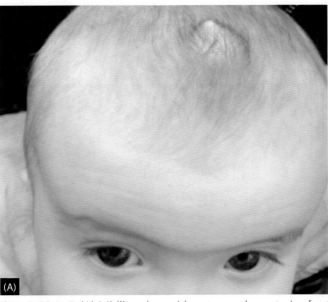

(A)

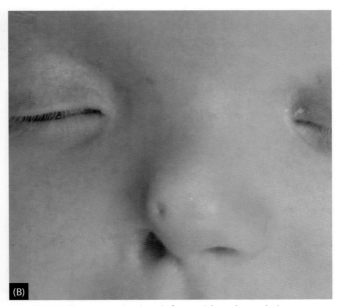

(B)

Figs. 3.23A, B (A) Midline dermoid cyst over the anterior fontanelle. (B) Midline neural tube defect with a dermal sinus extending from the tip of the nose to the frontal dura.

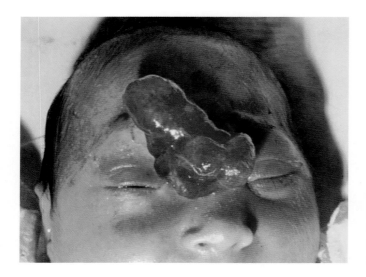

Fig. 3.24 The differential diagnosis of an encephalocele or nasal glioma includes a dermoid cyst of the nose, lateral nasal proboscis (tubular nose) and teratoma. In this example, the nasal lesion was an aborted conjoined twin (incomplete cephalopagus) and contained a skeleton.

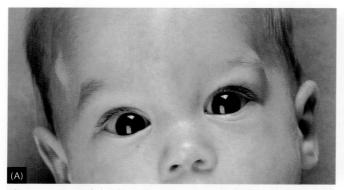

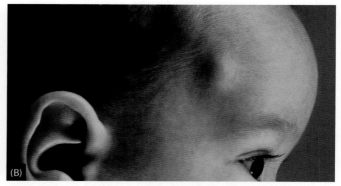

Figs. 3.25A, B (A) Bilateral external angular dermoid cysts. Both the lesion on the left, which is in the common position under the lateral end of the eyebrow, and the lesion on the right are situated on the line of fusion between the frontonasal process and the maxillary processes. The cyst forms when a few cells of ectoderm are caught beneath the surface during fusion as the embryo rolls from 2 to 3 dimensions to form the head and face. The cyst may lie beneath the pericranium, which makes it feel much firmer and more adherent to the bone than may be expected. It contains pultaceous, cheesy yellow material, caused by desquamation of the inner lining of the skin. (B) A lateral view of the same child, showing the more posterior location of this congenital inclusion dermoid cyst.

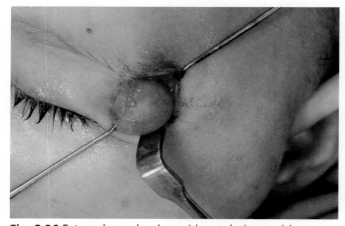

Fig. 3.26 External angular dermoid cyst during excision.

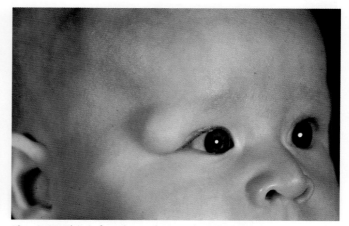

Fig. 3.27 This infant has a lesion that looks like an external angular dermoid cyst, but was in fact a neurofibroma. It is too large for the age of the infant to be a dermoid cyst.

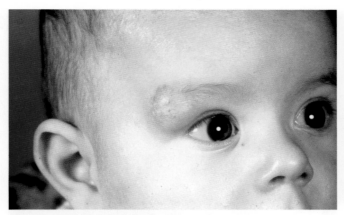

Fig. 3.28 Other lesions can occur in the same position as an external angular dermoid. This small child has a haemangioma of the eyebrow. The skin colouring and its softer consistency enable a clinical diagnosis to be made.

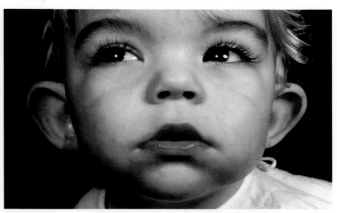

Fig. 3.29 Protruding ears is a common congenital abnormality caused by inadequate development of the antihelical fold in the pinna.

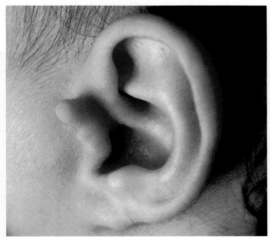

Fig. 3.30 Most preauricular skin tags are found anterior to the tragus and contain a central cartilaginous core, which must be removed for the lesion to be fully excised.

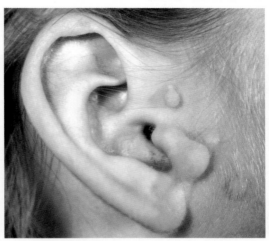

Fig. 3.31 In this more severe example of preauricular skin tags, there are multiple lesions of varying degrees of formation. They are often bilateral and asymmetrical. These lesions are sometimes associated with renal anomalies.

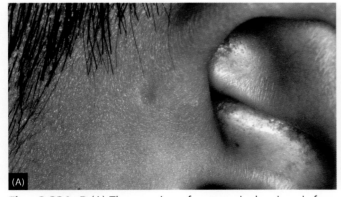

(A)

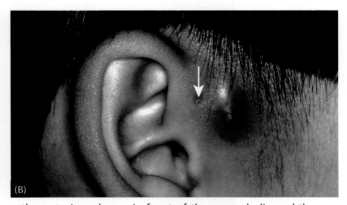

(B)

Figs. 3.32A, B (A) The opening of a preauricular sinus is found on the anterior edge or in front of the upper helix and the track extends downwards and forwards. Preauricular sinuses are often bilateral and may become infected to produce a preauricular abscess. (B) This infected preauricular sinus is on the same patient, but on the other side. Preauricular abscesses typically appear about 1 cm anterior and below the preauricular sinus opening (arrow).

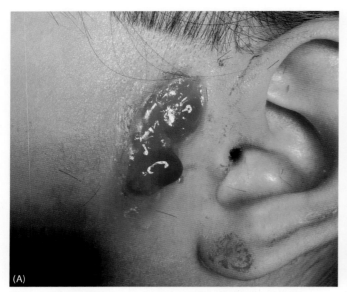
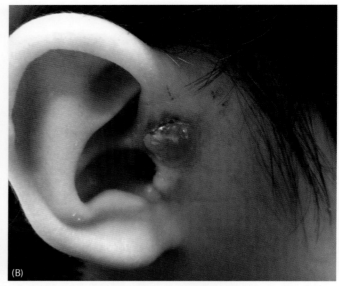

Figs. 3.33A, B (A) Preauricular abscess, which has been caused by infection in a preauricular sinus. (B) Chronic infection in a preauricular sinus with granulation tissue. In neither child will the lesion heal while the sinus persists.

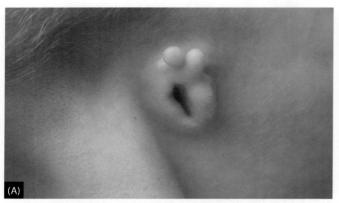
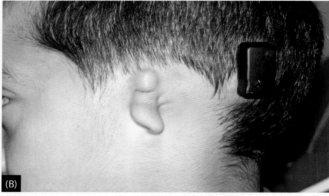

Figs. 3.34A, B (A) Severe deficiency (microtia) or agenesis of the external ear is seen in a number of syndromes. In many patients, the middle and inner ear are affected as well. (B) Microtia with a bone anchored hearing aid.

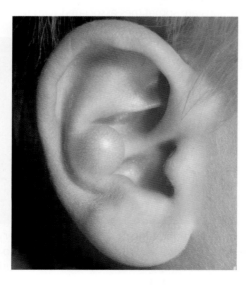

Fig. 3.35 An inclusion dermoid cyst of the pinna following an ear-piercing procedure.

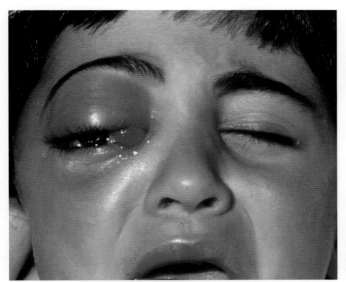

Fig. 3.36 Periorbital cellulitis with eyelid oedema and erythema, proptosis and chemosis. In this child, the affected eyelids are not closed. Children with periorbital cellulitis tend to be systemically ill, unlike those with preseptal cellulitis (see **Fig. 3.38**). Proptosis with painful limitation of eye movement is the classical sign. Orbital cellulitis is a sight-threatening infection. It usually arises from the contiguous sinuses and vision is threatened by compression of the optic nerve and compromise of intraocular circulation. Urgent CT scanning of the orbits and adjacent sinuses, followed by drainage of involved sinuses, is indicated. True orbital abscesses are relatively uncommon.

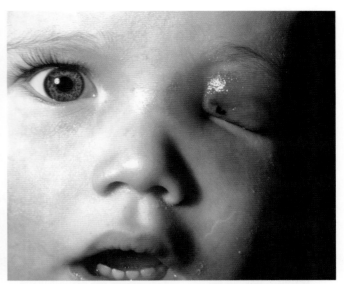

Fig. 3.37 Preseptal cellulitis is more common than orbital cellulitis. In this child it involves the upper eyelid and has caused complete closure of the palpebral aperture as a result of marked lid oedema. Eyelid retraction and inspection of the globe to exclude orbital involvement is vital. The commonest causative organism is *Haemophilus influenzae*. Rarely, there is a treatable focus in the lid, such as a tarsal gland abscess (acute hordeolum).

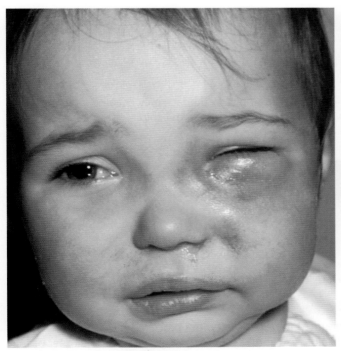

Fig. 3.38 Preseptal cellulitis involving the lower lid. Again, the lid oedema causes the eye to close.

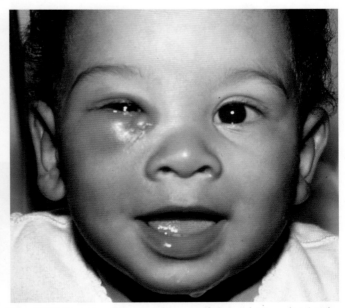

Fig. 3.39 Dacrocystitis. An abscess of the right nasolacrimal sac is about to point through the skin below and medial to the eye. It is associated with preseptal cellulitis. Following resolution of the acute infection, tear duct drainage needs to be re-established.

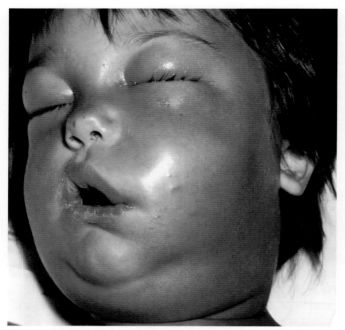

Fig. 3.40 Extensive facial cellulitis affecting the whole of the left side of the face, including the eyelids and neck, and causing distortion of the mouth. Note that the oedema has extended across to the right side and caused closure of the right eye.

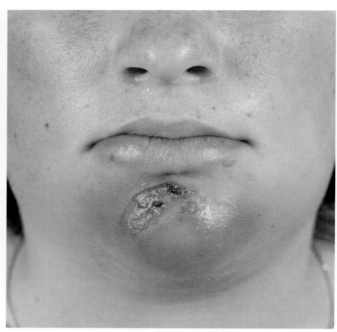

Fig. 3.41 Staphylococcal cellulitis (carbuncle) involving the chin.

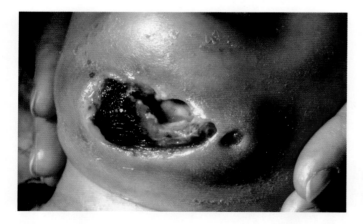

Fig. 3.42 A dog-bite to the face may become infected. In this child, the dog-bite to the chin is infected, producing extensive tissue necrosis.

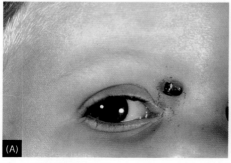
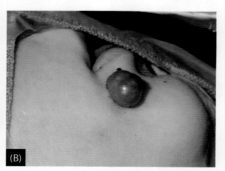
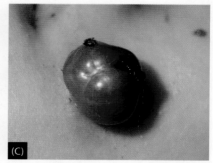

Figs. 3.43A–C (A) Pyogenic granuloma. Minor local trauma is presumed to have initiated this process, where there is localised overgrowth of granulation tissue supplied by an arteriole which bleeds readily. (B) Pyogenic granuloma near the corner of the mouth. (C) Close-up appearance of the pyogenic granuloma shown in B.

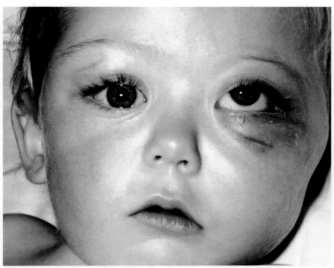

Fig. 3.44 This child has a neuroblastoma causing left orbital swelling and proptosis. This needs to be distinguished from periorbital cellulitis.

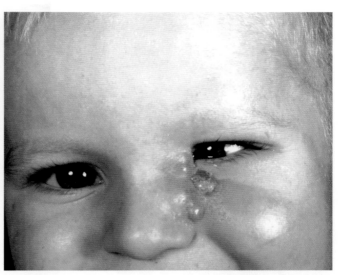

Fig. 3.45 Reticulum cell carcinoma in the region of the eye. Histology will provide the diagnosis.

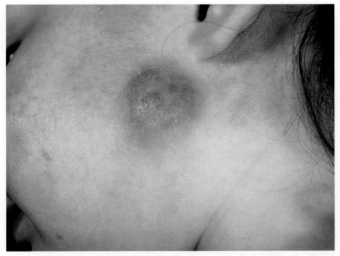

Fig. 3.46 MAIS infection is seen in pre-school children who are presumed to get the infection by putting their dirty hands in their mouth, as the atypical mycobacterium is found in soil, water or dust. Over a 3–6 week period there is painless enlargement of one or more cervical lymph nodes, often in the parotid region, which if untreated will ultimately ulcerate through the skin. This is because the infected nodes rupture into the subcutaneous tissue, producing a collar-stud abscess.

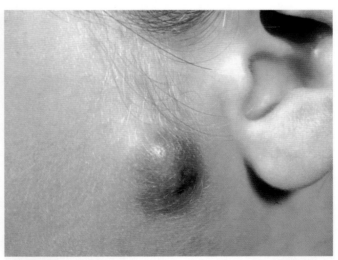

Fig. 3.47 Degenerating pilomatrixoma. Clinically, this lesion looked very similar to a MAIS infection, but felt harder.

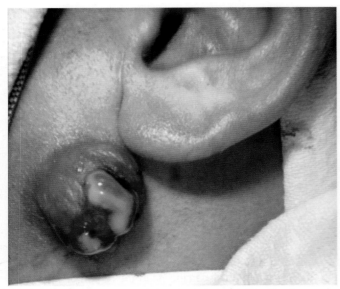

Fig. 3.48 First branchial cleft, which was incompletely excised at the first operation. Secondary infection has occurred, producing a chronic discharging sinus. Complete excision of the branchial remnant is curative. First branchial remnants open internally into the external auditory canal and are much less common than second branchial remnants.

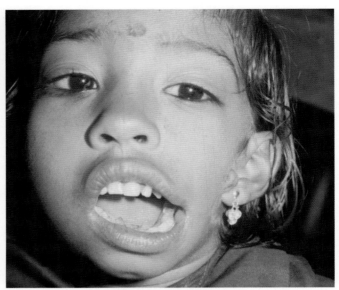

Fig. 3.49 First arch syndrome, showing macrostomia, mandibular hypoplasia and deformity anterior to, and involving, the left ear. The right side of the face was normal.

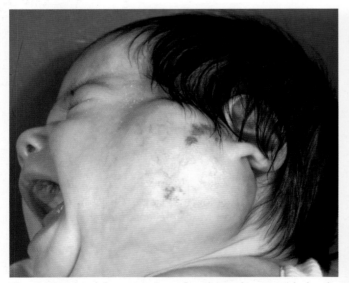

Fig. 3.50 A large haemangioma involving the parotid gland and causing distortion of the pinna. The lesion was soft and had skin changes consistent with a haemangioma.

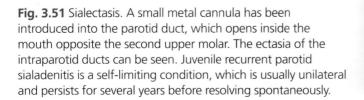

Fig. 3.51 Sialectasis. A small metal cannula has been introduced into the parotid duct, which opens inside the mouth opposite the second upper molar. The ectasia of the intraparotid ducts can be seen. Juvenile recurrent parotid sialadenitis is a self-limiting condition, which is usually unilateral and persists for several years before resolving spontaneously.

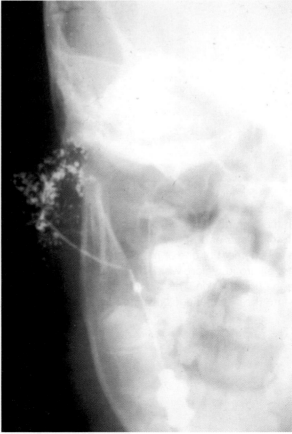

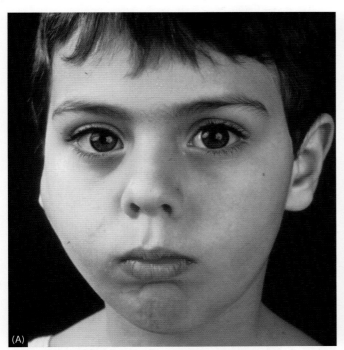

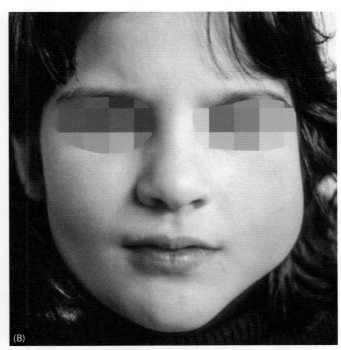

Figs. 3.52A, B (A) In sialectasis there is generalised enlargement of the affected parotid gland. The child suffers periods of discomfort, particularly prior to and during meals. Some relief can be obtained by regularly massaging the gland to assist drainage. This condition can be distinguished from mumps infection as the latter is always bilateral. (B) The typical appearance of parotitis.

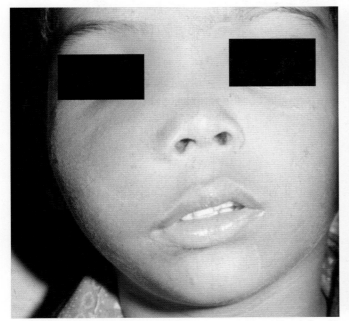

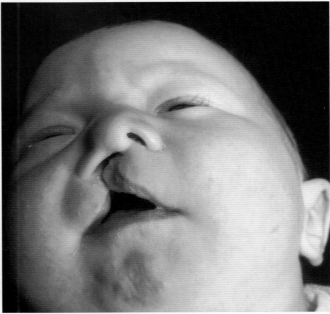

Fig. 3.53 Rhabdomyosarcoma of the right maxilla in a 10-year-old boy. The swelling is anterior to the parotid.

Fig. 3.54 Unilateral cleft lip producing significant distortion of the upper lip and nose.

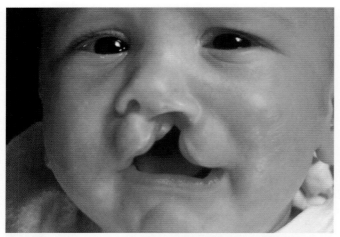

Fig. 3.55 Unilateral cleft lip with an associated defect in the alveolar margin.

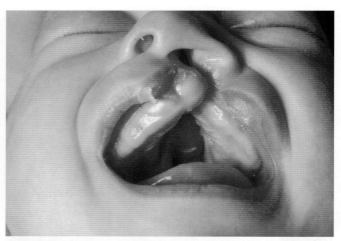

Fig. 3.56 Inilateral cleft lip combined with a cleft palate.

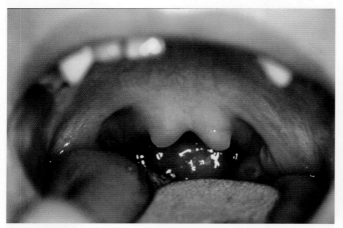

Fig. 3.57 A bifid uvula alone is relatively common. If this is associated with a notched hard palate and a midline mucosal lucency (representing midline palatal muscle diastasis), it amounts to a submucosal cleft.

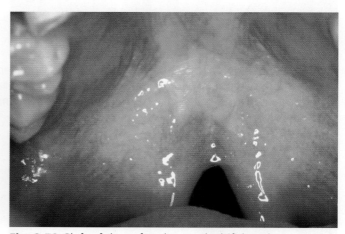

Fig. 3.58 Cleft of the soft palate and a bifid uvula, associated with a midline bony defect posteriorly.

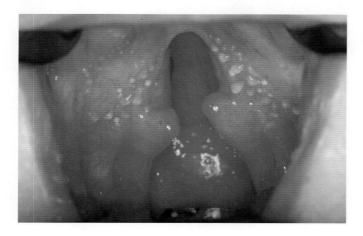

Fig. 3.59 Cleft of the soft and hard palates viewed through the mouth showing the nasopharynx deep to the cleft. Although the cosmetic defect is less obvious than in cleft lip, breast-feeding is impossible because of the infant's inability to achieve adequate oral suction.

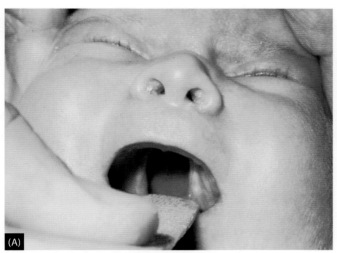

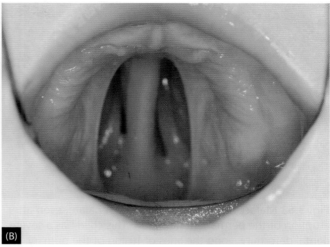

Figs. 3.60A, B (A) A wider cleft of the whole of the hard palate. The tongue has been depressed by the spatula. The defect in the secondary palate interferes with feeding, and causes poor speech development. Recurrent otitis media relates to the abnormal openings of the eustachian tubes. (B) Another view of the wide cleft palate in a patient with the Pierre-Robin sequence.

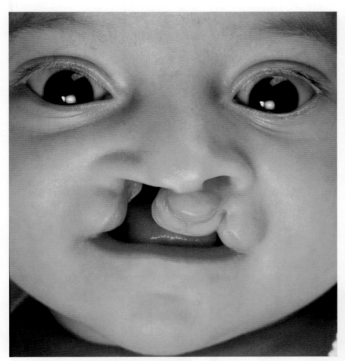

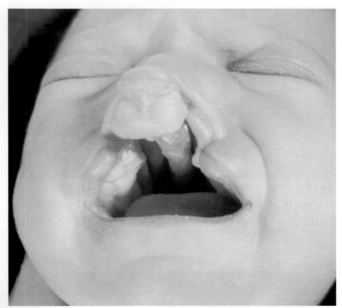

Fig. 3.61 Asymmetric bilateral cleft lip with deficiency of the alveolar margin.

Fig. 3.62 Serious deformity and upward rotation of the premaxilla in an infant with bilateral cleft lip and palate. The premaxillary ridge, which comprises the middle third of the upper lip and the alveolar margin containing the incisor teeth, is rotated forwards in an abnormal manner. This is caused by failure of the bilateral cleft in the lip to hold the skeletal elements in their correct alignment. The midline nasal septum and the inferior and middle conchae of the nasal cavity are visible through the open roof of the mouth.

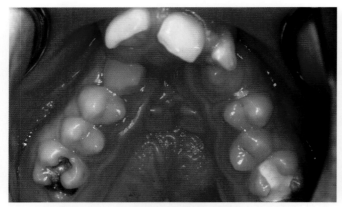

Fig. 3.63 Malocclusion is common in cleft palate, even after eruption of the permanent dentition. This child has a severe dental deformity along the lines of fusion of the primary palate. Teeth may be in excess, absent or deformed, along the line of fusion.

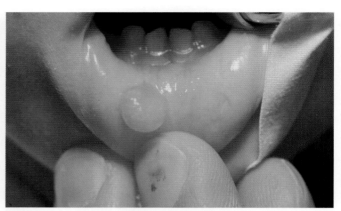

Fig. 3.64 Mucus retention cyst, commonly found on the inside of the lower lip.

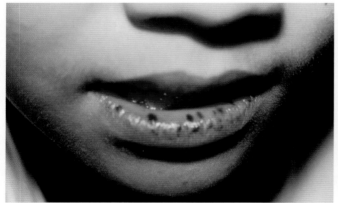

Fig. 3.65 The pigmentation of the lip is characteristic of Peutz-Jegher syndrome, which is associated with intestinal polyps. Pigmentation also may be seen in the perianal region and under the nails.

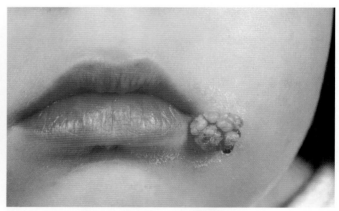

Fig. 3.66 Perioral warts.

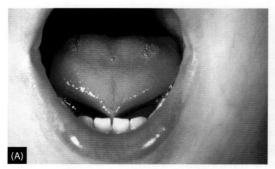
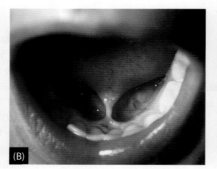
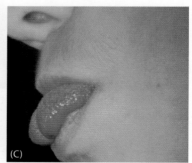

Figs. 3.67A–C (A) Tongue-tie. The tip of the tongue is tethered to the floor of the mouth by a tight band (frenulum). This prevents protrusion of the tongue beyond the lower incisors. The tongue is sometimes anchored so closely to the floor of the mouth that it is difficult to see the frenulum at all. (B) A less severe degree of tongue-tie. This child is attempting to lift the tongue to the roof of the mouth but cannot do so. Tongue-tie never interferes with swallowing, but may impair latching on to the breast during breast feeding and can affect speech. (C) When a child with tongue-tie attempts to protrude the tongue it tends to curl up. Minor degrees of tongue-tie do not need treatment.

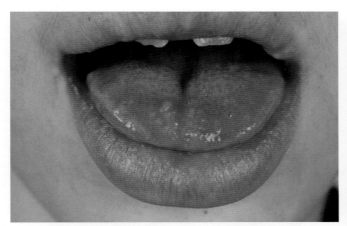

Fig. 3.68 Pathognomonic nodules in the tip of the tongue in a patient with MEN2B who presented with severe, chronic constipation. The nodules are overgrown autonomic nerves caused by a mutation in the RET gene leading to upregulation of its function.

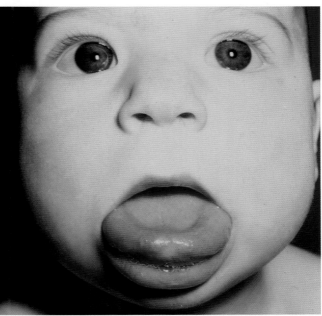

Fig. 3.69 Macroglossia occurs in association with a number of recognised syndromes. This infant has Beckwith–Weidemann syndrome, which is also associated with grooved ear lobes, hemihypertrophy and an increased incidence of Wilms tumour, hepatoblastoma and adrenal tumours.

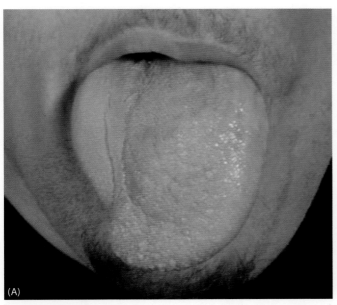

(A)

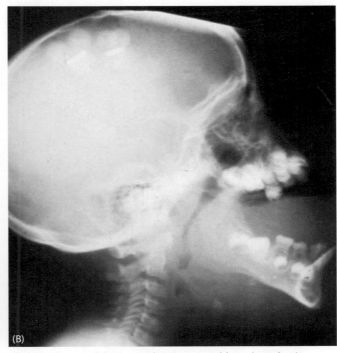

(B)

Figs. 3.70A, B (A) Hemihypertrophy of the tongue as part of Proteus syndrome. (B) Macroglossia caused by a lymphatic malformation of the tongue.

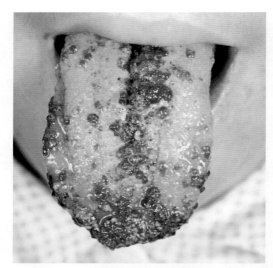

Fig. 3.71 Lymphatic malformation of the tongue, producing multiple small vesicles on its surface. They tend to weep and bleed and may become infected. Sometimes they have a 'warty' appearance. The malformation usually extends into the floor of the mouth.

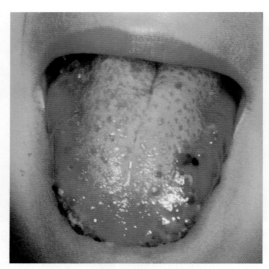

Fig. 3.72 Lymphatic malformation of the tongue, in which repeated episodes of inflammation and trauma have occurred. The tongue bleeds frequently and periodically enlarges. Gross lesions may cause mandibular deformity.

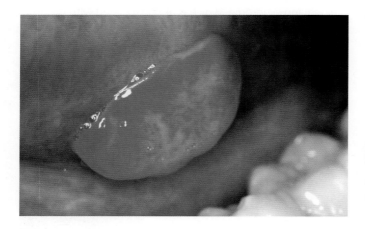

Fig. 3.73 A pyogenic granuloma on the side of the tongue. There was a similar lesion on the other side. It may have commenced with minor trauma from the teeth. It should be distinguished from a squamous papilloma, which appears more 'warty'.

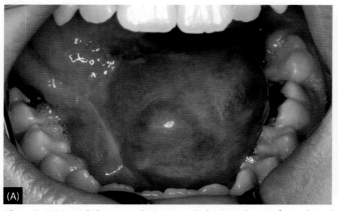

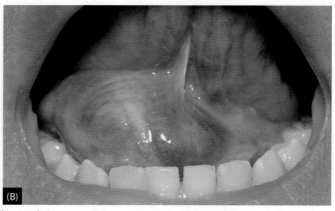

Figs. 3.74A, B (A) A ranula is a cystic lesion that is found in the floor of the mouth beneath the tongue. This ranula is on the left side of the mouth, pushing the tongue and frenulum to the right. It has a blue colour through the membrane. (B) Ranula in the floor of the right side of the mouth.

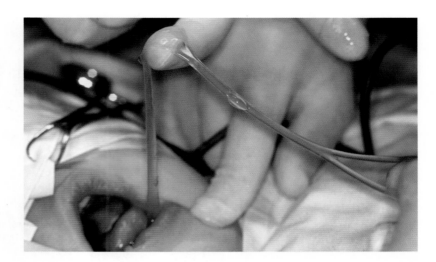

Fig. 3.75 A ranula contains opaque tenacious mucoid material, suggesting that the aetiology might be related to mucus retention.

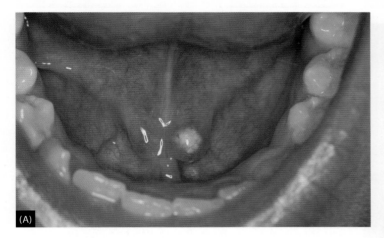

(A)

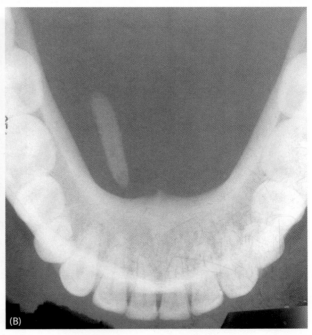

(B)

Figs. 3.76A, B (A) A calculus formed in the submandibular salivary gland may pass as far as the submandibular duct orifice. When it becomes arrested here, it produces intermittent pain and swelling of the gland. It can be seen and palpated. (B) The position of a submandibular calculus is confirmed on radiography.

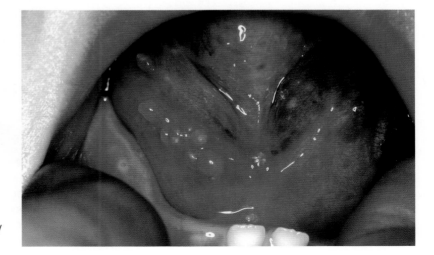

Fig. 3.77 Lymphatic malformations may involve the floor of the mouth and usually produce multiple small cystic lesions. In addition, there may be other evidence of the lymphatic anomaly in the neck.

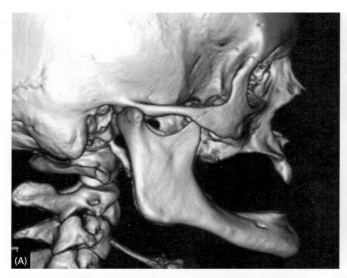

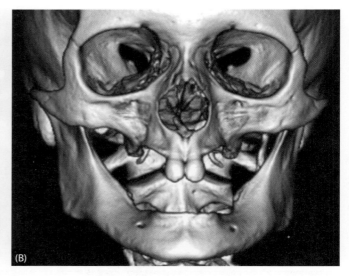

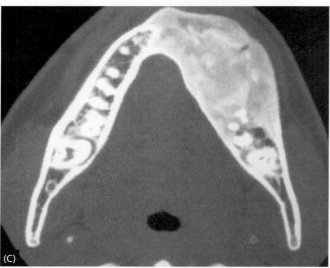

Figs. 3.78A–C (A, B) Ectodermal dysplasia in an adolescent on CT reconstruction, shown from the side and front. Ectodermal dysplasia comprises a group of rare genetic disorders that affect the skin and its appendages (hair follicles, eccrine glands, sebaceous glands and nails) and teeth. (C) Imaging of fibrous dysplasia of the mandible, showing its ground-glass appearance. In fibrous dysplasia, normal bone and marrow are replaced by fibrous tissue and abnormal woven bone. It may affect a single bone, multiple bones (polyostotic) or be part of McCune–Albright syndrome. It is caused by gene mutations affecting intracellular stimulatory G proteins.

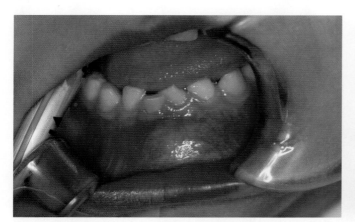

Fig. 3.79 A dentigerous cyst arising from a permanent incisor tooth germ and producing a swelling around the unerupted tooth on the external side of the alveolus. It is non-tender, causes no pain, and there are no signs of inflammation. Note the displacement of the primary incisor teeth.

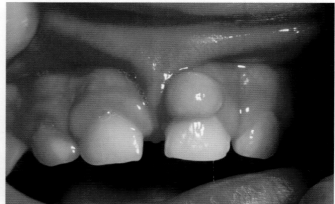

Fig. 3.80 An epulis presenting as a localised swelling attached to the gingival tissue. This child also has a low attachment of the upper frenulum (lip tie) and separation of the upper incisor teeth.

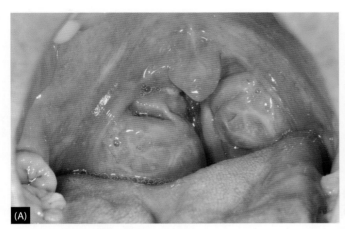
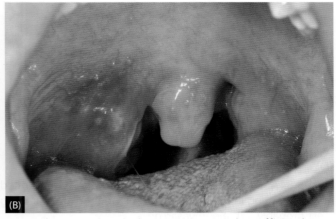

Figs. 3.81A, B (A) Purulent tonsillitis showing significant enlargement of the tonsils, which sometimes may be sufficiently large to cause airway obstruction. (B) Streptococcal pharyngitis with early microabscess formation in the tonsil.

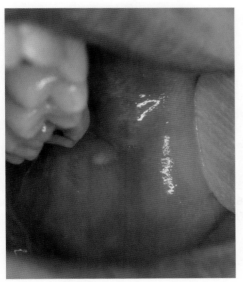

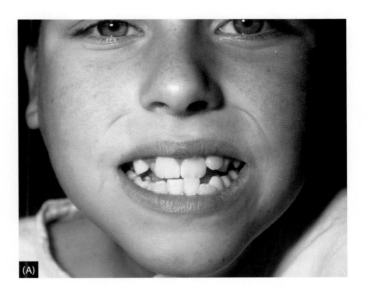

Fig. 3.82 Crohn disease may produce a buccal abscess. In this child pus is draining from the parotid duct opening from a buccal abscess. The child had other typical features of Crohn disease, including short stature and delayed puberty.

Figs. 3.83A, B (A) This chid presented with a partial seventh cranial nerve palsy and a mass in the right neck. Weakness of the right side of the face is evident when he attempts to smile. The deep-seated cervical lesion, which extended into the pharynx and mouth, was a lymphoma. (B) In the same patient, inspection of the inside of the mouth shows a protruding lesion in the region of the fauces and pharynx, which was the lymphoma.

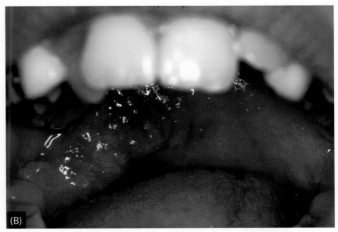

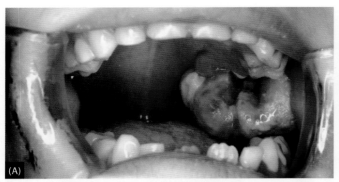
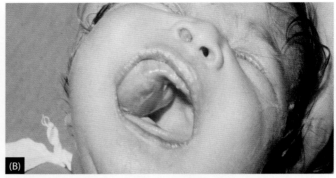

Figs. 3.84A, B (A) A rhabdomyosarcoma, which has ulcerated through the buccal mucosa into the mouth. (B) An irregular mass presenting in the mouth and replacing the alveolar margin, which on its clinical appearance is likely to be a tumour, most probably a rhabdomyosarcoma.

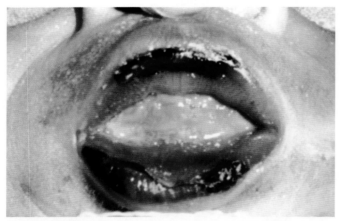
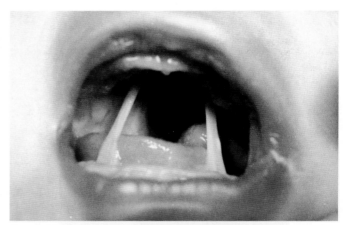

Fig. 3.85 Imperforate mouth due to failure of breakdown of the buccopharyngeal membrane. This membrane lies in the depths of an ectodermal depression, the stomatodeum, or primitive mouth. Normally, this membrane should break down, thereby establishing continuity between the stomatodeum and the foregut.

Fig. 3.86 Congenital bands from the lower jaw to the palate. There is an associated cleft palate.

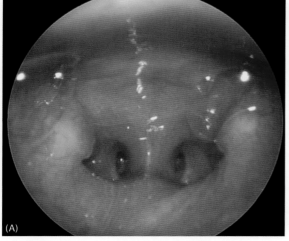
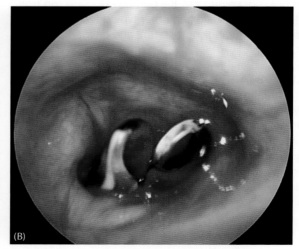

Figs. 3.87A, B (A) Bilateral choanal atresia on endoscopy in a baby with CHARGE association. (B) Choanal atresia after excision of the obstructing membrane.

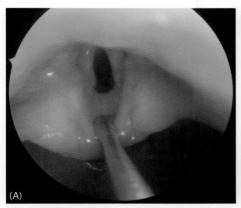
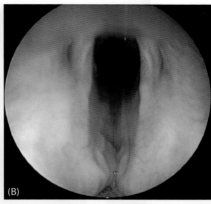
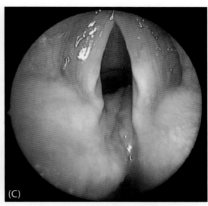

(A)   (B)   (C)

Figs. 3.88A–C (A) Endoscopic view of a normal larynx, demonstrating the normal interarytenoid region above the vocal cords. (B, C) A type 1 laryngeal cleft (B) extending down towards the vocal cords. A type II laryngeal cleft (C) extends below the vocal cords to the cricoid cartilage. Types III and IV clefts (not shown) extend down into the trachea.

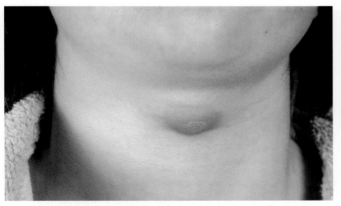

Fig. 3.89 Infected thyroglossal cyst, with signs of inflammation. The infection has tracked down from the foramen caecum. Untreated, the infection would ultimately extend to the overlying skin and produce a discharging sinus.

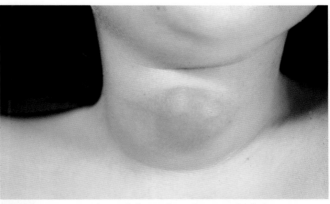

Fig. 3.90 Large infected thyroglossal cyst, which has produced an abscess. Note the erythema of the skin extending lateral to the abscess. In contrast, an infected submental lymph node produces a more circular inflammatory reaction.

Fig. 3.91 Recurrent thyroglossal cyst. This results from either incision and drainage of a thyroglossal cyst abscess or incomplete excision of the cyst and its tract. The risk of recurrence can be markedly reduced by performing a Sistrunk operation, which includes excision of the middle third of the hyoid bone and a suprahyoid core of tongue muscle.

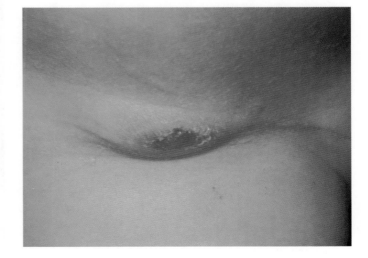

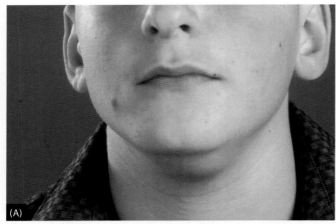
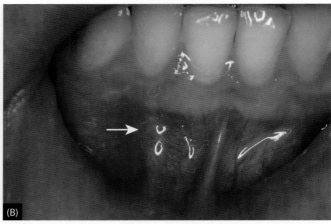

Figs. 3.92A, B (A) Enlargement of the submental nodes may appear similar to a thyroglossal cyst, except that the submental nodes are usually more anterior than a suprahyoid thyroglossal cyst, may be multiple and there may be an obvious source of infection. They move little on tongue protrusion or swallowing, suggesting that they are not attached to the hyoid bone. (B) Examination of the inside of the mouth in this same patient revealed an ulcer (arrow), which was the source of the submental nodal infection.

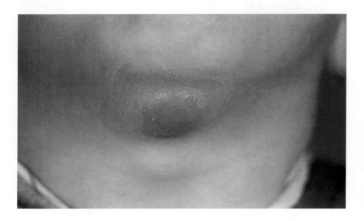

Fig. 3.93 Submental abscess pointing just behind the mandible. Inspection of the lower dentition revealed severe dental caries, almost certainly the origin of the infection. The inflammation of this lesion can be distinguished from an infected thyroglossal cyst because in lymph node infection, the area of erythema tends to be circular.

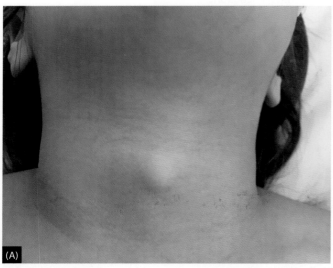
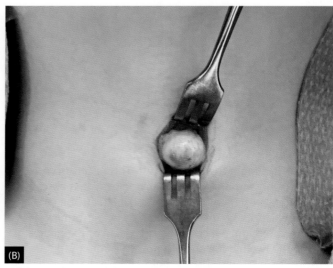

Figs. 3.94A, B A dermoid cyst may occur anywhere in the midline of the neck anteriorly. Dermoid cysts are mobile and often appear as slightly yellow, discrete swellings in the subcutaneous tissue, unattached to deeper structures. This distinguishes them from thyroglossal cysts. In practice, however, the distinction is not always clear-cut and can only be determined at operation.

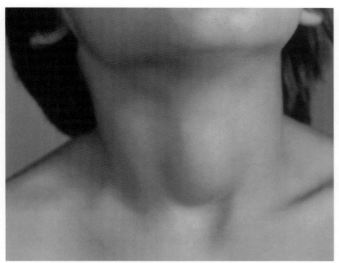

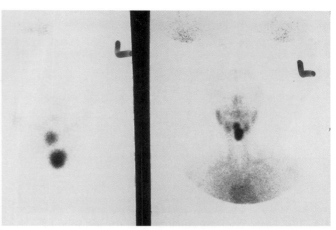

Fig. 3.95 An ectopic thyroid may present anywhere along the thyroglossal duct from the foramen caecum to the normal position of the thyroid in the lower neck. Most commonly, it is located in the infrahyoid region and may appear clinically indistinguishable from a thyroglossal cyst. It does not transilluminate, and may feel more solid. In addition, there is no normal thyroid palpable in the lower neck. Where there is clinical doubt as to the diagnosis, an ultrasound scan is helpful and a nuclear scan will identify the location of functioning thyroid tissue.

Fig. 3.96 Double ectopic thyroid with both functioning suprahyoid and lingual components. The child presented with a midline cervical mass and, on examination of the mouth, the lingual thyroid could be seen. A nuclear scan demonstrated that both areas contained functioning thyroid tissue with no normally located thyroid.

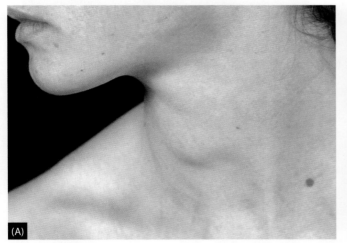

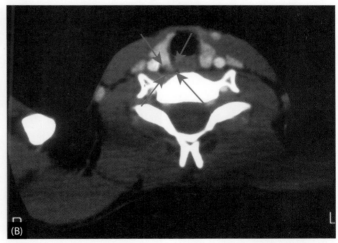

Figs. 3.97A, B (A) Adenoma of the thyroid may present as either a lower cervical midline or lateral neck swelling in the region of the thyroid gland. Clinically, it is indistinguishable from a papillary or follicular carcinoma of the thyroid, all of which are uncommon in childhood. (B) Thyroid adenoma (arrows) as revealed on a CT scan.

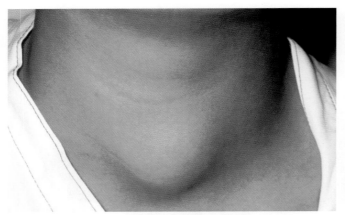

Fig. 3.98 Large papillary carcinoma of the left lobe of the thyroid.

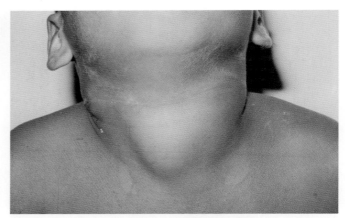

Fig. 3.99 Enlarged isthmus and left lobe of thyroid gland. The various causes of goitre need to be excluded.

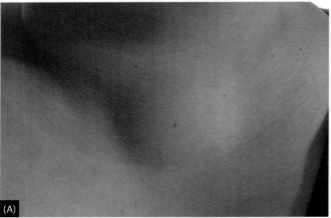

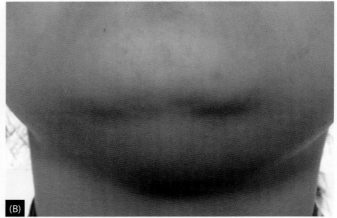

Figs. 3.100A, B (A) Ranula extending well down into the neck. (B) Ranula most obvious clinically in the submental region.

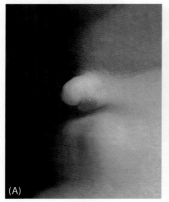

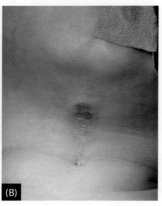

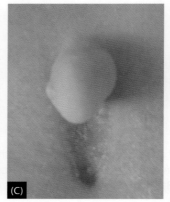

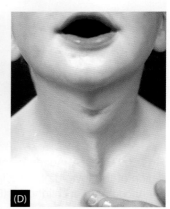

Figs. 3.101A–D Variations on the spectrum of median cervical cleft. Adjacent (usually superior) to the cleft, there is often a polypoid lesion (A–C). The sinus runs downwards towards the sternum for a variable distance, and may be associated with tethering of the skin in the midline (D).

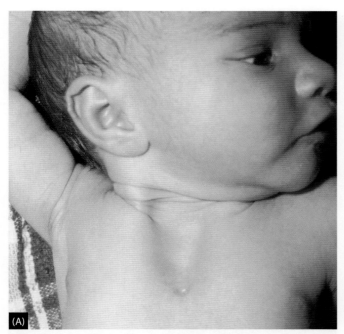
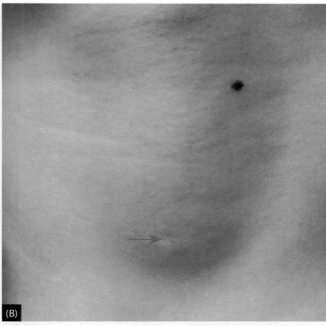

Figs. 3.102A, B (A) Superior sternal cleft in a neonate. Cardiac pulsation was visible through the U-shaped cleft. When the child cried herniation occurred. (B) Midline neck sinus connecting with a dermoid cyst (arrow).

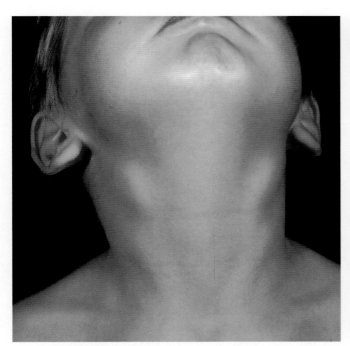

Fig. 3.103 Reactive hyperplasia involving the lateral cervical lymph nodes on both sides. This is the normal response to infection in the head and neck in children. The relative paucity of fat and the relatively large size of the lymph nodes in this age group make lymphadenopathy obvious, even without resorting to palpation.

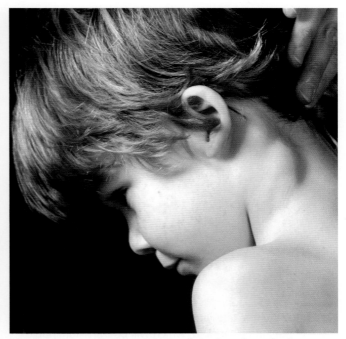

Fig. 3.104 Reactive hyperplasia of the lymph nodes in the posterior triangle of the neck. These nodes enlarge in response to infection of the scalp and ear.

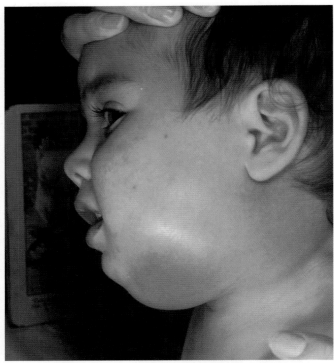

Fig. 3.105 Cervical abscess formation deep to the investing cervical fascia produces a poorly localised lesion and considerable cellulitis. Its location deep to the cervical fascia and the surrounding induration make it difficult to elicit the sign of fluctuation. It requires surgical drainage.

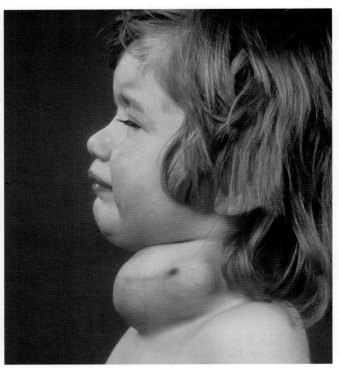

Fig. 3.106 Lymphatic malformation presenting at birth with a swelling in the neck, which increases in size over the first few months of life. Infection or haemorrhage into the cyst may cause it to enlarge rapidly. Note the scar from previous surgery.

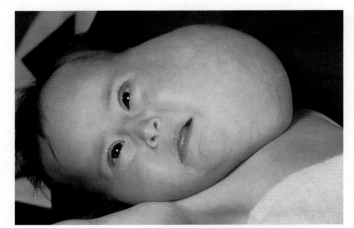

Fig. 3.107 A large left lymphatic malformation, at this stage containing clear fluid, which will be transilluminable. The size of the lesion is pushing the head to the right and involvement of the floor of the mouth and tongue may give the appearance of macroglossia and may cause respiratory obstruction. This child has Down syndrome as well, a known association with lymphatic malformations, and another factor contributing to macroglossia.

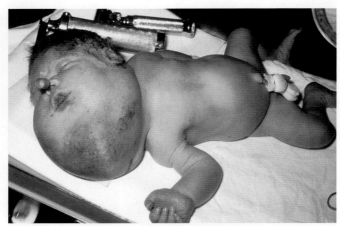

Fig. 3.108 A massive lymphatic malformation into which haemorrhage has occurred early. This child developed respiratory obstruction and required nasotracheal intubation. The abdominal distension is evidence of the difficulty experienced in obtaining an adequate airway.

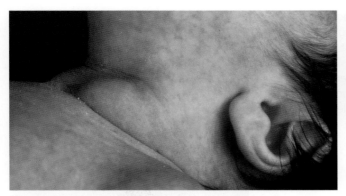

Fig. 3.109 A sternomastoid tumour, which typically appears at about 3 weeks of age, and which may be caused by fibrosis of a torn sternocleidomastoid muscle after a traumatic delivery. Sternomastoid tumour has become less common with breech presentations, which are now managed mostly by caesarean section.

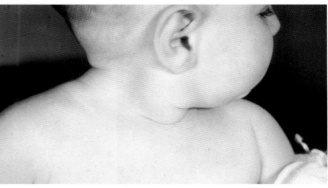

Fig. 3.110 A sternomastoid tumour presents with a hard, non-tender lump in one sternomastoid muscle, which causes limitation of neck movement. Characteristically, the infant's head is turned away from the side involved and tilted to the side of the tumour.

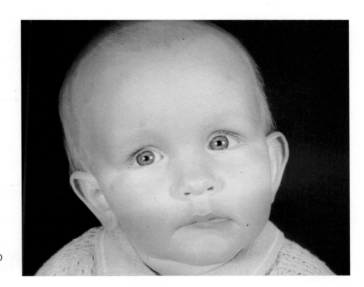

Fig. 3.111 Scarring of the sternomastoid muscle after resolution of the sternomastoid tumour may cause torticollis and lead to facial hypoplasia. This toddler has hypoplasia of the right side of the face. Note that the head is still turned to the contralateral side and there is ipsilateral head tilt.

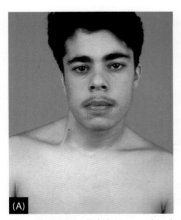
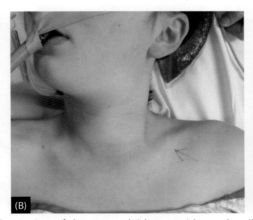
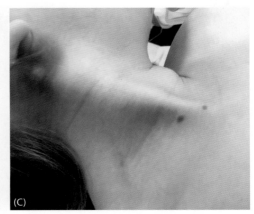

Figs. 3.112A–C (A) Unresolved shortening of the sternocleidomastoid muscle will lead to the classic torticollis of later childhood, with the head held level but the ipsilateral shoulder elevated in compensation to keep the eyes level. The affected muscle appears as a tight band. Full rotation of the head to the affected side is impossible. (B) A shortened left sternocleidomastoid muscle before surgical division. (C) Sternomastoid torticollis, where the muscle has been replaced with a tendinous scar.

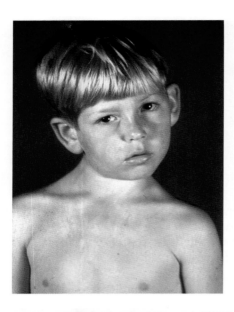

Fig. 3.113 Atlanto-occipital subluxation following a tonsillectomy. At first glance, the appearance may be similar to sternomastoid shortening, but there is no tightness of either sternomastoid muscle.

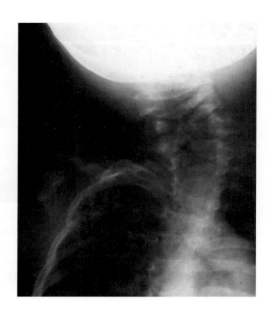

Fig. 3.114 Radiograph of the cervical spine showing hemivertebrae as the cause of torticollis.

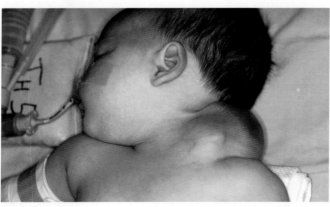

Fig. 3.115 Lymphangiosarcoma. This infant presented initially with a transilluminable lesion in the left neck, which was diagnosed as a simple cystic hygroma. Within 1 month, the lesion enlarged rapidly and developed malignant vascular markings on the skin surface.

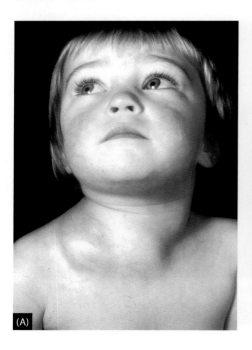

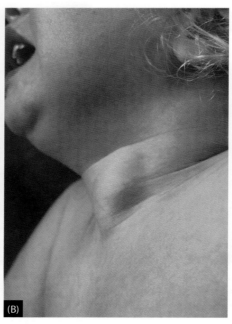

Figs. 3.116A, B Two examples of venous malformations involving the jugular vessels. The dilated venous 'lakes' of 'varices' fill and dilate on crying or the Valsalva manoeuvre.

(A)

(B)

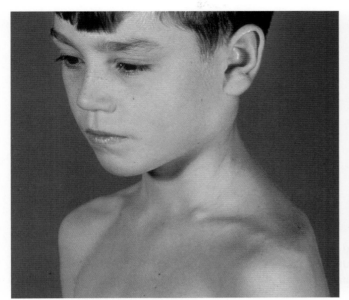

Fig. 3.117 Hodgkin disease. This boy has two masses in the left side of the neck: a large mass of jugulodigastric lymph nodes and a metastatic lymph node at the junction of the thoracic duct with the venous system. An enlarged lymph node at the base of the neck is a sinister sign of malignancy. This Virchow lymph node may be an indication of neuroblastoma or lymphoma.

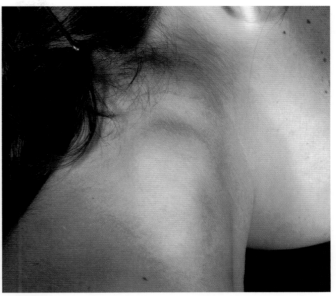

Fig. 3.118 Hodgkin disease in an adolescent who presented with painless enlargement of her right cervical lymph nodes, night sweats and fever. The nodes were non-tender and 'rubbery'.

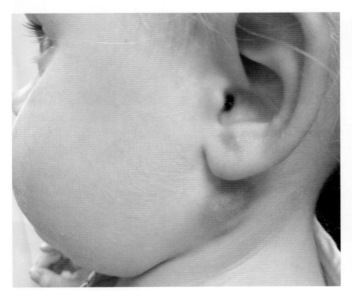

Fig. 3.119 Cervical abscess in a toddler.

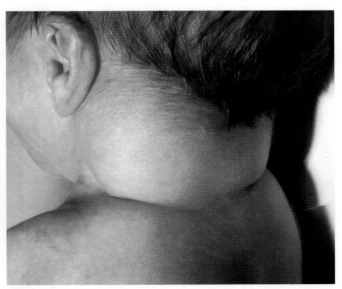

Fig. 3.120 Infantile fibrosarcoma involving the posterior cervical region.

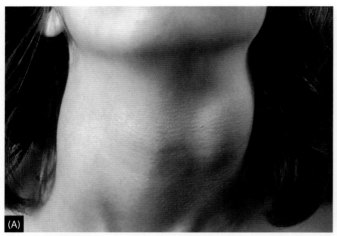

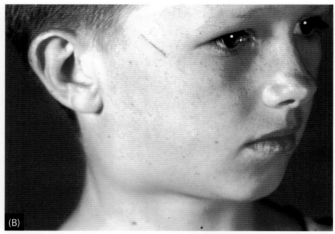

Figs. 3.121A, B (A) Branchial cyst may be seen in late childhood as a swelling deep to the sternocleidomastoid muscle, but protruding from its anterior surface. (B) A branchial cyst in a younger child is relatively uncommon. The deep location of the cyst may make it appear poorly localised on palpation, particularly if inflammation and secondary infection have occurred.

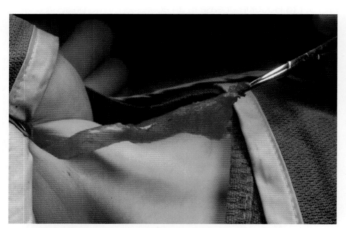

Fig. 3.122 Second branchial fistula during excision.

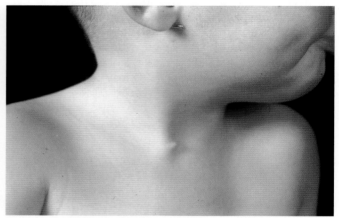

Fig. 3.123 A small cartilaginous lesion at the junction of the middle and lower thirds of the anterior border of the sternomastoid is suggestive of a second branchial remnant.

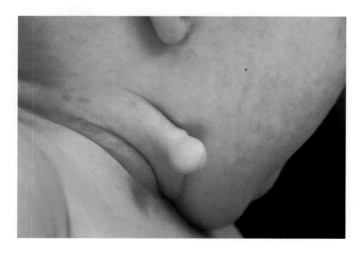

Fig. 3.124 A larger persistent cartilaginous remnant of the second branchial arch in an infant. There was a similar lesion on the other side.

Figs. 3.125A, B (A) Branchial sinus presents as an inconspicuous sinus opening at the junction of the middle and lower thirds of the sternomastoid muscle, here seen on the right side of the neck (arrow). Occasionally, a small amount of fluid is discharged from this opening. Discharge of saliva or ingested fluid suggests a communication with the pharynx, in which case the pathology is a branchial fistula. (B) Infection in a branchial cleft remnant, which could be a second or third branchial cleft.

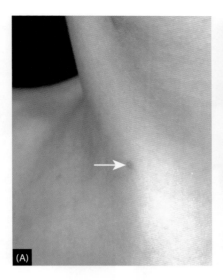

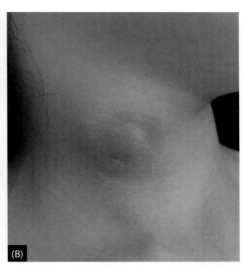

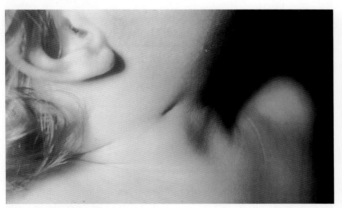

Fig. 3.126 A second branchial cleft sinus opening showing tethering of the underlying tissues on extension of the head. The sinus opening itself is tiny, but the skin around it becomes puckered with this manoeuvre as the fistula passes cranially to the tonsillar fossa.

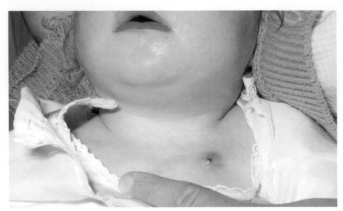

Fig. 3.127 An infected sinus opening of a fourth branchial cleft. Fourth branchial cleft anomalies are rare, usually left-sided and extend from the piriform fossa to the left thyroid lobe. They typically present with a lateral neck abscess or suppurative thyroiditis.

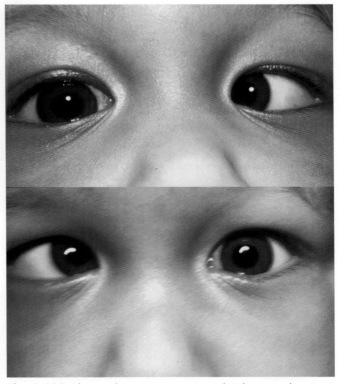

Fig. 3.128 Alternating convergent squint (concomitant strabismus) occurs when the deviation of the two visual axes is the same in all directions of gaze. This is the commonest problem encountered in paediatric ophthalmology. Consistent strabismus after 3 months of age requires assessment by an ophthalmologist to identify any underlying sensory defect, such as cataract, retinal abnormality or refractive error, and detection of amblyopia (reduced vision in one eye). Functional improvements that may follow surgery are improved stereopsis (depth perception) and an increased field of peripheral vision.

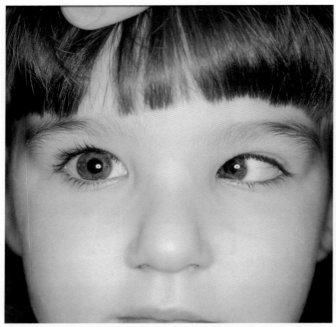

Fig. 3.129 Paralytic strabismus due to right sixth nerve palsy with failure of abduction of the right eye on gaze to the right. Paralytic strabismus results from damage to the third, fourth or sixth cranial nerves, or a combination thereof. Investigation is directed towards identifying the cause of the palsy.

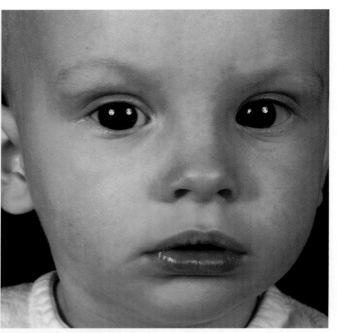

Fig. 3.130 Paralytic strabismus caused by a subdural haematoma.

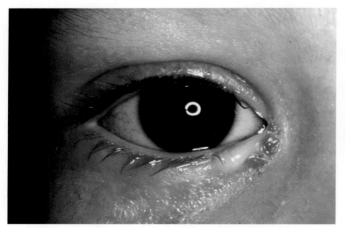

Fig. 3.131 Lacrimal duct obstruction producing a typical mucopurulent discharge and a 'wet-eyed look'. The lower eyelid is reddened secondary to chronic wetness. The majority of congenital nasolacrimal duct obstructions resolve spontaneously within 12 months of birth. The underlying problem is a mechanical obstruction of tear drainage.

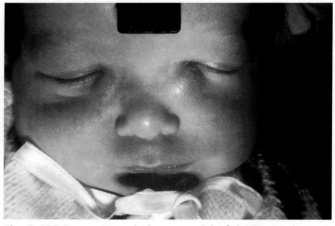

Fig. 3.132 Dacrocystocele (a mucocele) of the lacrimal sac may sometimes be confused with an infantile haemangioma. In mucoceles of the lacrimal sac their position is characteristic and the swelling feels tense on palpation. Many resolve spontaneously over the first few days of life with warm compresses and gentle pressure. Untreated, they often become infected. They are located beneath the medial canthal ligament and have a bluish hue. Rarely, the entire nasolacrimal drainage system may become dilated and cystic expansion of the lower end may cause obstruction of one nostril.

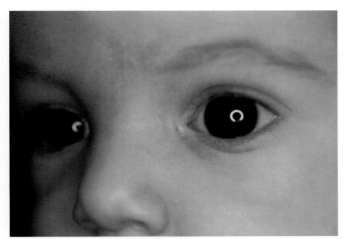

Fig. 3.133 Congenital lacrimal fistula produces a characteristic small dimple at the medial canthal ligament. Tears may be observed coming from this opening. Congenital lacrimal fistulae are frequently associated with nasolacrimal duct obstruction.

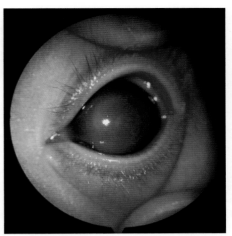

Fig. 3.134 Congenital glaucoma (idiopathic infantile glaucoma) produces a corneal haze and corneal enlargement (not readily apparent in this photograph). The four characteristic features of congenital or infantile glaucoma are: (1) enlargement of the eyeball (buphthalmos); (2) corneal haze (oedema); (3) epiphora (watery eye); and (4) photophobia. The diagnosis is confirmed by detection of optic disc cupping, increased corneal diameter and raised intraocular pressure.

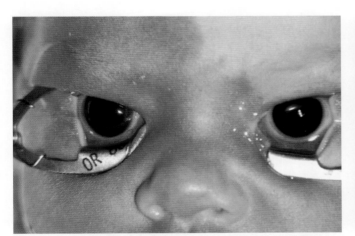

Fig. 3.135 Sturge–Weber syndrome and glaucoma. The presentation of glaucoma in association with Sturge–Weber syndrome is the same as for idiopathic infantile glaucoma. This infant has a bilateral capillary vascular anomaly (port-wine stain) of the face with corneal haze and enlargement on the right, secondary to the associated glaucoma. Glaucoma is much more likely to occur if both upper and lower eyelids are involved by the vascular malformation.

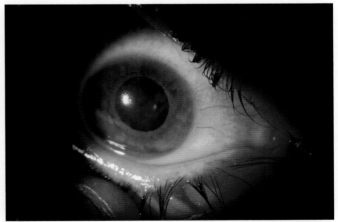

Fig. 3.136 Corneal abrasions are common and generally minor. This child has a linear abrasion of the cornea highlighted with fluorescein stain. If the abrasion is linear and vertically orientated, the under surface of the upper eyelid should be closely inspected for a subtarsal foreign body. Rarely, an abrasion may be associated with a deeper laceration of the corneal stroma. If the anterior chamber is shallow or the pupil distorted in shape, a full-thickness corneal laceration should be strongly suspected.

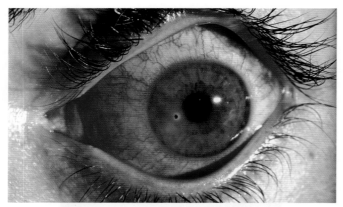

Fig. 3.137 Corneal foreign bodies cause pain on opening and shutting the eyelids. Note the surrounding corneal infiltrate (white area) and the conjunctival inflammation. In children under 5 years of age a brief general anaesthetic is often required to facilitate removal of the foreign body.

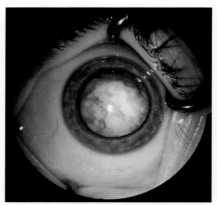

Fig. 3.138 Retinoblastoma in which the vascular tumour mass is obvious within the posterior segment of the eye once the pupil has been dilated. Retinoblastoma is the most common intraocular tumour in childhood and usually occurs in children under 5 years. It usually presents with leukocoria (white pupillary reflex) or strabismus. In some cases, retinoblastoma is inherited in an autosomal dominant pattern. In these patients, the tumours may be bilateral. Metastasis occurs along the optic nerve to the central nervous system.

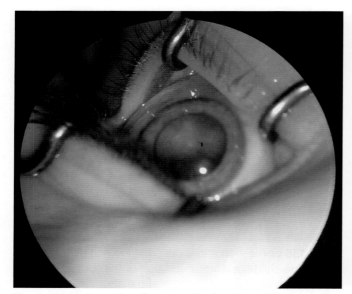

Fig. 3.139 Retinopathy of prematurity (retrolental fibroplasia). In end-stage retinopathy of prematurity, a fibrous membrane forms behind the lens. This is a disorder of retinal angiogenesis that follows birth prior to the maturation of the retinal blood vessels. It is seen most commonly in extremely premature infants (birth weight less than 1,000 g) and in those who have been exposed to increased concentrations of inspired oxygen. In the majority of affected infants, the disturbance of vascularisation is transient, and has no permanent sequelae. A small group develop more severe vascular changes and fibrovascular proliferation beyond the plane of the retina. As the fibrous component of this abnormal tissue matures, cicatricial changes develop, which result in retinal distortion and detachment.

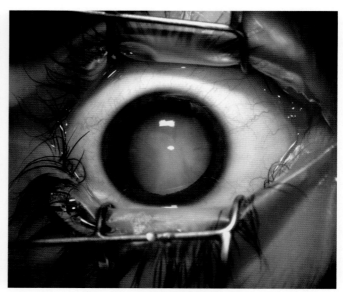

Fig. 3.140 Complete congenital cataract. The majority of bilateral congenital cataracts have an identifiable cause (e.g. genetic, metabolic or teratogenic). Most unilateral congenital cataracts are idiopathic. The final visual outcome in bilateral congenital cataracts is better than in unilateral cataracts, presumably because in unilateral cases, the normal eye has a marked advantage.

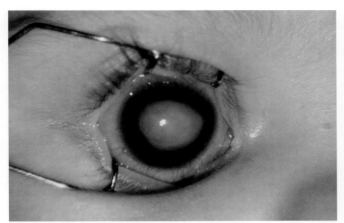

Fig. 3.141 Corneal opacity resulting from the Peter anomaly (a dysgenesis of the anterior segment of the eye). Corneal opacities in infancy may result from trauma (e.g. after forceps delivery), metabolic disorders (mucopolysaccharidoses) or isolated ocular malformations. In infants with isolated corneal opacity, the eye is frequently abnormal in other respects: it may be small (microphthalmos), have a lenticular malformation (cataract or lens adherent to the posterior surface of the cornea) or retinal or optic nerve malformations.

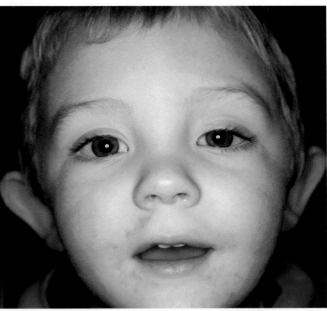

Fig. 3.142 Mild left congenital ptosis demonstrating the relative lack of the upper lid skin crease on the left side. Frequently, children with significant ptosis adopt a chin-up head posture to see beneath the lid margin.

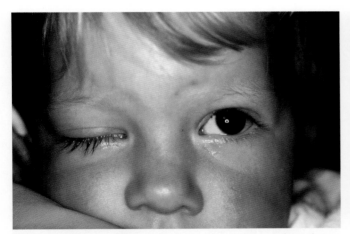

Fig. 3.143 Severe right congenital ptosis. The pupil on the right side is completely covered by the eyelid. Such occlusion of the pupil will cause amblyopia in a young child, which is why surgical correction should not be delayed.

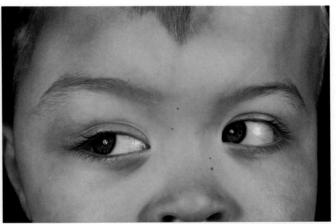

Fig. 3.144 Apparent ptosis of the right eyelid in association with left proptosis secondary to a ganglioneuroblastoma.

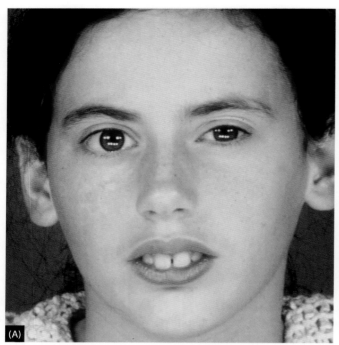

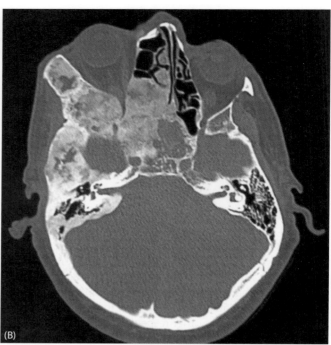

Figs. 3.145A, B (A) What appears to be ptosis of the left eyelid is in fact proptosis of the right eye, secondary to an optic glioma on that side. (B) CT of skull showing fibrous dysplasia of the orbit, causing proptosis.

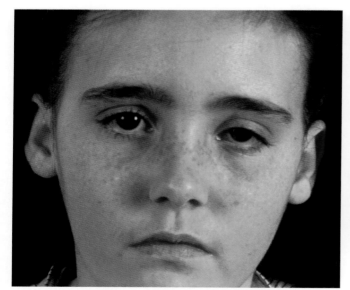

Fig. 3.146 Myasthenia gravis causing muscular weakness involving the eyelids. The ptosis, more marked on the left in this patient, is secondary to that weakness.

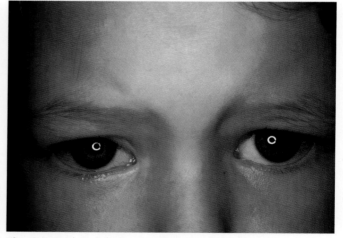

Fig. 3.147 This child has Horner syndrome, including right ptosis and a small right pupil. The syndrome is caused by interruption of the oculosympathetic pathway between the hypothalamus and the orbit. Trauma (including birth and iatrogenic trauma), tumours and infection are among the recognised causes.

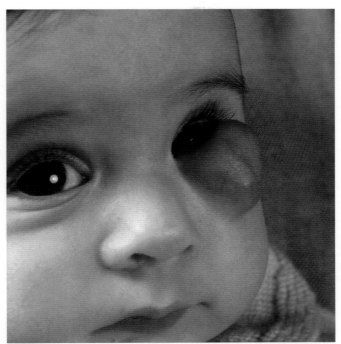

Fig. 3.148 A haemangioma obscuring the eye will result in amblyopia if not corrected promptly.

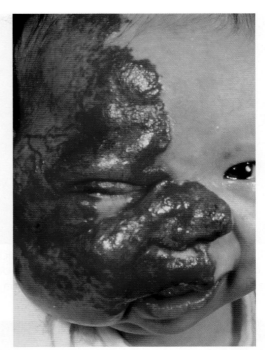

Fig. 3.149 Segmental haemangioma involving the right side of the face, causing occlusion of the visual pathway. This lesion needs investigation for PHACES syndrome: Posterior fossa brain malformations, Haemangiomas, particularly plaque-like facial lesions, Arterial anomalies such as coarctation of the aorta, Cardiac anomalies, Eye anomalies, and Sternal cleft.

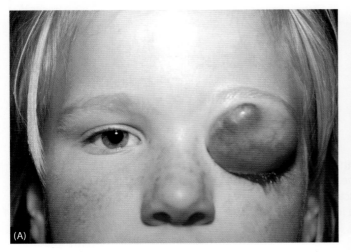

(A)

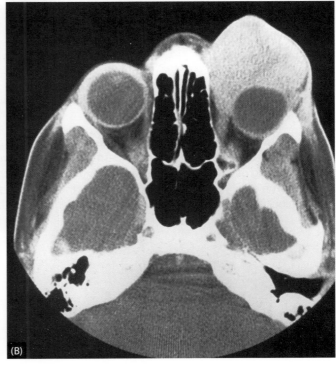

(B)

Figs. 3.150A, B (A) An orbital rhabdomyosarcoma with massive involvement of the roof of the orbit and upper lid. This child had a short history of a rapidly-developing orbital mass. (B) A CT scan of the same patient, showing extensive orbital and soft tissue involvement by the rhabdomyosarcoma, which has caused marked proptosis of the globe.

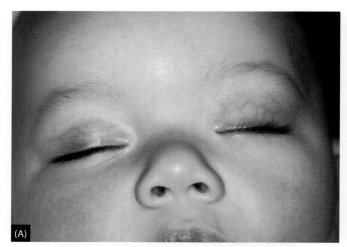
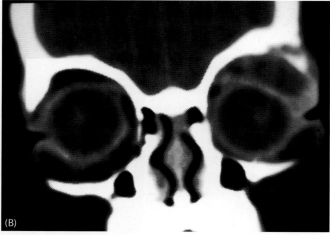

Figs. 3.151A, B (A) An infant with histiocytosis in which a small mass at the orbital rim superotemporally is associated with recent development of ptosis. Systemic assessment includes a bone scan and skeletal survey to exclude more generalised disease. (B) CT scan of the same child showing a lesion of the left orbital rim with erosion.

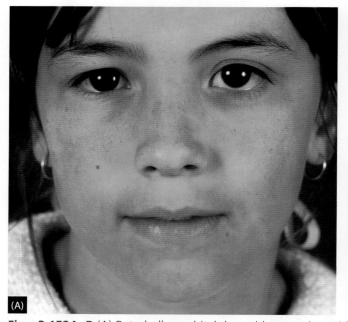
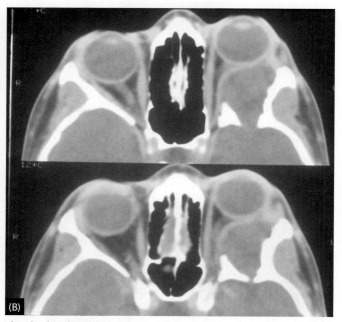

Figs. 3.152A, B (A) Retrobulbar orbital dermoid presenting with slowly developing proptosis of the left eye. Note the slight widening of the left palpebral aperture. (B) CT scan of the same patient, revealing the extensive nature of the orbital dermoid. The optic nerve has been distorted by the mass. CT scanning is mandatory to differentiate the dermoid from an encephalocele and to identify 'dumbell-shaped' dermoids with intracranial extension.

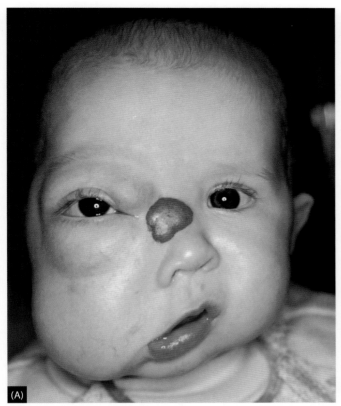
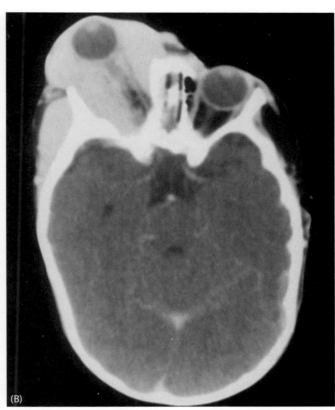

Figs. 3.153A, B (A) This infant presented at 3 weeks of age with progressive proptosis and lid and cheek swelling, secondary to an infantile haemangioma. An orbital haemangioma may result in visual loss if the blood supply of the optic nerve or the globe is compromised. A typical superficial capillary haemangioma is also present on the bridge of the nose. (B) Same patient: CT scan reveals the extensive mass involving the orbit, maxillary sinus and cheek.

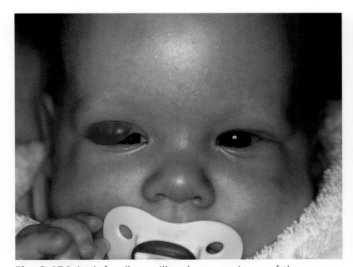

Fig. 3.154 An infantile capillary haemangioma of the upper lid which just spares the pupil. Most capillary haemangiomas of the lid are relatively superficial.

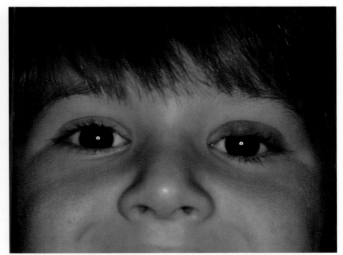

Fig. 3.155 Not all chalazia appear as inflamed as this lesion. The natural history of a chalazion (a cyst in the eyelid due to a blocked Meibomian gland) is of gradual resolution over many months, but they may recur. Occasionally, it will be the focus of a more severe preseptal cellulitis.

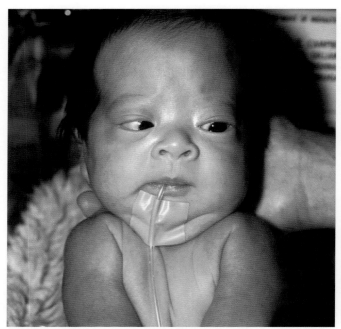

Fig. 3.156 Cleidocranial dysostosis, a generalised dysplasia of osseous and dental tissues. The child has brachycephaly, with bossing of the frontal, parietal and occipital bones. There is partial or complete aplasia of the clavicles with associated muscle defects, a small thorax and short oblique ribs. Hand anomalies include asymmetric finger lengths and a slow rate of carpal ossification. In this infant, the absence of the clavicles means that the shoulders can be rotated forwards to an excessive degree.

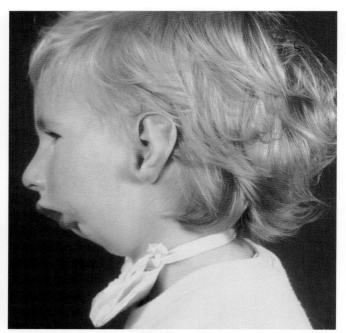

Fig. 3.157 Pierre-Robin sequence includes micrognathia, glossoptosis and a wide cleft of the hard and soft palates. Early failure of mandibular growth prevents descent of the tongue into the mouth and palatal closure. The tongue is too posterior at birth, causing airway obstruction, which may need tracheostomy. Pierre-Robin sequence may be part of trisomy 18 or a variety of named syndromes.

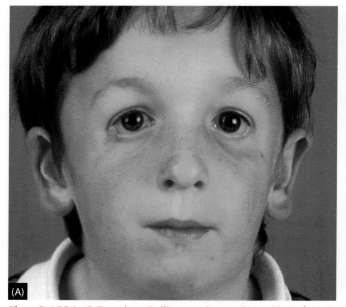

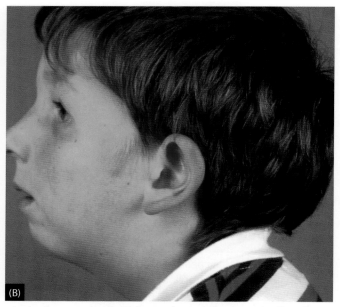

Figs. 3.158A, B Treacher Collins syndrome (mandibulofacial dysostosis; Franceschetti–Klein syndrome) is a genetic disorder involving malar hypoplasia with down-slanting of the palpebral fissures producing oblique-looking eyes. In this child there is a notch defect in the lower eyelid, which is more obvious on the right side.

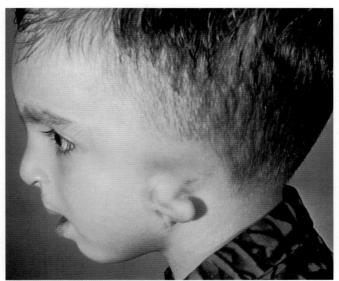

Fig. 3.159 A more severe example of Treacher Collins syndrome, in which there is also a malformed external ear. About 40% will have a conductive deafness.

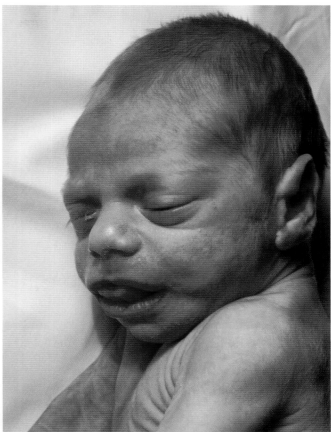

Fig. 3.160 Beckwith–Weidemann syndrome. There is macroglossia and a relative infraorbital hypoplasia and prominent occiput. The linear fissures in the lobule of the external ear can be seen. Neonatal hypoglycaemia occurs in about half, and sometimes can be severe. Exomphalos (omphalocele), cardiovascular defects and renal abnormalities often co-exist. Potential later development of Wilms tumour and hepatoblastoma necessitates ongoing surveillance.

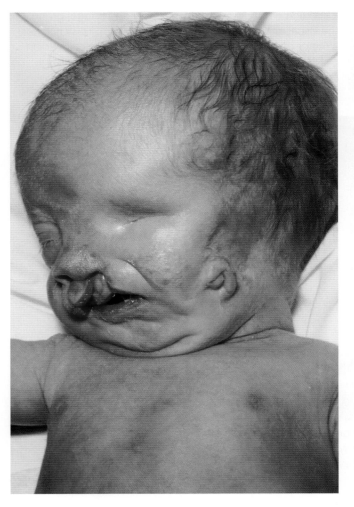

Fig. 3.161 Goldenhar syndrome is a severe form of the facio-auriculo-vertebral spectrum. Note the microtia, microphthalmia, cleft lip and hypoplasia of the maxillary and mandibular regions. These anomalies are associated with inner ear defects, deafness, intellectual impairment and major cardiac abnormalities including tetralogy of Fallot.

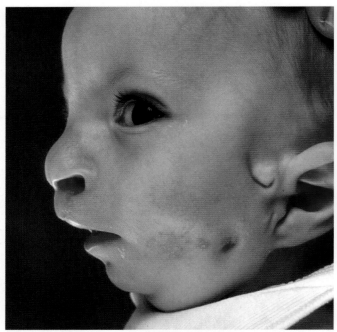

Fig. 3.162 Facio-auriculo-vertebral spectrum in which there is defective morphogenesis of the first and second branchial arches, often accompanied by vertebral abnormalities and ocular problems. These abnormalities may be largely unilateral, in which case they are described as 'hemifacial microsomia'.

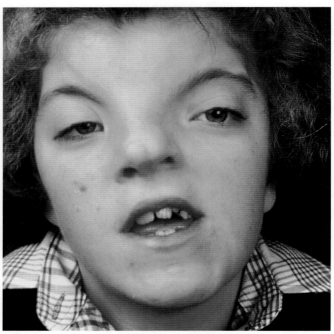

Fig. 3.163 Hypertelorism refers to widely spaced eyes. It should be distinguished from a low nasal bridge, giving the visual impression of ocular hypertelorism. This child has a minor degree of frontonasal dysplasia sequence (median cleft face syndrome). Hypertelorism is frequent in a large number of recognised syndromes.

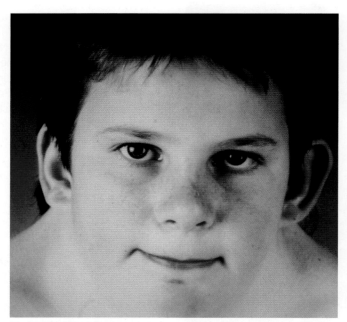

Fig. 3.164 Webbed neck is a common finding in a variety of conditions including Turner syndrome in girls, Noonan syndrome and the Klippel–Feil syndrome.

CHEST WALL DEFORMITIES

Chest wall deformities may be primary or secondary (acquired) and, from a clinical and cosmetic point of view, range from mild to severe. They rarely cause significant impairment of respiratory function, although minor deficiencies may be found on formal pulmonary function tests. Exercise tolerance may be reduced in severe pectus excavatum because of right ventricular compression by the sternal depression and mitral valve dysfunction. Some affected individuals have significant psychological distress because of the cosmetic deformity.

Primary chest wall deformities

Primary chest wall deformities can be classified as:

1 Depression deformities (pectus excavatum or 'funnel chest').
2 Protrusion deformities (pectus carinatum or 'pigeon chest').
3 Deficiency deformities (aplasia or dysplasia).

Pectus excavatum is the most common chest wall deformity and is typically seen in thin Caucasian males. It may be associated with Marfan syndrome. The sternal depression is often maximal at the xiphisternal junction but may extend up the sternum to a variable level. A localised depression is compatible with a well-developed upper chest. In asymmetrical lesions, the sternum is rotated around its longitudinal axis, producing prominence of the costal cartilages on one side and recession on the other. A shallow horizontal sulcus may extend on each side, corresponding to the attachment of the diaphragm to the lower costal cartilages, and the costal margin itself may protrude. Postural kyphosis and scoliosis often co-exist. The deformity may progress during childhood until growth ceases.

Protrusion deformities are less common. In high sternal protrusions, the sternum is angulated forwards at the level of the manubriosternal joint, below which it recedes. There may be 'pinching in' of the lower costal cartilages. Radiographs may reveal osseous fusion of the synchondroses of the sternum. This deformity tends to increase with age and does not regress spontaneously. Some affected individuals also have scoliosis. Low sternal protrusion deformities may be secondary to chronic asthma or mediastinal lesions and may improve spontaneously.

In deficiency deformities, the pectoral muscles are often absent on one side, and there is hypoplasia of the underlying ribs and costal cartilages. Breast tissue may be absent, and occasionally the nipple and areola are hypoplastic or absent as well. Hypoplasia of the ipsilateral upper limb and syndactyly suggest Poland syndrome, possibly caused by an impaired vascular supply during early development. A sternal cleft or bifid sternum is more often partial than complete and is another example of a deficiency deformity; paradoxical respiratory movements and subcutaneous cardiac contractions may be visible.

Secondary or acquired chest wall deformities

Acquired chest wall deformities may result from a variety of underlying causes including previous thoracotomy (e.g. for oesophageal atresia), intrathoracic tumours, after repair of congenital diaphragmatic hernia, asthma, spinal disease and vertebral malformations, chronic abdominal distension (causing flaring of the costal margins), avitaminosis D, achondroplasia, neurofibromatosis and the aftermath of radiotherapy.

THE LUNGS

Diseases of the lung or the pleural cavity range from being life-threatening to asymptomatic, with the diagnosis being made on incidental imaging. Lung conditions may be congenital or acquired but, with few exceptions, pleural problems are acquired. In children, the more common congenital pulmonary conditions include:

1 Congenital lobar emphysema.
2 Congenital pulmonary airway malformation.
3 Pulmonary sequestration (intralobar or extralobar).
4 Bronchogenic cyst.

Most of these lesions are now detected during routine prenatal ultrasound scans (see Chapter 1). While there is agreement that symptomatic pulmonary malformations require surgical excision, the management of asymptomatic lesions is controversial, with arguments in favour of a non-operative observational approach and of primary definitive surgery.

Congenital lobar emphysema

Congenital lobar emphysema (synonym: congenital lobar hyperinflation) is a potentially serious condition, particularly in infancy, manifesting as overdistension of one or more lobes, most often the left upper lobe. Three clinical presentations can be recognised: life-threatening respiratory distress in the newborn; symptomatic lobar emphysema in older children;

and asymptomatic congenital lobar emphysema detected on pre- or postnatal imaging. Lobectomy is curative for symptomatic disease.

Congenital pulmonary airway malformation

Previously called congenital cystic adenomatoid malformation, this is the most common congenital lung abnormality. It is characterised by cystic change at the level of the terminal bronchioles; macrocystic, microcystic (solid) and mixed varieties are recognised. The right or left lower lobe is most often affected. Some lesions are 'hybrid', having features of both cystic disease and pulmonary sequestration. Affected patients may present with respiratory distress, infection in the cyst, recurrent chest infections or as an incidental finding.

Pulmonary sequestration

Pulmonary sequestration occurs where lung tissue is separated from the tracheobronchial tree and pulmonary vessels. It is a congenital malformation comprising nonfunctioning lung tissue with an abnormal or absent bronchial communication and a blood supply from anomalous systemic arteries, which usually arise from the aorta. The abnormal lung tissue may be incorporated within normal lung (intralobar sequestration) additional to the normal pulmonary segments. When the abnormal pulmonary tissue has its own pleural covering, it is called extralobar sequestration. It may lie below, within or above the diaphragm and receives a blood supply directly from the aorta. The pulmonary structures (bronchial and alveolar elements with mucus-secreting epithelium) without normal communications may develop static accumulations of secretions, which are prone to infection. The vessels may form significant arteriovenous shunts, especially in the first year of life. In older children, sequestration becomes apparent when there are persistent radiological changes after respiratory infection. A correct diagnosis before thoracoscopy or thoracotomy enables the abnormal systemic artery that supplies the sequestered segment to be identified more easily at surgery.

Bronchogenic cyst

These cysts are a consequence of abnormal tracheal and foregut budding during development. They mostly occur in the mediastinum (paratracheal, carinal, hilar) but sometimes are found within the lung parenchyma.

Pulmonary interstitial emphysema

Pulmonary interstitial emphysema is an acquired condition seen in premature infants with severe hyaline membrane disease (respiratory distress syndrome) who require high pressure respiratory support for prolonged periods. Many go on to develop bronchopulmonary dysplasia. Advances in neonatology, including surfactant therapy, mean that this condition is now relatively rare.

Miscellaneous pulmonary conditions

There are several pulmonary conditions that are seen occasionally. These include hamartoma of the lung, staphylococcal pneumonia, pneumatocele, spontaneous pneumothorax, inflammatory pseudotumour, bronchiectasis, hydatid disease and pulmonary metastases (e.g. from Wilms tumour or osteosarcoma).

THE PLEURAL CAVITIES

Fluid may accumulate in the pleural cavities secondary to a variety of primary conditions, which include pulmonary infection, intrathoracic malignancy, ascites and trauma. Air in the pleural cavities may come from the lungs, bronchi, trachea or the oesophagus, or from outside the chest after trauma.

THE MEDIASTINUM

The important pathological conditions that affect the mediastinum are cysts and tumours (Table 4.1), although surgical emphysema (pneumomediastinum) and infection (mediastinitis) occur. The site of a tumour or cyst is frequently the key to its nature, although sometimes the final diagnosis is made only at operation. When a superior and/ or anterior mediastinal tumour is present, a pleural effusion is suggestive of lymphoma and examination of the pleural aspirate may enable a diagnosis without the need for direct biopsy of the tumour. Some tumours are asymptomatic and detected incidentally by radiographic examination, while in other cases the size and position of the tumour may lead to compression of vital structures (particularly the airway) and a life-threatening situation. This is particularly true in patients with non-Hodgkin lymphoma.

TABLE 4.1 Mediastinal conditions in childhood

- Thymic tumours
- Teratoma (benign or malignant)
- Dermoid cysts (superior mediastinal or intrapericardial)
- Mediastinocervical lymphatic malformation
- Lymphomas (Hodgkin and non-Hodgkin lymphoma)
- Paravertebral tumours (e.g. neural crest tumours: ganglioneuroma or neuroblastoma)
- Neurofibroma (with von Recklinghausen disease, neurofibromatosis type 1)
- Aggressive fibromatosis (desmoid fibromatosis)
- Chordoma
- Para-oesophageal (duplication) cyst

THE OESOPHAGUS

The common paediatric diseases of the oesophagus are oesophageal atresia (see Chapter 2), oesophagitis (e.g. reflux or eosinophilic oesophagitis), corrosive oesophagitis (see Chapter 10) and ingested foreign bodies (see Chapter 10). Unusual manifestations of oesophageal atresia include:

1 An unusually long upper oesophageal segment.
2 Oesophageal atresia with a proximal or double fistula.
3 Oesophageal atresia with distal oesophageal stricture from an intramural bronchial remnant.
4 Postmyotomy diverticulum.

A number of rare conditions that affect the oesophagus are listed in *Table 4.2*.

TABLE 4.2 Rare conditions involving the oesophagus
• Aggressive fibromatosis (desmoid fibromatosis)
• Scleroderma
• Oesophagitis in the immunocompromised patient
• Explosive rupture of the oesophagus
• Congenital stricture of the oesophagus
• Iatrogenic oesophageal perforation (e.g. from a nasogastric tube or post stricture dilatation)
• Achalasia
• Oesophageal varices
• Vascular ring

THE DIAPHRAGM

Congenital diaphragmatic hernia can be divided as follows:

1 Posterolateral hernia – the Bochdalek hernia; presents most frequently in the neonatal period and is discussed in more detail in Chapter 2.
2 Anterior hernia – the Morgagni hernia.
3 Eventration of the diaphragm.
4 Hernia through or alongside the oesophageal hiatus (hiatal or para-oesophageal hernia).

The late-presenting Bochdalek hernia often presents difficulties in diagnosis, which may lead to inappropriate treatment. The prime example is when the gas-filled stomach in the chest is mistaken for a tension pneumothorax. Strangulation is a rare, but important, complication of Bochdalek hernias. The majority of Morgagni hernias are asymptomatic and these strangulate rarely. Some Morgagni hernias may present in early infancy with respiratory symptoms.

Eventration of the diaphragm may be difficult to distinguish preoperatively from congenital diaphragmatic hernia with a sac. Fortunately, such distinction is frequently unimportant, as the decision for intervention is based on an evaluation of clinical and radiological features. Paralysis of the diaphragm due to phrenic nerve palsy recovers spontaneously in the majority of cases; occasionally diaphragmatic plication may be indicated.

The diagnosis of traumatic diaphragmatic hernia often is overlooked in the presence of other major injuries (see Chapter 10). The danger of strangulation of the hernial contents is ever present, and repair should be undertaken without delay once the diagnosis is made.

THE BREAST

Apart from neonatal infection, there are few serious conditions involving the breast in either sex in children, although a number of minor conditions may give rise to anxiety or inconvenience. Absence of the breast may be seen in isolation or as part of a regional dysplasia (Poland syndrome). Multiple nipples are more common, and occur along the 'milk line'. Supernumerary breasts are seen in the axilla. Transplacental passage of lactogenic hormones may lead to hyperplasia and the secretion of breast milk in neonates. This resolves spontaneously, but the engorgement predisposes to infection (mastitis) and occasionally a breast abscess will form.

Precocious puberty in a young girl presenting with bilateral breast enlargement and menstruation suggests the possibility of an underlying lesion – intracranial or ovarian tumour or adrenal anomalies. A more common aberration is premature hyperplasia occurring in one or both breasts of girls in mid-childhood, who present with a firm discoid lump about 1–2 cm in diameter behind the nipple. It may become tender. There are no other signs of puberty, which develops at the usual time.

In boys, during early adolescence (12–13 years) it is common for transient breast development to occur (gynaecomastia). Direct pressure on the breast may cause pain.

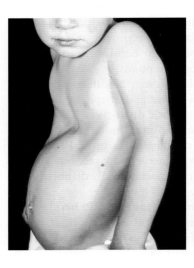

Fig. 4.1 Pectus excavatum in a 6-year-old girl. She has marked sternal depression extending laterally to the ribs, with costal margin eversion. The girl's facies and posture reflect her embarrassment and unhappiness with her deformity. The chest wall deformity has produced an apparent 'pot-belly'.

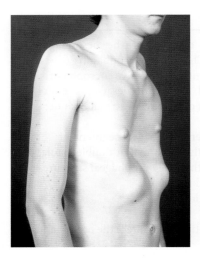

Fig. 4.2 Severe pectus excavatum in an adolescent boy. The deformity is symmetrical and there is no rotation of the sternum. Note the marked 'flaring' of the costal margin.

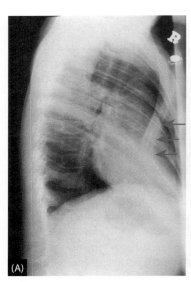

(A)

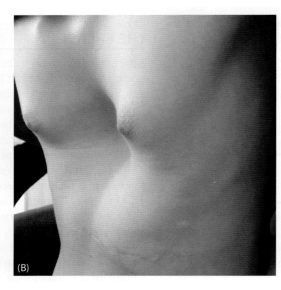

(B)

Figs. 4.3A, B (A) Lateral chest radiograph of severe pectus excavatum showing the pronounced sternal depression (arrows). The deformity rarely causes cardiorespiratory symptoms. (B) Pectus excavatum after congenital diaphragmatic hernia repair in infancy.

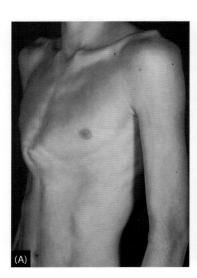

(A)

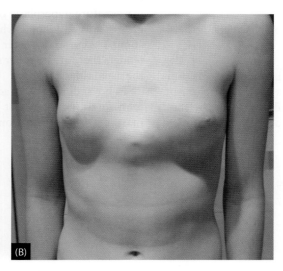

(B)

Figs. 4.4A, B (A) A low protrusion deformity ('pigeon chest'). The main feature is the sternal protrusion. 'Pinching-in' of the costal cartilages is common. (B) Pectus carinatum in an older girl.

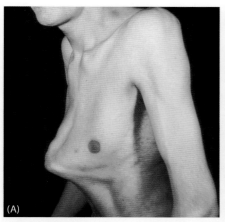

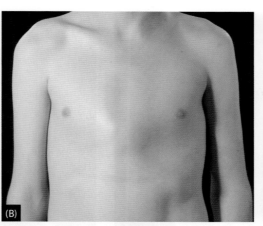

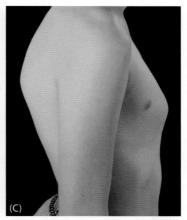

(A)

(B)

(C)

Figs. 4.5A–C (A) Gross protrusion deformity. (B) A less common form of pectus carinatum with a low sternal protrusion. In this circumstance chest x-ray is useful to exclude any abnormality in the mediastinum. (C) Lateral view of low protrusion in the same patient as in (B).

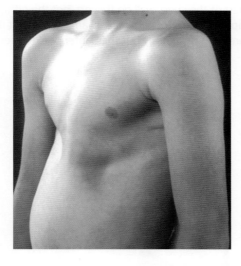

Fig. 4.6 Pectus carinatum ('pigeon chest') with marked 'pinching-in' of the lower costal cartilages.

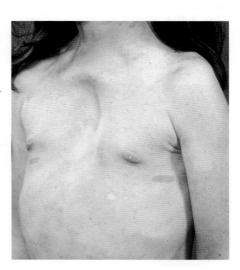

Fig. 4.7 High protrusion deformity in a girl with neurofibromatosis. This girl had a plexiform neurofibroma in the cervical region and multiple café-au-lait spots. On x-ray there was a short fused sternum with absence of sternebrae.

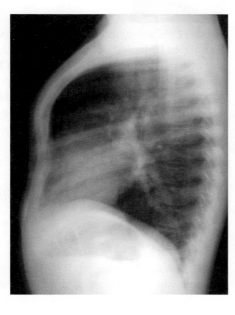

Fig. 4.8 Lateral radiograph of a high protrusion deformity with fused sternum and absence of sternebrae. A pseudodepression is present.

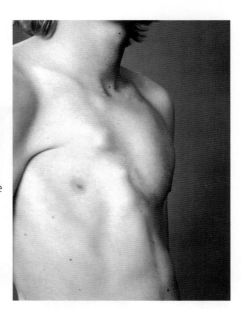

Fig. 4.9 This adolescent has deficiency of the sternocostal component of the right pectoralis major muscle and absence of the pectoralis minor muscle. The nipple is hypoplastic and there is deformity of the rib cage. This is not necessarily part of the deficiency but often co-exists.

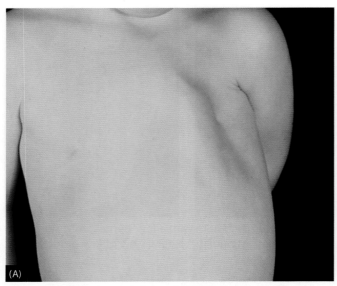

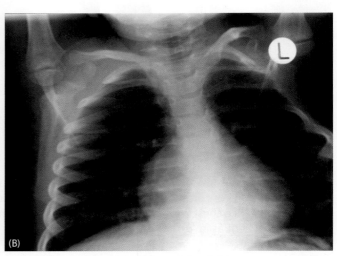

Figs. 4,10A, B (A) A deficiency deformity involving absence of part of the chest wall on the left, not the right, as appears at first. This resulted in a lung hernia which, on inspiration, caused the appearance shown here. (B) Same boy: chest radiograph shows hypoplasia of the upper ribs on the left side anteriorly. The ribs are seen posteriorly but their anterior extension is absent.

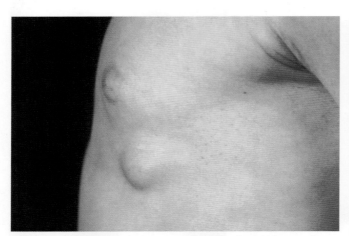

Fig. 4.11 Localised lung herniation through a defect in the rib cage. Lung herniation can be either congenital or post traumatic.

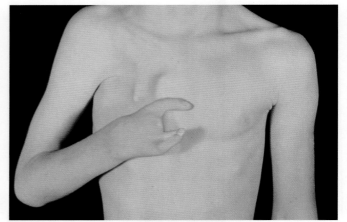

Fig. 4.12 Poland syndrome is characterised by unilateral absence or hypoplasia of the pectoral muscles and breast and abnormally short webbed fingers on the same side. Some individuals have ipsilateral rib or upper limb skeletal anomalies. The syndrome may be caused by a vascular insult to the developing upper limb in the embryo. It is more common on the right side and in boys.

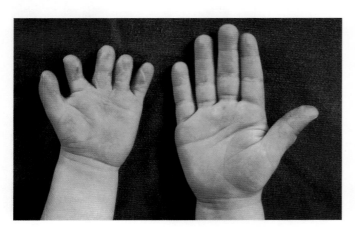

Fig. 4.13 Poland syndrome. The main limb abnormality in this boy with a deficiency deformity of the chest wall was hypoplasia and syndactyly (repaired) of the hand and digits.

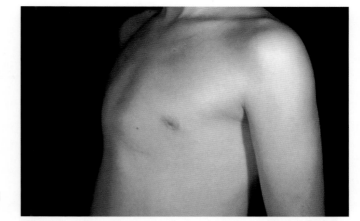

Fig. 4.14 Chest wall deformity secondary to asthma. Acquired chest wall deformities usually produce protrusion deformities.

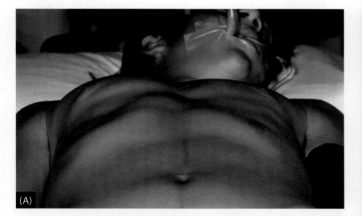

(A)

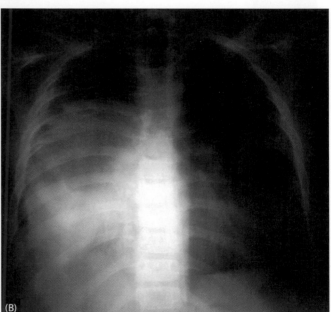

(B)

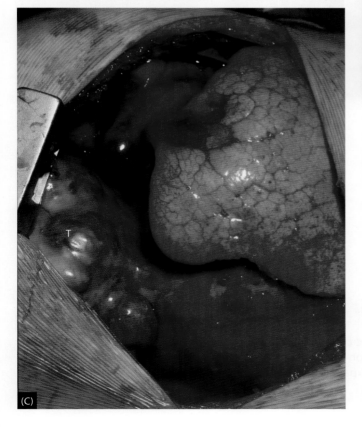

(C)

Figs. 4.15A–C Malignant thoracic teratoma causing right chest wall protrusion. Investigation of this 10-year-old boy with precocious puberty and Kleinfelter syndrome revealed a chest wall deformity (A) which, on chest x-ray, was shown to be due to a large intrathoracic tumour (B). At operation, a large malignant thoracic teratoma (T) was excised (C). The boy subsequently developed malignant histiocytosis and died.

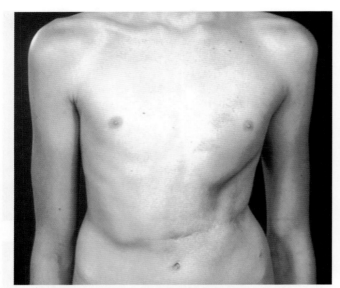

Fig. 4.16 Secondary chest wall deformity following radiotherapy earlier in childhood for a Wilms tumour. The nephrectomy scar can be seen. This type of deformity has led to less frequent use of radiotherapy in young children.

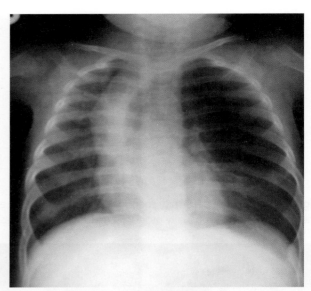

Fig. 4.17 Congenital lobar emphysema of the left upper lobe causing displacement of the mediastinum.

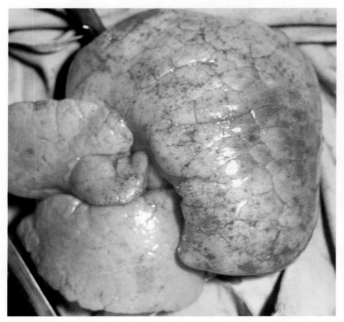

Fig. 4.18 Congenital lobar emphysema. At operation, the involved lobe appears emphysematous and hyperexpanded. The normal lobes are relatively collapsed. Many cases of congenital lobar emphysema are due to deficiency of cartilage in the bronchial tree.

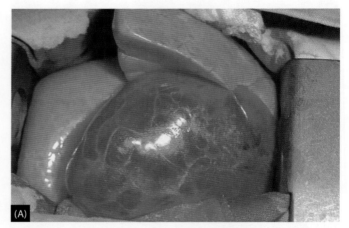

(A)

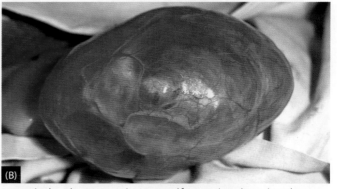

(B)

Figs. 4.19A, B (A) The operative appearance of macrocystic congenital pulmonary airway malformation (previously known as congenital cystic lung). This cyst was diagnosed on an incidental radiograph. (B) Same patient: inflation of the lungs by the anaesthetist at operation caused the cyst to expand to more than twice its previous size. This confirms its communication with the main bronchial tree.

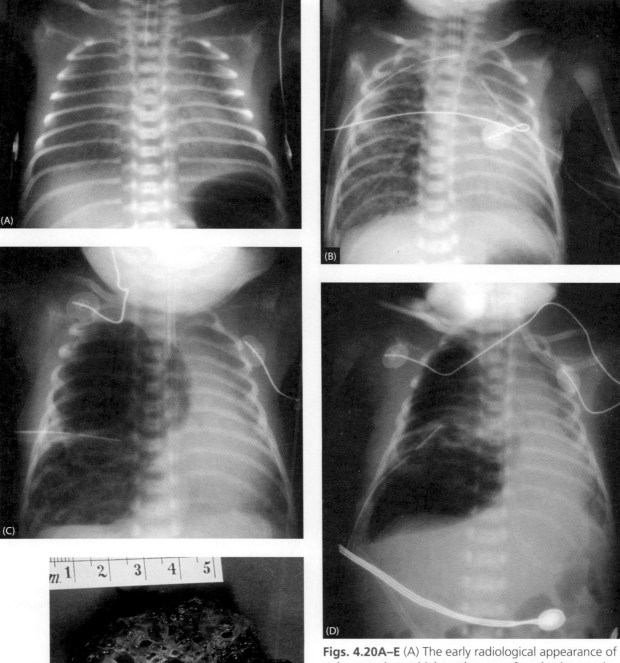

Figs. 4.20A–E (A) The early radiological appearance of pulmonary interstitial emphysema. On a background of hyaline membrane disease, small cysts develop in the lung parenchyma. Note the air bronchogram. Pulmonary interstitial emphysema may be localised to a single lobe or be diffuse throughout both lung fields. (B) Progression of pulmonary interstitial emphysema in the same patient. The cysts developing in the right lung have increased in size and have a space-occupying effect, pushing the mediastinum to the left. (C) There is now severe pulmonary interstitial emphysema with gross interstitial cystic dilatation of the right upper and lower lobes, and marked mediastinal deviation. (D) Pneumothorax has occurred, which is a common complication of severe pulmonary interstitial emphysema. (E) Autopsy specimen of pulmonary interstitial emphysema showing multiple interstitial cysts of varying sizes.

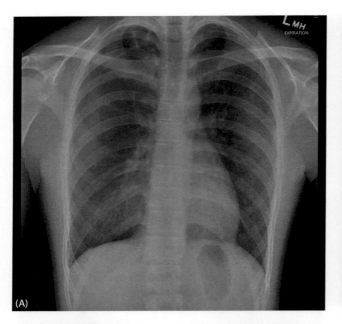

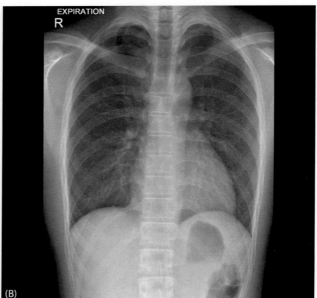

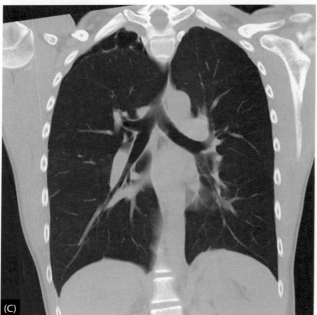

Figs. 4.21 A–C (A) Chest radiograph in an adolescent with a spontaneous pneumothorax on the right caused by rupture of apical blebs. (B, C) Same patient: plain chest radiograph and CT. The right pneumothorax has resolved and the right apical blebs can be clearly seen. This patient subsequently underwent stapled apical resection and apical pleurectomy for a good result.

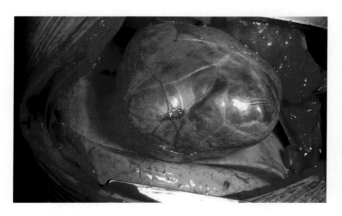

Fig. 4.22 Spontaneous pneumothoraces in children are usually secondary to rupture of an apical cyst. This is an operative photograph of an apical cyst in a 12-year-old boy who had a spontaneous pneumothorax. The cyst is often a manifestation of localised pulmonary dysplasia.

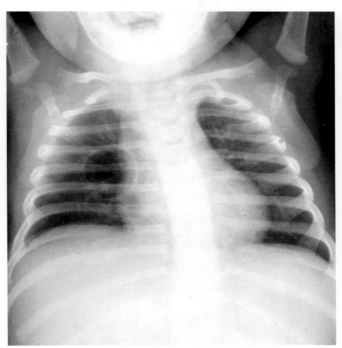

Fig. 4.23 Pneumatocele, following staphylococcal pneumonia. These may resolve over many months.

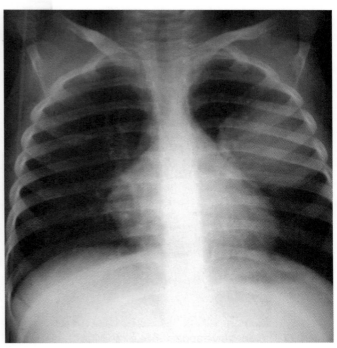

Fig. 4.24 Inflammatory myofibroblastic tumour (inflammatory pseudotumour) of the left lung.

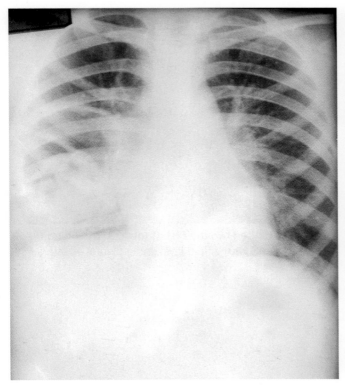

Fig. 4.25 'Water-lily sign' on a chest radiograph in a child with hydatid disease. Detachment of the endocyst membrane within the pericyst mimics the appearance of a water lily.

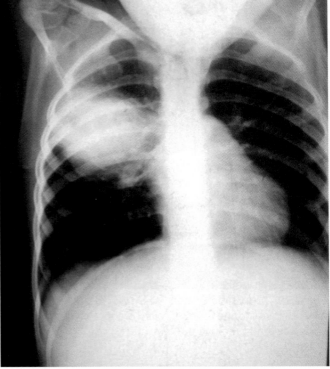

Fig. 4.26 Hydatid cyst of the right upper lobe with surrounding pneumonitis.

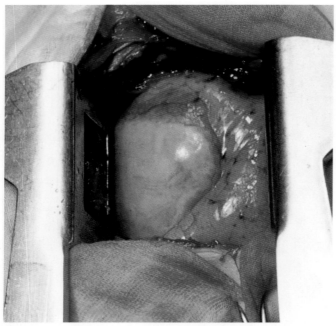

Fig. 4.27 The operative appearance of an intact hydatid cyst in the lung.

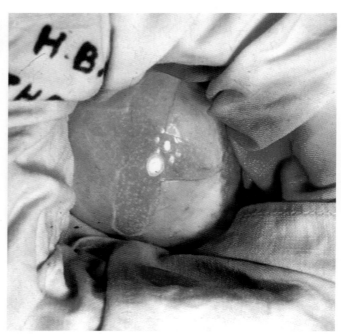

Fig. 4.28 A cruciate incision has been made into the adventitia of a pulmonary hydatid cyst. Inflation of the lungs by the anaesthetist is helping to extrude the cyst.

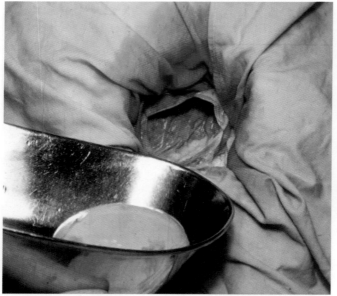

Fig. 4.29 The hydatid cyst has been 'blown out' by the anaesthetist and the residual cavity is about to be closed. Care is taken to remove the cyst intact.

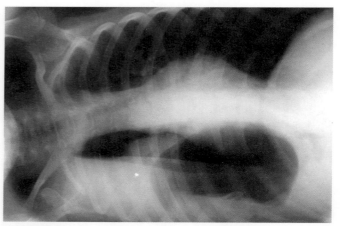

Fig. 4.30 Ruptured hydatid cyst of the lung exhibiting the 'water-lily sign', with a fluid level and a pleural effusion.

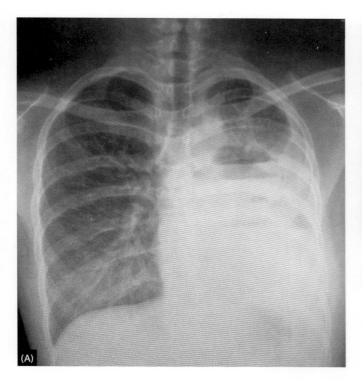

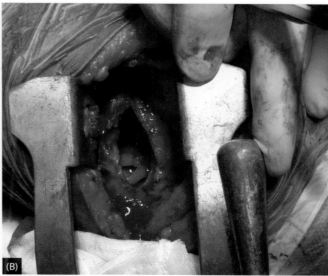

Figs. 4.31A, B (A) Chest radiograph showing a large abscess in the left lung with a fluid level, as the cavity communicates with the airway. (B) Operative view at thoracotomy showing the large abscess cavity in the lung.

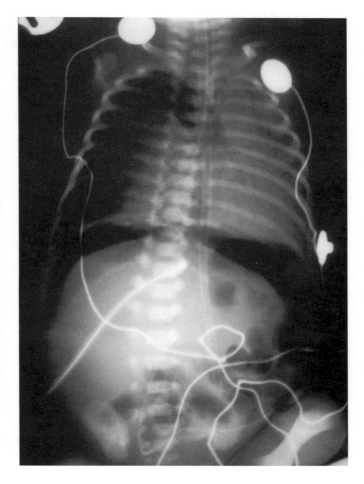

Fig. 4.32 Pneumothorax, pneumomediastinum and pneumoperitoneum in a neonate, as a result of mechanical ventilation.

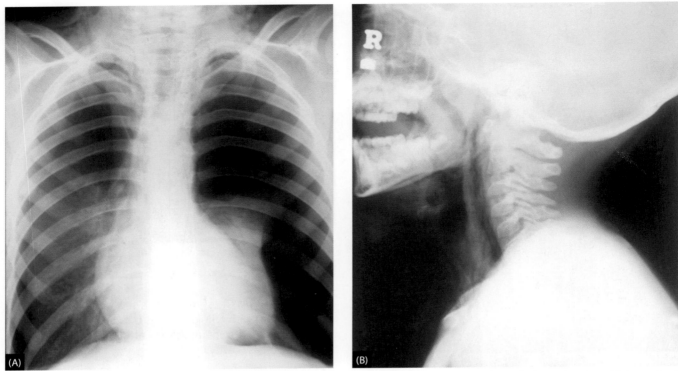

Figs. 4.33A, B (A) Explosive rupture of the oesophagus with bilateral pneumothoraces and surgical emphysema. This resulted from barotrauma after biting the inflated inner tube of an old fashioned tyre. (B) Same patient: lateral cervical radiograph showing retropharyngeal surgical emphysema in a child with a ruptured oesophagus.

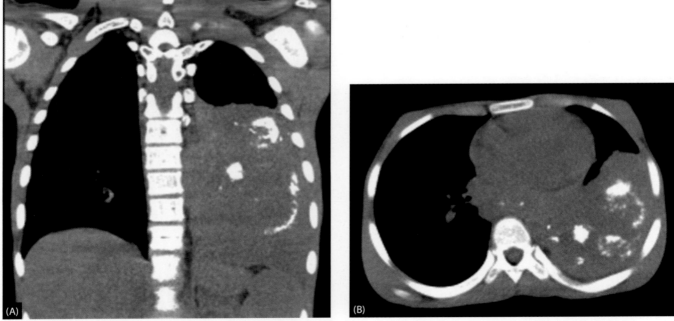

Figs. 4.34A, B This inflammatory myofibroblastic tumour involved the posterior mediastinum and extended into the left thoracic cavity. The emaciated 13-year-old girl presented with vomiting (from oesophageal involvement) and weight loss.

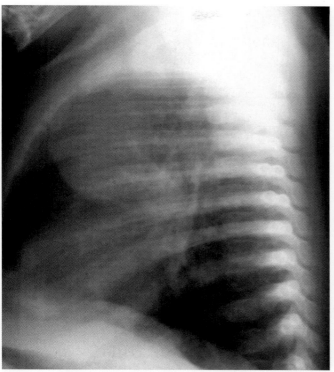

Fig. 4.35 Normal thymic enlargement of infancy. The infantile thymus is a substantial structure and is occasionally confused as being a superior mediastinal tumour.

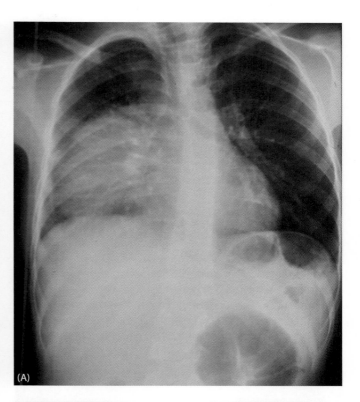

(A)

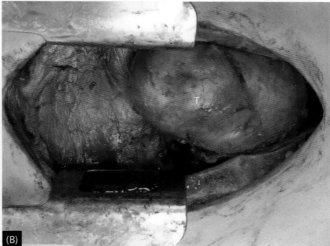

(B)

Figs. 4.36A, B (A) Benign mediastinal teratoma in a 12-year-old girl. (B) Same patient: mediastinal teratoma (T) exposed by median sternotomy.

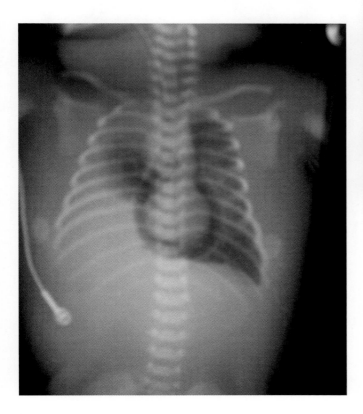

Fig. 4.37 Pneumopericardium, with air outlining the heart.

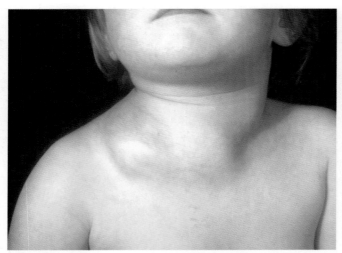

Fig. 4.38 A cervical lymphatic malformation with mediastinal extension. The cervical component can be seen as a mass low in the neck. The mediastinal component may cause diminished air entry and be percussible in the upper chest. Its extent may be determined on a plain radiograph of the chest.

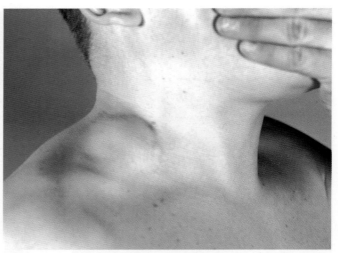

Fig. 4.39 A lymphatic malformation in a boy. The lesion becomes more obvious on forced expiration. A chest radiograph will diagnose any mediastinal component.

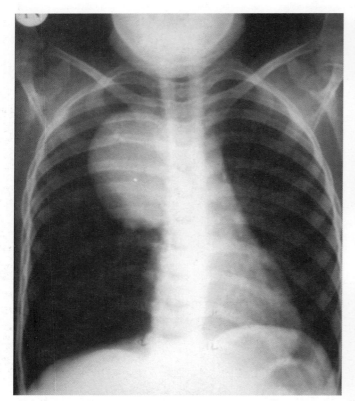

Fig. 4.40 Mediastinal neuroblastoma showing calcification.

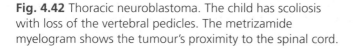

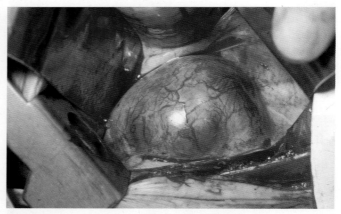

Fig. 4.41 Operative photograph of neural crest tumour (neuroblastoma). The tumour is lying in the paravertebral gutter.

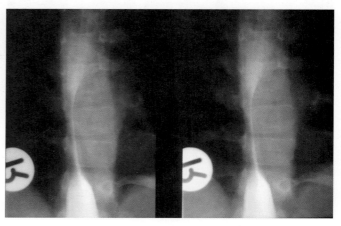

Fig. 4.42 Thoracic neuroblastoma. The child has scoliosis with loss of the vertebral pedicles. The metrizamide myelogram shows the tumour's proximity to the spinal cord.

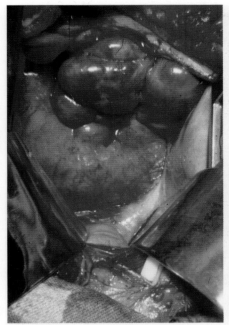

Fig. 4.43 Subpleural plaques of neuroblastoma in the paravertebral gutter, highlighting their close relationship to the intervertebral foramina.

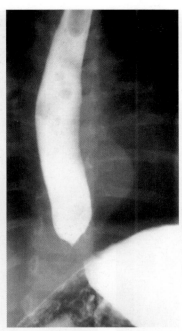

Fig. 4.44 Paraspinal ganglioneuroma causing deviation of the oesophagus on contrast study. Note the widening of the ribs, a distortion caused by the tumour.

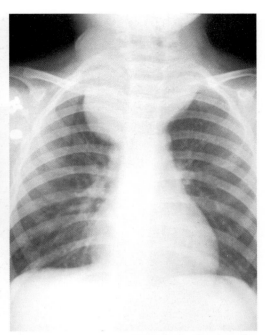

Fig. 4.45 Bilateral neural crest tumours in a patient with neurofibromatosis type 1 (NF1, von Recklinghausen disease).

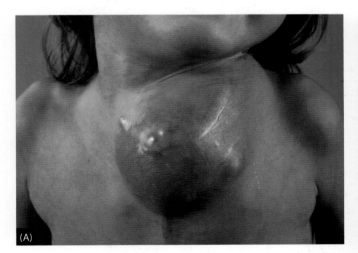

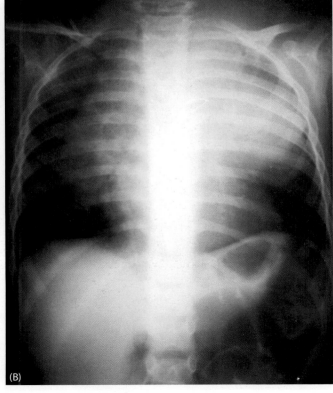

Figs. 4.46A, B (A) Aggressive fibromatosis (desmoid fibromatosis), which became apparent following median sternotomy for repair of a ventricular septal defect. (B) The chest radiograph reveals the mediastinal component of the aggressive fibromatosis.

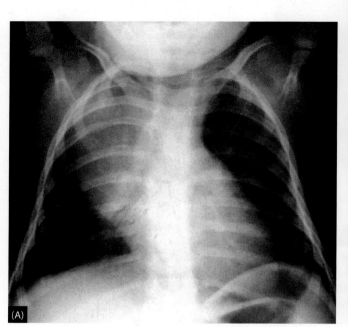

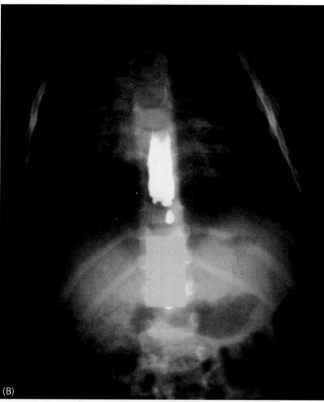

Figs. 4.47A, B (A) Chordoma. This child presented with paraplegia and was originally thought to have a neural crest tumour. At operation, the paravertebral tumour was found to be a chordoma. (B) Same patient: the myelogram shows an intraspinal block secondary to the tumour.

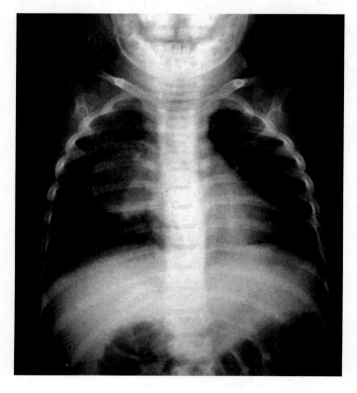

Fig. 4.48 Bronchogenic cyst. This forms one extreme of the spectrum of foregut duplications.

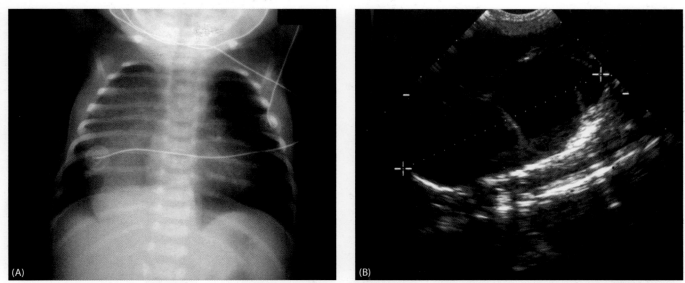

Figs. 4.49A, B (A) Oesophageal duplication. This infant presented at 2 weeks with increasing respiratory distress, which was misdiagnosed as a right pneumothorax. Insertion of a chest drain did not improve the respiratory embarrassment. The oesophageal duplication extended from the root of the neck to the diaphragm and caused compression of surrounding structures. (B) Same patient: ultrasound examination (longitudinal view) of the oesophageal duplication. Note the hyperechogenic material ('sludge') in the oesophageal duplication.

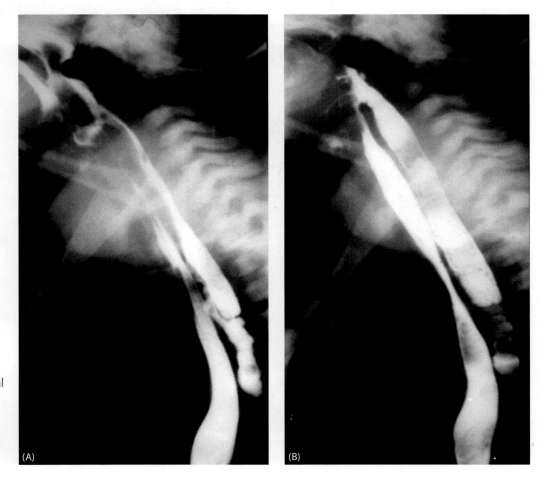

Figs. 4.50A,B Oesophageal duplication, which was initially thought to be oesophageal atresia. The contrast study revealed the true diagnosis.

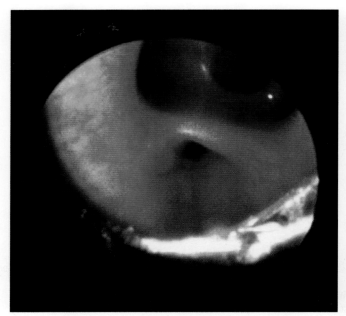

Fig. 4.51 Bronchoscopic view of a distal tracheo-oesophageal fistula, leaving the trachea posteriorly, immediately above the carina. Just within view is the take-off of the right upper lobe bronchus with the right bronchus intermedius continuing beyond.

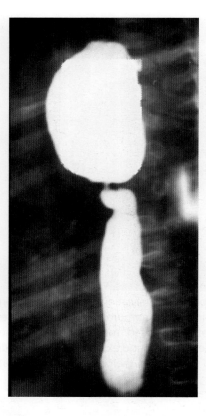

Fig. 4.52 Postanastomotic oesophageal stricture in repaired oesophageal atresia. Gastro-oesophageal reflux contributed to the formation of the stricture.

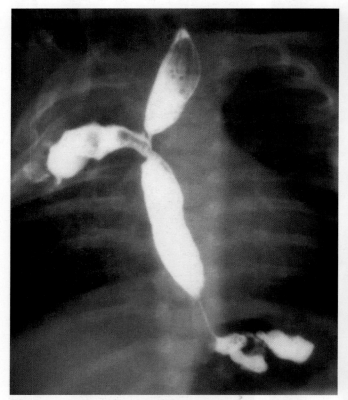

Fig. 4.53 Major postanastomotic disruption after repair of oesophageal atresia. There is an anastomotic stricture with a major leak of contrast into the right hemithorax.

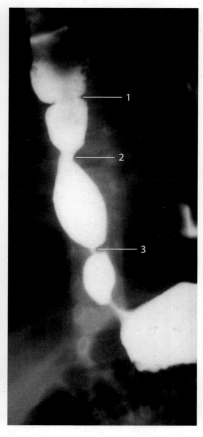

Fig. 4.54 Contrast swallow following repair of oesophageal atresia showing several areas of narrowing: (1) slight narrowing at the anastomotic site; (2) a non-constant narrowing associated with oesophageal peristalsis; (3) a fixed narrowing in the lower third of the oesophagus due to a tracheobronchial remnant causing oesophageal stenosis.

Fig. 4.55
Congenital tracheo-oesophageal fistula ('H' fistula). These infants present in the first few weeks or months of life with choking on feeds, recurrent respiratory tract infections or abdominal distension. The fistula is higher on the tracheal side than the oesophageal side. The diagnosis can be made on contrast study (as shown here) or on endoscopy (bronchoscopy).

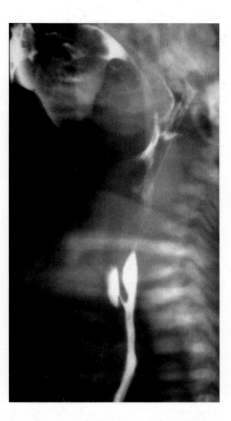

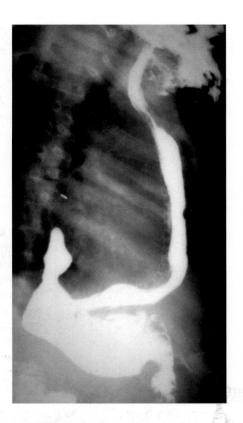

Fig. 4.56
Retrosternal placement of the greater curve of the stomach for oesophageal replacement in a patient who had long-gap oesophageal atresia. Note the contrast filling of the distal oesophagus.

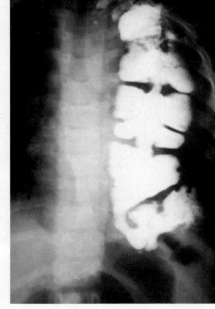

Fig. 4.57 Oeso-phagocoloplasty performed for a long corrosive stricture of the oesophagus, which could not be dilated.

Fig. 4.58
Postmyotomy diverticulum (arrow) of the oesophagus. This infant had long-gap oesophageal atresia and in order to achieve an oesophageal anastomosis a Livaditis circular myotomy of the upper oesophageal segment was performed.

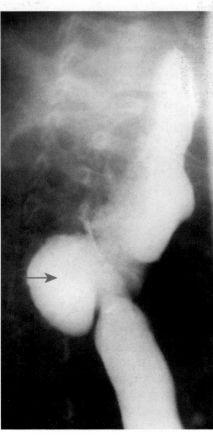

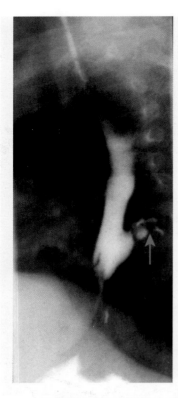

Fig. 4.59
Oesophagobronchial
fistula (arrow), a
complication that
occurred following
repair of long-gap
oesophageal atresia,
a repair that included
circular myotomies of
both the upper and lower
oesophageal segments.

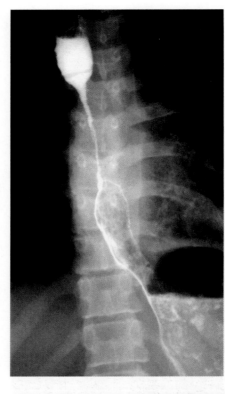

Fig. 4.60 Gastro-
oesophageal reflux
with a long peptic
oesophageal
stricture
and Barrett
oesophagus. This
child required
oesophageal
replacement.

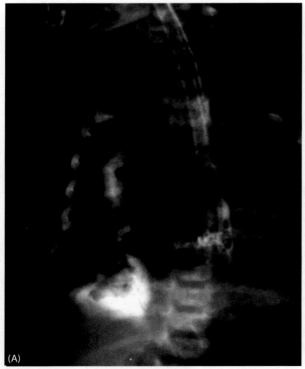

(A)

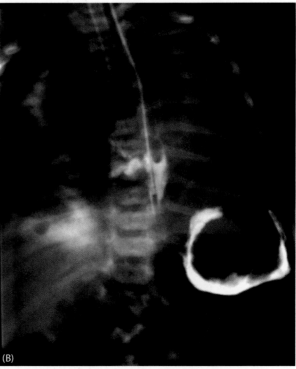

(B)

Figs. 4.61A, B (A) Spontaneous neonatal rupture of the oesophagus. This infant presented at 17 hours with respiratory distress and a right tension pneumothorax. Salivary fluid was obtained from the right pleural cavity and on contrast oesophagogram he was shown to have rupture of the oesophagus into the right pleural cavity. (B) Same patient: the contrast in the stomach outlines a space-occupying lesion, which was a blood clot. Iatrogenic perforation of the oesophagus is more common than spontaneous rupture and may occur as a complication of orogastric tube insertion in a premature infant.

Fig. 4.62
Traumatic intramural pseudodiverticulum of the oesophagus in a premature infant who had a difficult intubation. Note the long length of the upper oesophageal segment and paucity of gas in the alimentary tract, which helped to distinguish it from oesophageal atresia.

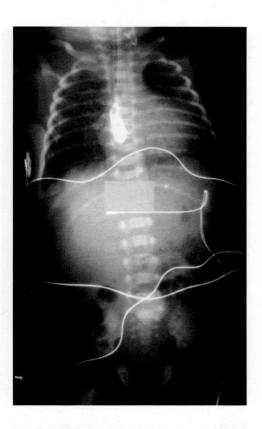

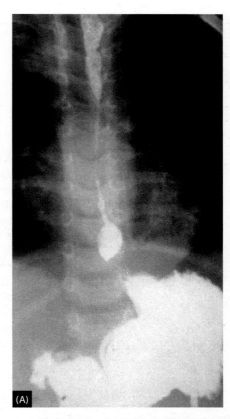

(A)

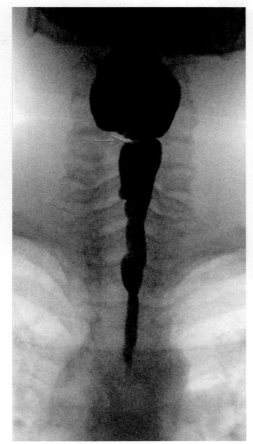

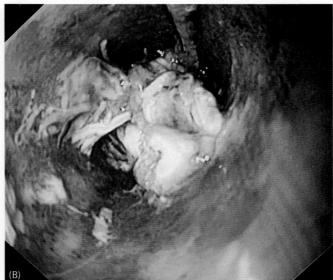

(B)

Figs. 4.63A, B (A) Contrast swallow demonstrating a caustic oesophageal stricture. (B) Endoscopic view of severe oesophageal injury after caustic ingestion.

Fig. 4.64 Contrast study showing an oesophageal stricture (arrow) in a child with epidermolysis bullosa.

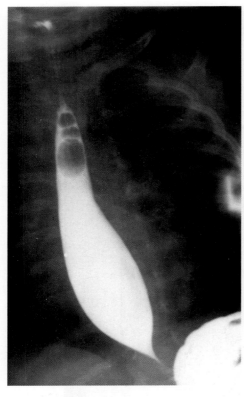

Fig. 4.65 Achalasia of the oesophagus showing narrowing of the lower end of the oesophagus with dilatation above the obstruction. This baby, aged 5 months, had dysautonomia (Riley–Day syndrome).

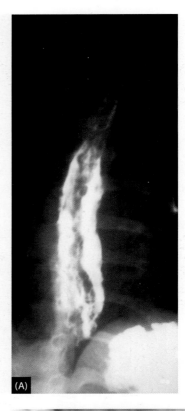

(A)

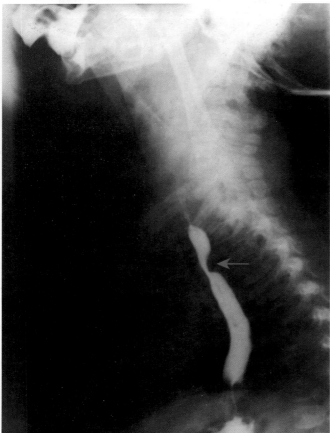

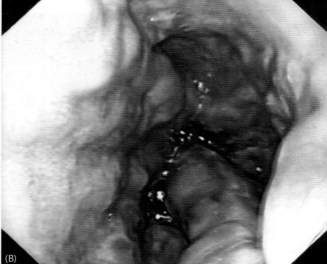

(B)

Figs. 4.66A, B (A) Gross oesophageal varices in a patient with extrahepatic portal hypertension. The dilated veins appear as filling defects in the lower half of the oesophagus. (B) Endoscopic view of oesophageal varices demonstrating the worm-like distended veins in the wall of the lower oesophagus.

Fig. 4.67 Contrast swallow of a baby with a vascular ring (arrow). This infant presented with dysphagia.

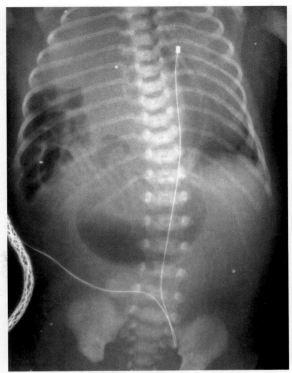

Fig. 4.68 Right-sided congenital diaphragmatic hernia presenting in a neonate.

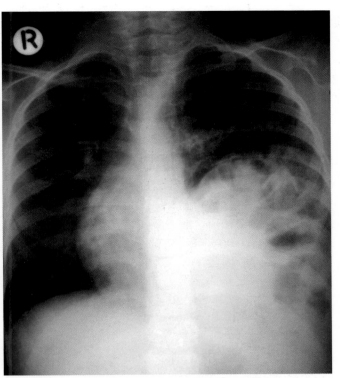

Fig. 4.69 Recurrent left diaphragmatic hernia. This child with a history of left-sided congenital diaphragmatic hernia developed new symptoms of respiratory distress and cough.

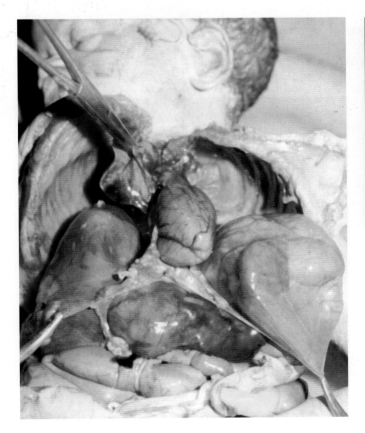

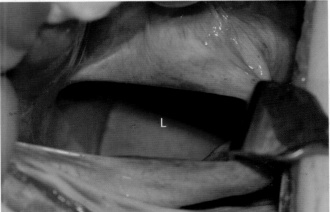

Fig. 4.71 Diaphragmatic defect in an infant with delayed presentation of congenital diaphragmatic hernia, shown at open operation. The left lung (L) is clearly visible through the defect.

Fig. 4.70 Bilateral diaphragmatic herniae seen at post mortem. There is a thin membrane on each side in lieu of the diaphragm. The lungs on either side are severely hypoplastic (and held up by the forceps).

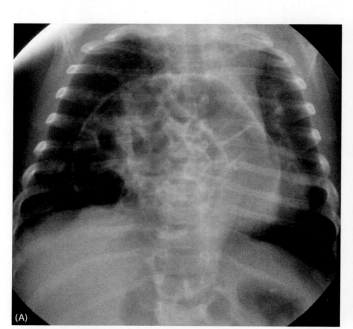

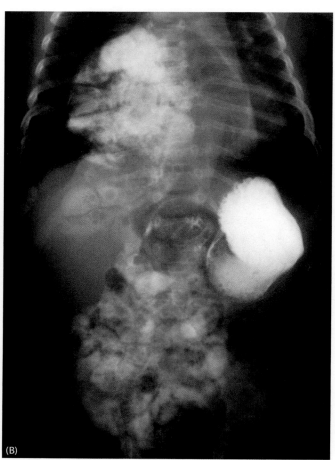

Figs. 4.72A, B (A) Chest radiograph showing distended bowel loops in the lower mediastinum in a child with a Morgagni hernia. The distension suggests there may be closed loop obstruction with the bowel incarcerated in the hernia. (B) Contrast study showing normally located stomach and small bowel loops in the chest in a Morgagni hernia.

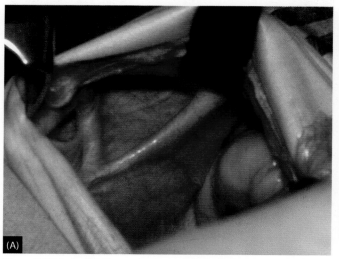

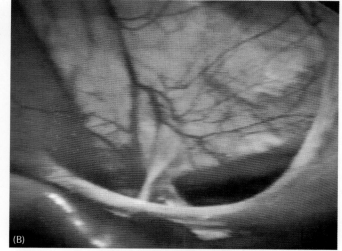

Figs. 4.73A, B (A) Operative appearance of a Morgagni hernia at open operation. (B) Laparoscopic view of a Morgagni hernia.

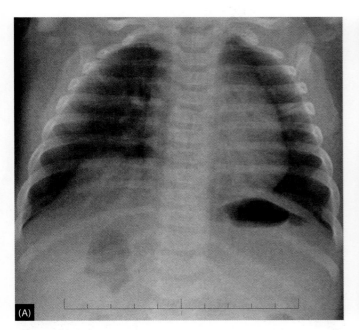

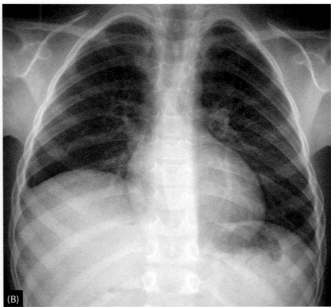

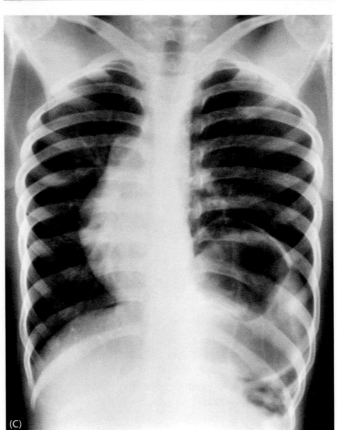

Figs. 4.74A–C (A) Eventration of the right hemidiaphragm. The differential diagnosis includes a congenital diaphragmatic hernia containing liver and paralysis of the diaphragm. (B) Another patient with a right-sided eventration. (C) A patient with left-sided eventration.

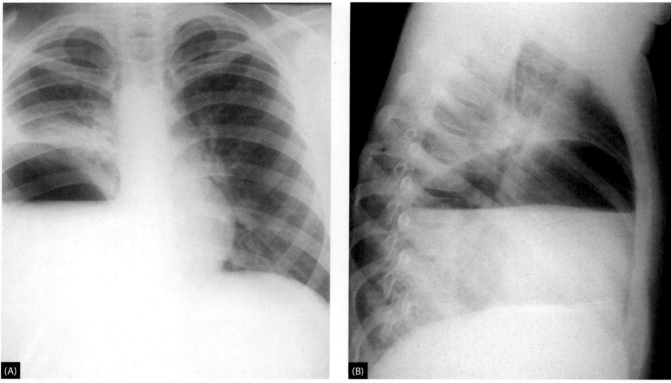

Figs. 4.75A, B (A) Traumatic diaphragmatic hernia through the right hemidiaphragm following a 'bear hug'. (B) Same patient: lateral radiograph of the traumatic rupture of the diaphragm following a 'bear hug'. The fluid level is in the stomach.

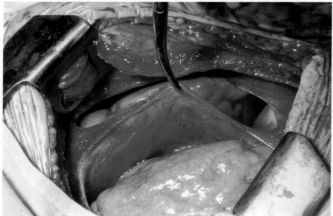

Fig. 4.76 Accessory diaphragm showing lung both above and below the structure. An incidental radiograph revealed an unexplained 'shadow'.

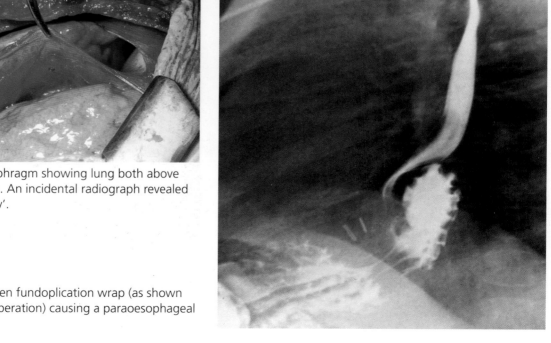

Fig. 4.77 Prolapsed Nissen fundoplication wrap (as shown by clips from previous operation) causing a paraoesophageal hernia.

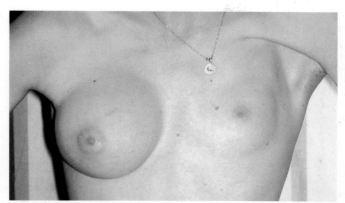

Fig. 4.78 Hypoplasia of the left breast in a girl with Poland syndrome. Note the absence of the sternocostal head of the pectoralis major muscle. The left nipple is small and hypoplastic.

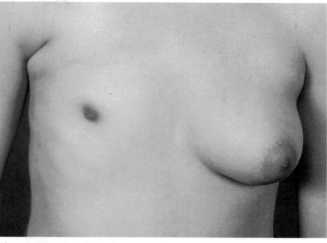

Fig. 4.79 Poland syndrome with complete absence of the right breast and a poorly formed right nipple.

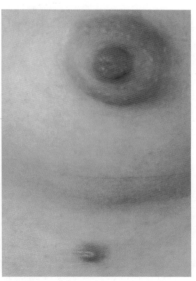

Fig. 4.80 Accessory nipples are a common abnormality and occur along the 'milk line'.

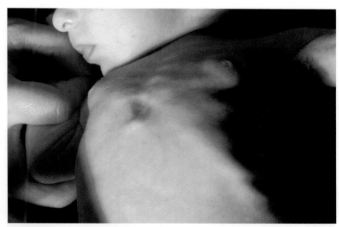

Fig. 4.81 Neonatal breast hypertrophy secondary to transplacental passage of lactogenic hormones.

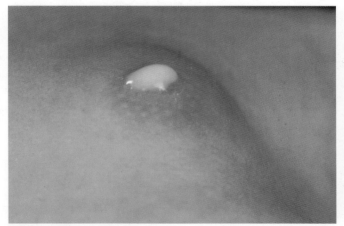

Fig. 4.82 Neonatal secretion of breast milk is a physiological response to transplacental passage of lactogenic hormones. It is sometimes called 'witch's milk', and can occur in both girls and boys.

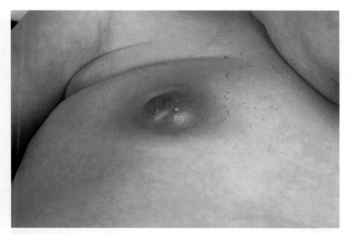

Fig. 4.83 Neonatal breast engorgement predisposes to infection (mastitis) and may result in a breast abscess.

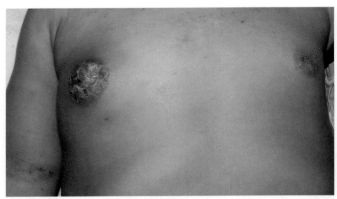

Fig. 4.84 Eczema with secondary breast abscess in an older child.

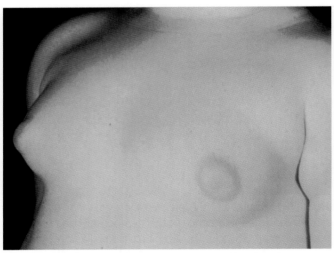

Fig. 4.85 Precocious puberty in a 5-year-old girl with an intracranial tumour.

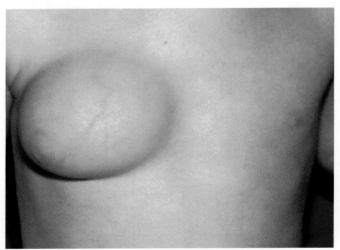

Fig. 4.86 Possible lipoblastoma in the region of the right breast in a 2-year-old girl.

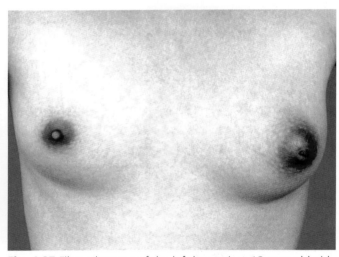

Fig. 4.87 Fibroadenoma of the left breast in a 13-year-old girl.

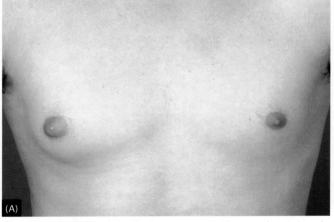

(A)

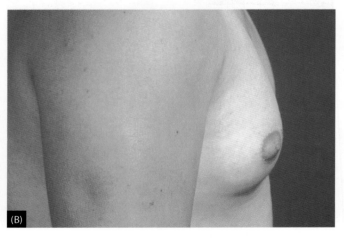

(B)

Figs. 4.88A, B Physiological gynaecomastia at puberty in a boy.

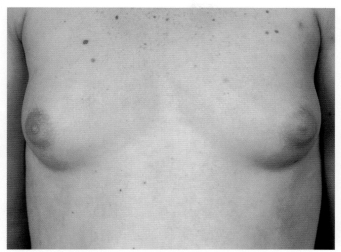

Fig. 4.89 This child presented at birth with a severe penoscrotal hypospadias and was raised as a boy. At puberty he developed breast enlargement secondary to ovarian tissue. He had a disorder of sexual development, and an ovotestis was removed from his abdomen.

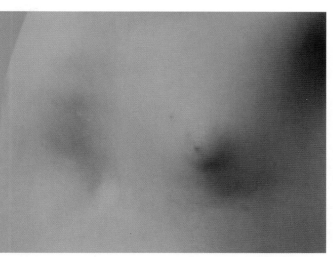

Fig. 4.90 Unilateral breast enlargement in a prepubertal child. The differential diagnosis includes congenital (vascular) anomalies and tumours, as well as premature, asymmetrical thelarche.

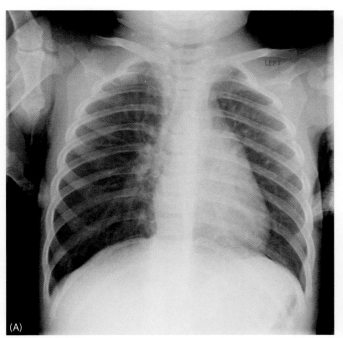

(A)

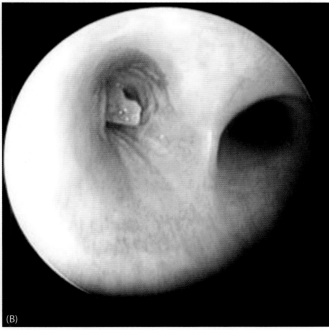

(B)

Figs. 4.91A, B (A) Overexpansion of the right lung with air trapping in a toddler who aspirated a piece of apple. (B) Airway foreign body: this different child has inhaled food lodged in the left main bronchus, which is clearly seen at tracheoscopy.

The abdomen | CHAPTER 5

Many of the intra-abdominal conditions that occur in children are age-specific. For example, pyloric stenosis usually occurs between 3 and 6 weeks of age, and for practical purposes is never seen beyond 3 months. Intussusception generally occurs between 3 and 12 months, although occasionally it is seen outside this age range. The commonest cause of abdominal symptoms requiring surgical correction is appendicitis, which is uncommon under the age of 5 years.

PYLORIC STENOSIS

Non-bile-stained vomiting in infants can be due to a wide variety of causes, ranging from sepsis (e.g. urinary tract infection, meningitis) to mechanical causes, such as gastro-oesophageal reflux and pyloric stenosis. However, the most frequent cause is related to feeding problems. Where the mother is inexperienced or the baby greedy, excessive feeding may lead to gastric distension and vomiting. Knowledge of the infant's age and a careful history will usually provide clues as to the correct diagnosis, even before physical examination has commenced. It should be determined whether the infant is otherwise well and active and keen to feed. If the vomiting is due to a septic cause, the infant is often listless and lethargic, and disinterested in feeds. If severe vomiting has a short history (i.e. a few days), it is less likely to be due to gastro-oesophageal reflux, which will have been present since birth.

Forceful or projectile vomiting is suggestive of pyloric stenosis. The infant is hungry and feeds with enthusiasm. The vomiting occurs after every feed and does not contain bile. Eventually, with progressive dehydration and electrolyte disturbance, the infant loses weight, has fewer wet nappies and becomes listless. The diagnostic sign of pyloric stenosis is palpation of a pyloric 'tumour', which can be felt either in the midline between the rectus abdominis muscles, or around the lateral border of the right rectus muscle, just below the liver edge, where the tumour can be compressed against the vertebral column. Once the tumour has been palpated, no other diagnostic test is required. However, the thickened pylorus may be difficult to palpate, particularly if the infant is not relaxed or has a full stomach. Some clinicians find it useful to empty the stomach with a nasogastric tube and to palpate the tumour with the child sucking on a dummy or at the commencement of a feed, before the stomach re-fills. Other confirmatory signs include visible gastric peristalsis, which is best seen when there is oblique lighting. Examination should also include assessment of dehydration, as this will influence fluid resuscitation prior to surgery. Ultrasonography can be done to confirm the diagnosis.

INTUSSUSCEPTION

Intussusception occurs when one part of the bowel acting as a 'lead-point' invaginates into the lumen of the adjacent distal bowel. Compression of the mesenteric vessels leads to lymphatic and venous obstruction with secondary oedema. The lumen of the intussuscepted bowel (intussusceptum) becomes occluded, causing a bowel obstruction and leading to dilatation of the proximal bowel. Most cases of intussusception occur in infants between 3 and 12 months of age. The infant presents with vomiting, lethargy, pallor and colicky abdominal pain. There may be episodes of screaming and pulling up of the knees, between which the infant appears pain-free for an interval of up to 10–20 minutes. The early vomiting that occurs is probably reflex and autonomic in origin, whereas later vomiting is the result of bowel obstruction. There may be passage of a few loose motions representing evacuation of the bowel distal to the intussusception. The presence of blood in the stools may be a relatively late sign, and is due to venous congestion of the intussusceptum. Such blood-stained stools have a characteristic appearance, the so-called 'red-currant jelly stool'.

On examination of the abdomen, the mass of the intussusception is most readily palpable early in the course of the disease. It is usually found lying beneath the rectus abdominis muscles on either side, depending on how far the intussusception has progressed. It lies midway between the normal line of the colon and the umbilicus, because as the intussusception advances, it is pulled towards the root of the small bowel mesentery. In the absence of signs of peritonitis or septicaemia, intussusception is usually confirmed by ultrasound scan and treated by enema reduction. Pathological lesions are identified at the lead-point in only 10% of patients, and include an inverted Meckel diverticulum, an intestinal polyp or, occasionally, a duplication cyst of the small bowel, lymphoma or submucosal haemorrhage with Henoch–Schönlein purpura.

APPENDICITIS

The classical presentation of appendicitis, involving central abdominal pain shifting to the right iliac fossa, nausea and vomiting with general malaise and anorexia, is well known. However, some children present atypically and may prove difficult to diagnose.

In preschool children, appendicitis tends to be advanced by the time a diagnosis is made. This results from many factors, including rapid progression of disease, a greater omentum that is less effective at limiting the spread of peritonitis, difficulties in communication and a low index of suspicion. Vomiting generally commences several hours after the onset of pain, although in the very small child, where the time of onset of the pain may be difficult to ascertain, vomiting may appear to be the first symptom.

The key to diagnosis is the demonstration of peritoneal irritation. Inflammation of the parietal peritoneum causes severe pain, which is exacerbated by movement such as walking and coughing. Percussion tenderness is a useful sign to elicit peritonism. Rebound tenderness is an unreliable sign in children, and better information can be obtained by gentle percussion. Increased involuntary muscular tone is called guarding. Guarding persists even when the child is asleep or distracted. A child with peritonitis will usually look unwell and prefer to lie still, will dislike being disturbed or handled, and will walk slowly, bent forward with the hands holding the abdomen, in an attempt to prevent movement of the inflamed peritoneum. Micturition may cause an exacerbation of the lower abdominal pain. The child will be reluctant to cough. Auscultation of the abdomen is of limited usefulness because the presence of bowel sounds does not exclude peritonitis. The combination of guarding and marked localised tenderness is strongly suggestive of peritonitis. The tenderness tends to be most pronounced in the region of the primary pathology, but as the peritonitis becomes more widespread in the abdomen, so too does the tenderness. In a non-perforated retrocaecal or pelvic appendicitis, the ventral abdominal wall tenderness may be relatively unimpressive.

MECKEL DIVERTICULUM

Meckel diverticulum can cause a variety of problems in childhood, and is the most frequent cause of major gastrointestinal bleeding. The child presents with pallor (anaemia) and painless dark red rectal bleeding. In other situations, the Meckel diverticulum may become inflamed and mimic acute appendicitis. If there is a band running from the diverticulum to the underside of the umbilicus, a loop of bowel can be caught around it, causing a bowel obstruction or even a localised volvulus of the small bowel. Occasionally, a Meckel diverticulum becomes inverted and acts as the lead-point in intussusception.

OTHER CAUSES OF THE ACUTE ABDOMEN

Although acute appendicitis is the most common surgical cause of the 'acute abdomen', there are numerous other conditions that may cause abdominal pain. Colicky abdominal pain followed by vomiting and abdominal distension in a child who has had previous intra-abdominal surgery (e.g. appendicectomy) is suggestive of an adhesive bowel obstruction. The danger is that when one or more loops of bowel become trapped beneath a band adhesion, their vascular supply can be compromised, leading to gangrene of that part of the bowel.

The clinical features include those of intestinal obstruction with (usually) marked localised tenderness and, with further progression of disease, signs of peritonitis develop. Plain radiographs will reveal small bowel obstruction.

Appendicitis may produce an inflammatory mass in the right iliac fossa. In the acute phase, the overlying guarding may make it difficult to palpate the mass, at least until the patient is anaesthetised. The mass is tender, has ill-defined margins and is immobile. It should be distinguished from a large ovarian cyst, which tends to be non-tender and mobile, and can be manipulated in and out of the pelvis. However, if an ovarian cyst has undergone torsion, it too may be difficult to palpate on account of overlying guarding and other signs of peritonism. In a child under 3 years of age, the possibility of an intussusception mass must be considered. In these children, there will be colicky pain and vomiting. In the older child, a relatively painless immobile mass is more suggestive of a lymphoma; other supporting features may include weight loss, fever, lymphadenopathy and hepatosplenomegaly. Less common causes include Meckel diverticulitis, *Yersinia* lymphadenitis, duplication cyst, lymphangioma, omental cyst, mesenteric cyst, omental infarction, tuberculosis or actinomycosis. In children with cystic fibrosis, severe constipation or distal intestinal obstruction syndrome from inspissated luminal gut content or appendiceal pathology may produce a palpable abdominal mass.

The rapid development of bile-stained vomiting, with or without colicky abdominal pain, should raise the possibility of intestinal malrotation with volvulus, particularly in an infant. This diagnosis must be proved or excluded promptly by contrast study, preferably a contrast meal, because if volvulus has occurred, complete infarction of the midgut may ensue.

Infection by a variety of enteric organisms (e.g. viruses, *Yersinia* spp. or *Campylobacter* spp.) may cause enlargement of the mesenteric lymph nodes and produce fever with diffuse tenderness of the abdomen. These signs may be confused with acute appendicitis. Tenderness is often most pronounced in the right iliac fossa, reflecting the location of the majority of the mesenteric lymph nodes. Associated features may include headache, generalised aches and pains and other manifestations of viral infection.

CONSTIPATION

In Western societies, constipation remains an endemic problem in children, affecting 3–8% of the population. Constipation often results from a poor diet, low in fibre, and may be exacerbated by a constitutional predisposition and poor bowel training. A minority of patients will be affected by slow transit constipation; in these patients the colonic motility is uniformly slowed, as can be demonstrated using radiopaque markers or on nuclear transit studies.

Often, constipation leads to colicky abdominal pain that may be subsequently relieved by a bowel action. In addition to abdominal pain, chronic constipation may lead to faecal soiling, the creation of anal fissures, and rectal prolapse.

The normal rectum is empty the majority of the time. Rectal distension, caused by the passage of faecal material from the colon, stimulates pressure receptors in the rectum to initiate the efferent arc of the defecation reflex. Evacuation is achieved by contraction of the rectum with coordinated relaxation of the anal sphincters. In chronic constipation, the rectum often fails to empty adequately, and the rectal walls may become chronically overstretched. It is believed that the sensory receptors are dulled and the rectal wall is unable to contract effectively. With absorption of water from the stool, the stools become harder and more difficult to pass. This may split the anal mucosa (anal fissures), producing further unwillingness to defecate. Eventually, the child may develop spurious diarrhoea around the large rectal faecal mass, and will present with soiling. If this leakage is continuous, it causes irritation to the perianal skin, which may become severely excoriated, leading to bleeding. The diagnosis may be made on clinical examination of the abdomen, with rectal examination reserved for rare cases. When constipation becomes chronic, treatment (both medical and surgical) may be required to assist emptying of the rectum.

Organic causes of constipation are rare, but include anorectal malformations, Hirschsprung disease, spinal lesions (e.g. spina bifida) and severe developmental delay.

GASTRO-OESOPHAGEAL REFLUX

Almost all babies have gastro-oesophageal reflux, which becomes less pronounced during the first year of life. Severe gastro-oesophageal reflux in the first month of life may be pronounced enough to raise suspicion of pyloric stenosis, but no pyloric tumour will be palpable or seen on ultrasonography. Severe gastro-oesophageal reflux may produce complications, which in themselves demand surgical correction of the reflux. The most important are life-threatening apnoeic episodes. An oesophageal stricture may develop secondary to oesophagitis from the corrosive effect of gastric acid reflux into the lower oesophagus. In infants, gastro-oesophageal reflux may lead to respiratory problems such as pneumonia from aspiration of gastric contents. Oesophagitis may produce dysphagia, bleeding – either haematemesis or melaena – and iron-deficiency anaemia. In a small group of infants, reflux is responsible for failure to thrive. Gastro-oesophageal reflux may occur in isolation or be associated with other conditions, both medical (e.g. severe neurological impairment, Down syndrome) and surgical (e.g. congenital hiatal hernia or after repair of oesophageal atresia, exomphalos major or congenital diaphragmatic hernia).

INTRA-ABDOMINAL TUMOURS

The three main malignant intra-abdominal tumours are neuroblastoma, Wilms tumour and hepatoblastoma. Neuroblastoma arises from fetal neural crest cells, usually from the adrenal gland but potentially in any site where sympathetic ganglion cells are normally found. Thus, a neuroblastoma may also arise from sympathetic ganglia in the abdomen, mediastinum, pelvis or, less commonly, from other sites. These tumours metastasise early to the bone marrow, lymph nodes and liver. Sometimes, metastases may be their first indication. For example, skin metastases and proptosis with periorbital ecchymosis and pain is a recognised pattern in the presentation of neuroblastoma. When an abdominal mass is suspected to be a neuroblastoma, the diagnosis can be confirmed by obtaining: a marrow biopsy for evidence of metastatic neuroblastoma (positive in about 70%); urine for tumour catecholamine metabolites; and biopsy of the tumour or metastases. A metaiodobenzylguanidine (MIBG) radioisotope scan highlights active metastases when radioactive iodine-labelled MIBG is incorporated into functioning neuroblastoma tissue. The patient's age, stage of the tumour and its biological features are major prognostic factors used for risk stratification and guiding treatment.

Wilms tumour (nephroblastoma) usually presents in preschool children as a painless smooth mass in the abdomen, which reaches but seldom crosses the midline. It may extend from the costal margin to the iliac fossa. In a few children, haematuria following minor trauma is the presentation. The blood pressure may be elevated. Ultrasonography will provide information on the site, size and extent of the tumour, and a chest x-ray or CT scan will identify pulmonary metastases (see Chapter 7). Prognosis relates to the stage of the tumour, its biology and whether the tumour is linked to an underlying syndrome/genetic condition.

The most common malignant liver tumour in children is hepatoblastoma, which usually presents in children younger than 3 years of age. Most such tumours are sporadic but some are associated with genetic abnormalities. Hepatoblastoma has to be distinguished from hepatic vascular malformations (which may be accompanied by thrombocytopaenia) and mesenchymal hamartoma, both of which are benign. In hepatoblastoma, the tumour marker, alpha-fetoprotein, is usually elevated. Imaging techniques include ultrasonography, CT scan and MRI; these are used to provide further information on the anatomical location of the tumour. Prognosis is related to the pretreatment extent of the disease (PRETEXT group) and tumour histology; combined treatment with chemotherapy and surgery is highly effective.

INFLAMMATORY BOWEL DISEASE

The incidence and prevalence of inflammatory bowel disease is increasing in many parts of the world. Crohn disease is more common than ulcerative colitis in childhood. Approximately 25% of all patients with Crohn disease present during the first two decades of life. Crohn disease may involve any part of the gastrointestinal tract, from the mouth to the anus, and 10–15% of affected children have perianal disease. Crohn disease typically shows discontinuous or segmental involvement and different disease phenotypes are recognised (e.g. ileal, ileocolonic, colonic), with stricturing and penetrating (fistulising) subtypes. In contrast, ulcerative colitis involves the large bowel mucosa in a diffuse and continuous manner and almost always affects the rectum; children are more likely than adults to have panproctocolitis.

There is considerable variability in the mode of presentation of inflammatory bowel disease in children, a fact that often causes a delay between the onset of symptoms and diagnosis. Crohn disease usually presents with recurrent abdominal pain and weight loss. There may be no change in bowel habit or the patient may have diarrhoea – with or without blood – similar to that seen in ulcerative colitis. In the older child, a striking feature is growth failure and delayed onset of puberty. The development of Crohn disease may be heralded or accompanied by extraintestinal symptoms or perianal disease. Occasionally, the child may present with an acute abdomen suggestive of acute appendicitis. The increasing diarrhoea with blood and mucus seen in ulcerative colitis may be associated with weight loss, fever and pallor. Children with suspected inflammatory bowel disease are best investigated by blood and stool tests, gastroscopy and colonoscopy with serial biopsies of the gut mucosa and, in Crohn disease in particular, by abdominal imaging (ultrasound, MRI, CT). Crohn disease is characterised histologically by transmural chronic inflammation with granuloma formation, whereas ulcerative colitis shows a florid mucosal infiltration by neutrophils forming crypt abscesses.

THE ANUS AND PERINEUM

Anal fissures are common in infants and toddlers and occur when passage of a stool splits the anal mucosa. There is a sharp anal pain and a few drops of bright blood may be seen on the surface of the stool or nappy. Acute anal fissures tend to be superficial and heal rapidly. They can be demonstrated by gently parting the perianal skin in a lateral direction with the baby lying supine with the legs elevated. The fissure appears as a breach in the mucosa running longitudinally within the anal canal, usually in the midline posteriorly or anteriorly. Chronic anal fissures often have whitish margins and an associated sentinel skin tag.

Perianal abscesses are common in infant boys and arise from infection of the anal glands, which open into the crypts or anal valves. The abscess presents superficially, but there is usually a fistulous tract passing through to the level of the anal valves. If this tract is not laid open, the abscess is likely to recur.

RECTAL BLEEDING

Rectal bleeding is a relatively common symptom in childhood and rarely signifies serious disease. Small amounts of fresh blood from an anal fissure may follow an acute episode of constipation (or diarrhoea). The child avoids further defecation, and the faeces become hard and more difficult to pass. When the stools are passed eventually, further trauma to the anal canal causes a small amount of bleeding, which can be seen as red streaks on the stool or spots of blood on the nappy. In the well baby with small streaks of blood and mucus in the stool, cow's milk protein intolerance is often the cause. In the sick premature infant, necrotising enterocolitis must be considered in the differential diagnosis of rectal bleeding.

An uncommon but extremely important cause of small-volume rectal bleeding is ischaemia of the bowel with impending gangrene, as is seen in volvulus secondary to intestinal malrotation and in advanced ileocolic intussusception. The child is in pain and may have bile-stained vomiting. With midgut volvulus there is rapid progression of symptoms and signs. Eventually the abdomen becomes distended, with widespread abdominal tenderness and guarding. By the time signs of peritonitis occur, there is almost certainly dead bowel already.

Henoch–Schönlein purpura is a rare cause of rectal bleeding with an acute abdomen. At the time the abdominal pain commences the characteristic Henoch–Schönlein rash and arthralgia may not be present. The abdominal pain and rectal bleeding are the result of vasculitis (and sometimes intussusception) affecting the bowel.

A Meckel diverticulum containing ectopic gastric mucosa may cause major haemorrhage. Secretion of hydrochloric acid produces an ulcer in adjacent ileal mucosa. The rapid blood loss that ensues may be painless. It is dark red in colour, reflecting the time it takes to reach the anus. A juvenile polyp may produce moderate bright red lower gastrointestinal bleeding, which is usually self-limiting. Haemorrhoids are rare in children. Congestion of the external haemorrhoidal venous plexus during straining at stool sometimes produces a bluish sessile perianal bulge, but bleeding from this source is extremely rare.

Bleeding associated with persistent diarrhoea is usually caused by infective organisms (e.g. *Campylobacter* or *Salmonella* spp.). In the absence of gastroenteritis, chronic bloody diarrhoea in older children is suggestive of inflammatory bowel disease.

RECTAL PROLAPSE

In rectal prolapse part or all of the rectum protrudes through the anal canal. Rectal prolapse may occur in association with myelomeningocele (from paresis of the pelvic floor), exstrophy of the bladder (from disturbance of the structural support of the rectum), cystic fibrosis (chronic cough with increased intra-abdominal pressure), following pelvic surgery, in chronic diarrhoea or severe malnutrition, but most often occurs without any obvious underlying cause. It tends to be seen in toddlers during the second year of life, and occurs after straining during defecation and may follow either constipation or acute diarrhoea. The prolapsed rectal mucosa has a pink/red glistening surface which, with chronic prolapse, may become congested and ulcerated. It may bleed readily on contact with nappies. Rectal mucosal prolapse rarely extends a few centimetres beyond the anal orifice; full-thickness rectal prolapse can extend much further. Usually the prolapse reduces spontaneously but occasionally it may require manual reduction. A rectal polyp can be distinguished by the demonstration of its pedunculated stalk. Rectal prolapse can be distinguished from anal prolapse of an intussusceptum in that the child is otherwise well and the prolapse causes eversion of the anal canal.

JAUNDICE

'Physiological' jaundice is seen frequently in the first 2 weeks of life and is secondary to functional immaturity of the neonatal liver. Deep or rapidly developing jaundice implies that haemolysis, infection or an inborn error of metabolism may be present, and demands urgent investigation and treatment.

Jaundice that appears later, or persists into the third week of life, is not likely to be 'physiological' jaundice. If accompanied by pale acholic stools, dark urine and an elevated serum conjugated (direct) bilirubin, a surgical cause must be considered (*Table 5.1*). In these infants haemolytic disease and congenital infections of the fetus (e.g. rubella, herpes, cytomegalovirus, syphilis and toxoplasmosis) need to be excluded. In breast milk jaundice, suppression of glucuronyl transferase by substances in the milk causes an unconjugated hyperbilirubinaemia. Alpha-1 antitrypsin deficiency may cause cholestasis, which can mimic

TABLE 5.1 Some major causes of non-physiological neonatal jaundice

Surgical	Medical
Biliary atresia	Breast milk jaundice
Choledochal cyst	Neonatal hepatitis
Inspissated bile	Sepsis (e.g. urinary tract infection)
	Inborn errors of metabolism (e.g. galactosaemia, alpha-1-antitrypsin deficiency)
	Endocrine disorders (e.g. hypopituitarism, hypothyroidism)
	Bile duct paucity syndromes (e.g. Alagille syndrome and progressive familial intrahepatic cholestasis)

obstruction of the bile ducts; it can be excluded by estimating the serum alpha-1 antitrypsin concentration and checking the alpha-1-antitrypsin protein phenotype. It may be difficult to distinguish biliary atresia from neonatal hepatitis and cholestatic liver disorders associated with intrahepatic bile duct paucity. Minor enlargement of the liver and spleen can occur in both. Liver function tests, an abdominal ultrasound scan, hepatobiliary scintigraphy, needle biopsy of the liver and, occasionally, laparotomy with intraoperative cholangiography will distinguish these pathologies. Coagulation must be checked (and treated appropriately) in any baby with prolonged jaundice to avoid major complications such as intracranial haemorrhage. Similarly, hypoglycaemia must be detected and treated promptly.

Biliary atresia is a progressive obliterative disorder of the biliary tract that presents in the first few weeks of life. The infant is often well but has a persistent conjugated hyperbilirubinaemia, pale stools and dark urine. The diagnosis is made by excluding other causes of neonatal conjugated jaundice and supported by findings consistent with the diagnosis (e.g. a small irregular gallbladder on ultrasound scan, no gut excretion on a biliary isotope scan and histological features on liver biopsy).

A choledochal cyst is a congenital dilatation of the common bile duct. Various types of the abnormality are described depending on the appearance of the extrahepatic and intrahepatic bile ducts. There is frequently an associated malunion of the terminal pancreatic and bile ducts. The presenting features are those of obstructive jaundice and/or abdominal pain; an upper abdominal mass and fever may be present. The diagnosis can be confirmed on ultrasonography, magnetic resonance cholangiopancreatography (MRCP) and/or endoscopic retrograde cholangiopancreatography (ERCP).

PORTAL HYPERTENSION

Portal hypertension may develop as a result of liver fibrosis or cirrhosis (e.g. from biliary atresia or metabolic liver disease) or from occlusion of the portal vein as a consequence of faulty development or thrombosis. High pressure in the portomesenteric venous system causes dilatation of collateral veins, particularly at sites of portosystemic anastomoses such as that around the lower end of the oesophagus (oesophageal varices). Variceal bleeding is a cause of major haematemesis and melaena.

The child with cirrhosis and secondary portal hypertension if often wasted, jaundiced and has a distended abdomen. The spleen is palpable and there may be ascites. The liver may or may not be palpable depending on whether its size has decreased because of the cirrhosis. Dilated collateral veins may be visible in the subcutaneous tissues radiating from the umbilicus, the so-called 'caput medusae'.

CHOLELITHIASIS

Gallstones may develop in children for a variety of reasons. Black pigment calculi composed of calcium bilirubinate may develop in newborn babies, particularly in those requiring total parenteral nutrition. In the newborn, there is an increased pigment load associated with the change from a high fetal haemoglobin to a lower newborn level, and in the setting of neonatal intensive care (with potential blood transfusion, transient dehydration and impaired enteral feeding) this may predispose to biliary sludge and gallstone formation. Black pigment calculi are also seen in haemolytic anaemia (e.g. spherocytosis and thalassaemia), where there is increased red cell turnover. Cholelithiasis may develop in congenital obstructive abnormalities of the bile duct, such as a choledochal cyst, as a consequence of biliary stasis. Finally, cholesterol stones are typically seen in overweight adolescent girls with a family history of gallstone disease.

Gallstones may be asymptomatic or cause biliary colic, cholecystitis, obstructive jaundice and/or acute pancreatitis. The pain of biliary colic is usually located in the epigastrium or right upper quadrant. Vomiting is common and there is tenderness in the right upper quadrant, with a positive Murphy sign. If the gallstone obstructs the common bile duct, the child will become jaundiced and pass dark urine and pale stools. Occasionally, the child will present with gallstone pancreatitis.

THE SPLEEN

A number of haematological diseases involve the spleen. In spherocytosis, there is chronic anaemia, episodic haemolytic jaundice and a tendency to form black pigment gallstones. These complications are due to premature destruction of the abnormally spherical red cells in the spleen. The haemolysis can be controlled by splenectomy.

In idiopathic thrombocytopaenic purpura a low platelet count may persist, despite maximal medical therapy, and may necessitate a splenectomy. In past years, thalassaemia was associated with hypersplenism, but modern treatments, including blood transfusions and regular iron chelation therapy, can avoid the need for splenectomy. In sickle cell anaemia splenectomy is usually contraindicated, as a higher haemoglobin tends to be associated with increased 'sickling' of the red cells. In sickle cell anaemia splenic infarcts may occur.

Splenic trauma is discussed in Chapter 10. Rare abnormalities of splenic development include splenic cysts, splenogonadal fusion, asplenia and polysplenia. Asplenia and polysplenia are both associated with heterotaxy (abnormal left-right axis thoracoabdominal visceral location) and cardiac malformations, and polysplenia is part of the biliary atresia splenic malformation syndrome.

THE PANCREAS

Pancreatitis is relatively uncommon in children. The leading causes of acute pancreatitis in children are trauma (including non-accidental), biliary diseases (e.g. gallstones and choledochal cysts), drugs (e.g. asparaginase and sodium valproate), viral infections and systemic disease. In contrast, chronic pancreatitis is most often caused by mutations in genes encoding pancreatic proteins. A pancreatic pseudocyst may develop following acute or chronic pancreatitis (see Chapter 10 for pancreatic pseudocyst complicating blunt abdominal trauma).

Other structural pancreatic pathologies in children include annular pancreas, duplication cysts and pancreatic tumours.

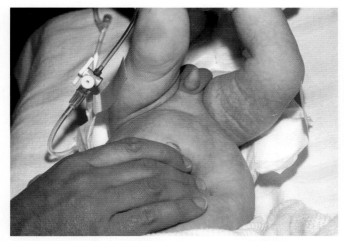

Fig. 5.1 The diagnosis of pyloric stenosis is confirmed by palpation of a pyloric tumour. This is best felt from the left side of the patient, palpating either in the midline between the rectus abdominis muscles, or around the lateral border of the right rectus muscle just below the liver edge. The tumour is most easily palpated when the stomach is empty and the infant is relaxed.

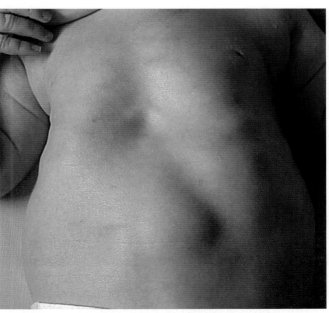

Fig. 5.2 Visible gastric peristalsis can be dramatic in pyloric stenosis. A wave of gastric peristalsis can be seen crossing the left hypochondrium and progressing towards the antrum.

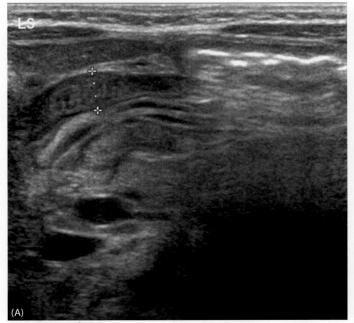

(A)

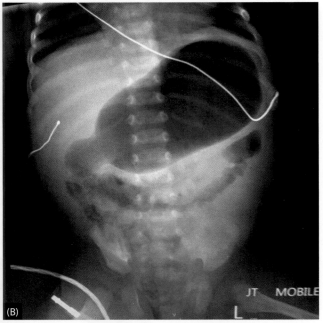

(B)

Figs. 5.3A, B (A) Ultrasonography is helpful in confirming the diagnosis of pyloric stenosis. This longitudinal section of the pylorus shows shows thickened circular muscle (marked with cursors) surrounding the obstructed pyloric canal. (B) Pyloric stenosis causing dilatation of body and antrum of stomach on abdominal x-ray.

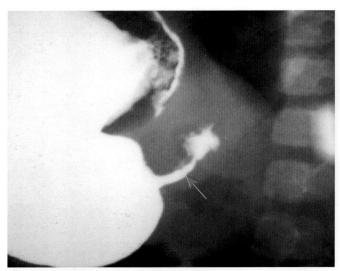

Fig. 5.4 A contrast study (which is rarely required now that ultrasonography is available) will show gastric outlet obstruction with a thin streak of contrast passing through the narrowed pylorus (arrow). This is sometimes called the 'string sign'.

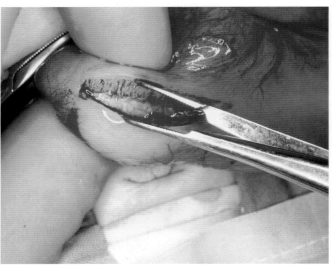

Fig. 5.5 The operative appearance of a pyloric tumour. After splitting the grossly thickened circular muscle, the submucosa can be seen bulging at the base of the split.

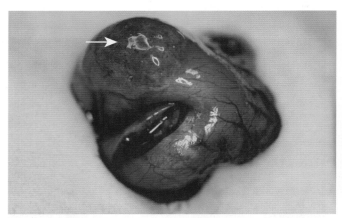

Fig. 5.6 Heterotopic pancreatic tissue in the antrum of the stomach (arrow), proximal to a pyloromyotomy wound in an infant with pyloric stenosis. This was an incidental finding.

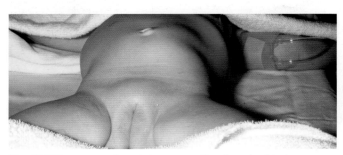

Fig. 5.8 The mass of an intussusception is palpable in more than 50% of patients. In this preoperative photograph of a paralysed child following a failed air enema, the mass can be seen in the left upper quadrant.

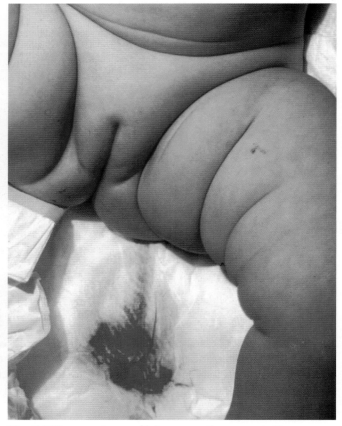

Fig. 5.7 The symptoms of intussusception are vomiting, lethargy, pallor and colicky abdominal pain. In up to 50% of cases, a small volume of blood-stained stool may be passed.

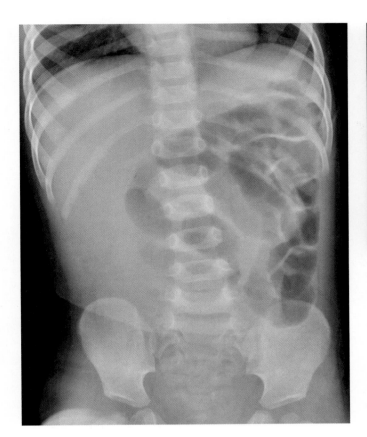

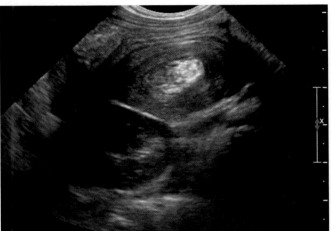

Fig. 5.10 A transverse abdominal ultrasound scan showing the 'target' or 'doughnut' sign of an ileo-colic intussusception.

Fig. 5.9 A plain abdominal radiograph in an infant with intussusception. There is evidence of small bowel obstruction and a paucity of gas in the lower right quadrant. The soft tissue mass of the intussusceptum is not clearly visible.

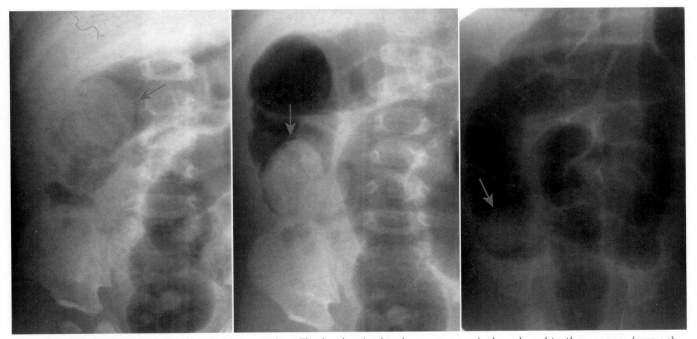

Fig. 5.11 Air-enema reduction of an intussusception. The lead-point has been progressively reduced to the caecum (arrows). This was followed by complete reduction of the intussusception with free passage of air into the small bowel.

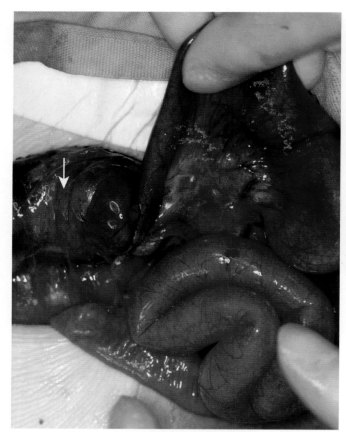

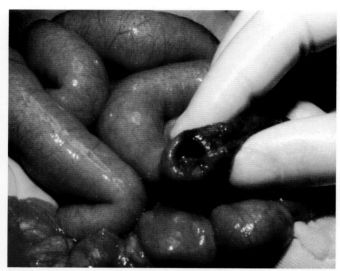

Fig. 5.13 Following successful reduction of ileocolic intussusception, a dimple is frequently encountered at the lead-point. There is no identifiable pathological lesion at this lead-point in 90% of patients with intussusception.

Fig. 5.12 Operative appearance of intussusception. The surgeon is holding the ileum. The intussusception can be reduced by gently squeezing the intussuscipiens (arrow), which contains the intussusceptum.

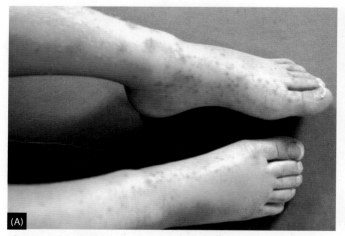

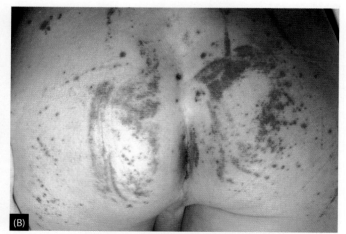

Figs. 5.14A, B Henoch–Schönlein purpura may produce submucosal haemorrhage, which acts as a lead-point for intussusception. The other features of Henoch–Schönlein purpura (e.g. a cutaneous vasculitic rash as seen here) are not always present at the time the intussusception occurs.

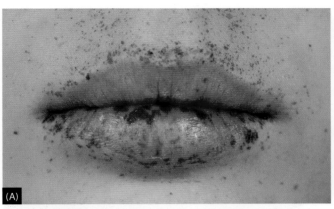
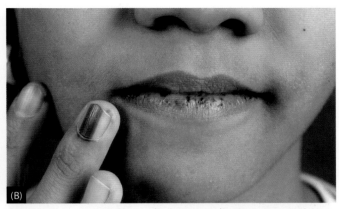

Figs. 5.15A, B Peutz–Jegher syndrome is associated with intestinal hamartomatous polyps, which may cause intussusception. Extragastrointestinal manifestations include perioral pigmentation (A), perianal pigmentation and subungual pigmentation (B).

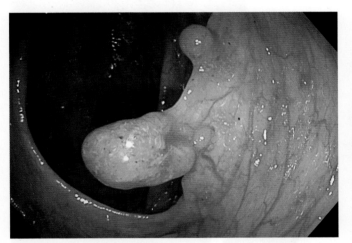

Fig. 5.16 Caecal polyps in Peutz–Jegher syndrome seen at colonoscopy.

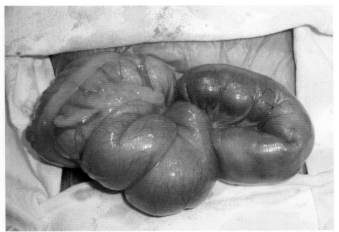

Fig. 5.17 Operative image of small bowel intussusception, in this case caused by a small bowel polyp. After Meckel diverticula, polyps are the commonest pathological lesion causing intussusception.

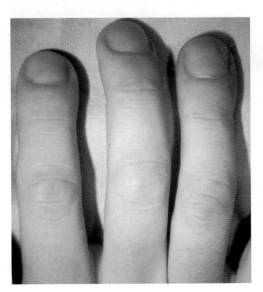

Fig. 5.18 This boy with finger-clubbing had familial adenomatous polyposis and presented with repeated episodes of intussusception and gastrointestinal haemorrhage.

Fig. 5.19 Gardner syndrome (a variant of familial adenomatous polyposis). The epidermoid cysts and sebaceous cysts on the face, scalp and back are characteristic. These children develop adenomatous polyps of the colon, and occasionally of the small intestine, which may intussuscept. Other features include dentigerous cysts, osteomata and desmoid tumours.

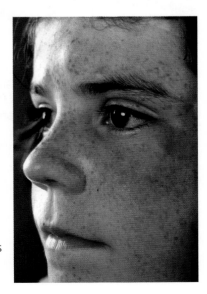

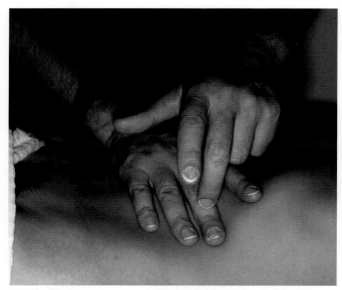

Fig. 5.20 In acute appendicitis, percussion tenderness is the most sensitive way of eliciting peritonism. All areas of the abdomen are percussed in turn. This is a reliable sign in marked contrast to rebound tenderness, which is inappropriate in children.

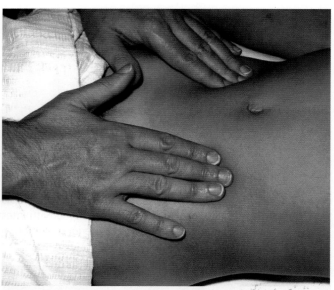

Fig. 5.21 Guarding is demonstrated by assessing the tone of the ventral abdominal wall muscles. It is useful to compare both sides, but this must be done symmetrically, as the tone over the rectus abdominis muscle is greater than lateral to it.

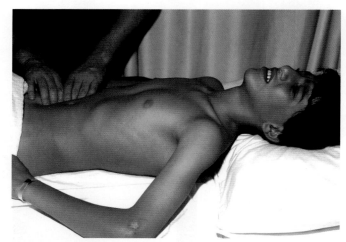

Fig. 5.22 The demonstration of guarding – and the concomitant response in the child's facies – will give clues to the presence of intraperitoneal inflammation.

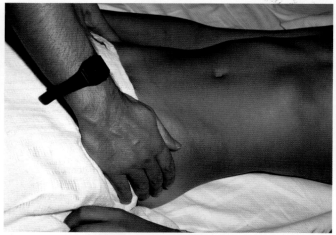

Fig. 5.23 Gently shaking the abdomen by side-to-side rocking of the pelvis (as shown here) or chest will cause the child obvious discomfort when peritonitis is present.

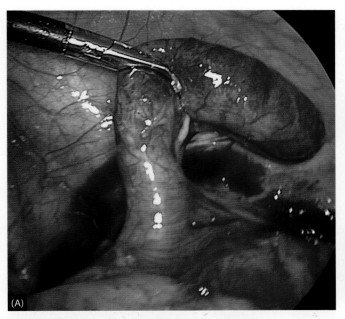

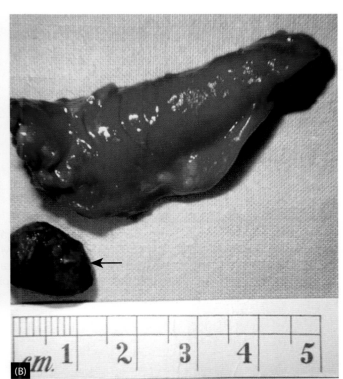

Figs. 5.24A, B (A) Acute appendicitis at laparoscopy.
(B) Appendicitis may develop secondary to the presence of
a faecolith (arrow) obstructing its lumen, as shown in this
appendicectomy specimen.

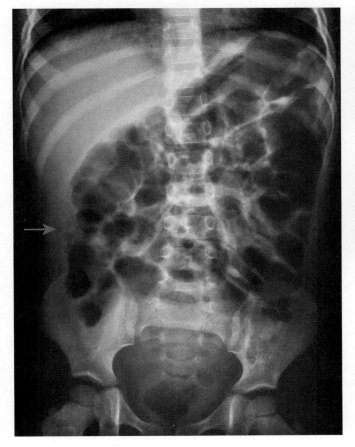

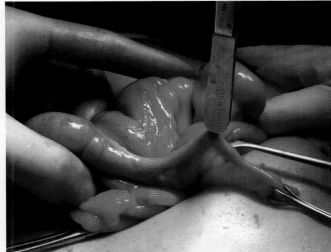

Fig. 5.26 Magnet in appendix.

Fig. 5.25 Plain radiographs of the abdomen are not
normally taken in a child presenting with suspected acute
appendicitis. However, occasionally they will reveal a
calcified faecolith (arrow).

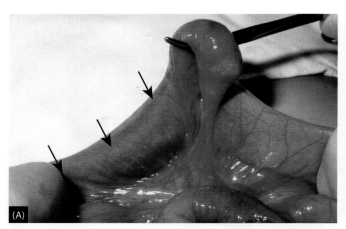
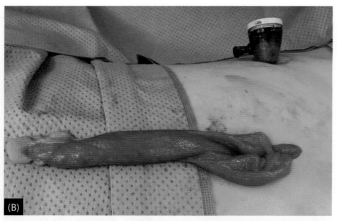

Figs. 5.27A, B (A) A Meckel diverticulum lined with ectopic gastric mucosa may cause ulceration of the adjacent ileum and lead to major gastrointestinal bleeding. This child presented with lethargy, pallor and bright red rectal bleeding. At operation, the blood within the ileum distal to the Meckel diverticulum can be seen by its blue–purple appearance through the bowel (arrows). (B) Meckel diverticulum specimen prior to laparoscopic-assisted excision.

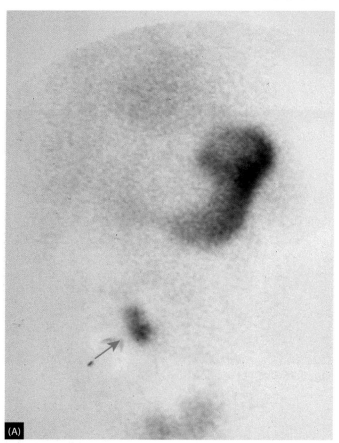
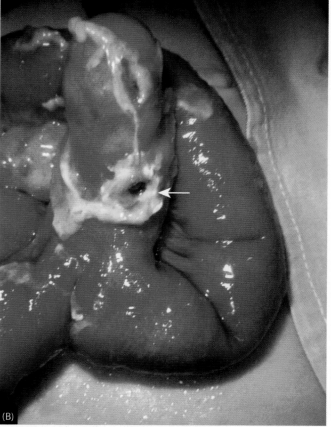

Figs. 5.28A, B (A) A technetium-99m pertechnetate scan, also called a Meckel scan, is used to detect heterotopic gastric mucosa in a Meckel diverticulum in the right lower quadrant (arrow). The normal gastric mucosa is also highlighted by the isotope. (B) A Meckel diverticulum may become inflamed, presenting in a manner similar to appendicitis and peritonitis. This Meckel diverticulum had perforated (arrow), causing peritonitis.

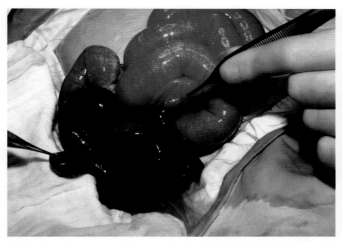

Fig. 5.29 A band may run from a Meckel diverticulum to the underside of the umbilicus. A loop of bowel can twist and become strangulated around this band, which is a remnant of the vitello-intestinal duct. This child had a localised volvulus with gangrene of the bowel secondary to a Meckel band.

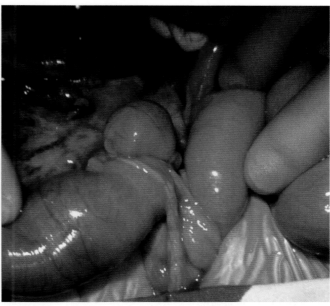

Fig. 5.30 Acute intestinal obstruction secondary to a band adhesion from the greater omentum following an appendicectomy.

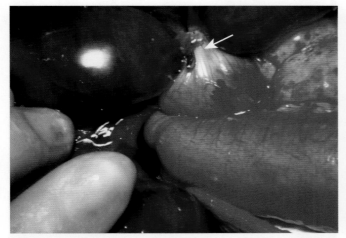

Fig. 5.31 A dense band adhesion (arrow) with a loop of ileum trapped beneath it. The loop of ileum distal to the band is ischaemic.

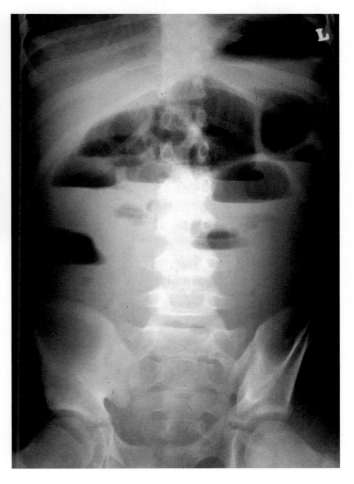

Fig. 5.32 Multiple air-fluid levels in an erect abdominal plain radiograph showing small bowel obstruction secondary to a band adhesion.

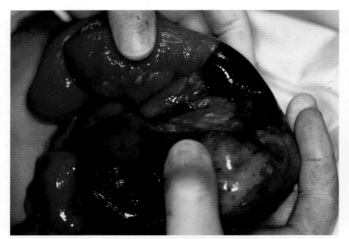

Fig. 5.33 This child presented with features suggestive of appendicitis but with a history of weight loss and general malaise. Clinically, a mass was palpable in the right iliac fossa. At operation, the lesion was identified as a lymphoma of the ileum.

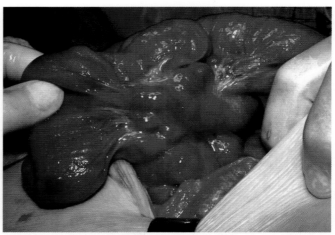

Fig. 5.34 Malignant histiocytosis involving mesenteric lymph nodes in a child who also had a malignant thoracic teratoma and Kleinfelter syndrome.

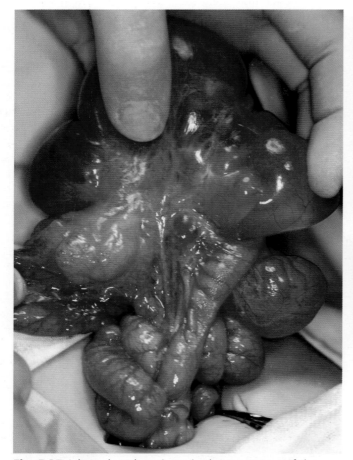

Fig. 5.35 A large lymphangioma in the mesentery of the small bowel.

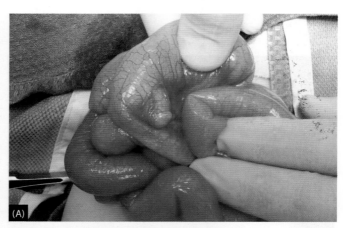

(A)

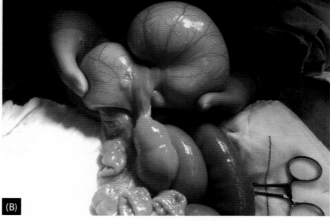

(B)

Figs. 5.36A, B (A) A duplication cyst of the terminal ileum. (B) A large lymphatic malformation causing bowel obstruction, as seen at laparotomy.

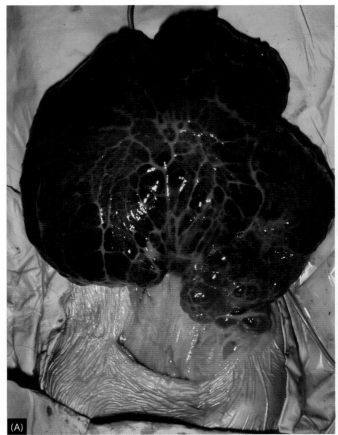

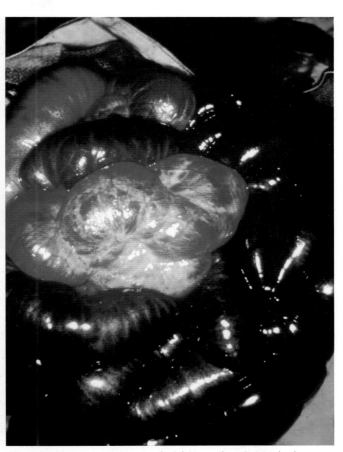

Fig. 5.38 A mesenteric cyst that has undergone volvulus, causing gangrene of much of the small bowel.

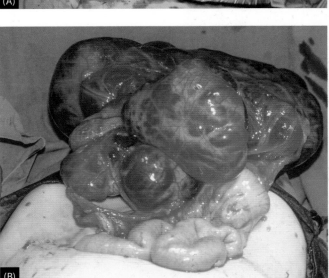

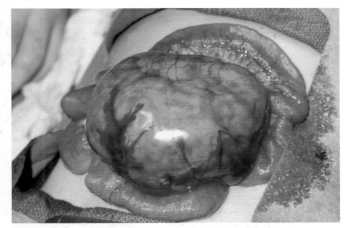

Figs. 5.37A, B (A) A massive omental cyst with secondary haemorrhage and infarction. (B) Another very large omental multiloculated cyst that caused an acute abdomen.

Fig. 5.39 Mesenteric lipoblastoma, which presented as a painless abdominal mass.

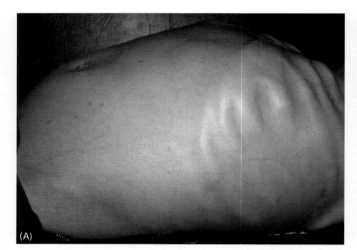

Figs. 5.40A, B Distended abdomen in a child with neurofibromatosis type 1 (NF1) (note the cafe-au-lait spots) who presented with a bowel obstruction from a plexiform neurofibroma affecting the small bowel, as shown in the CT scan (B).

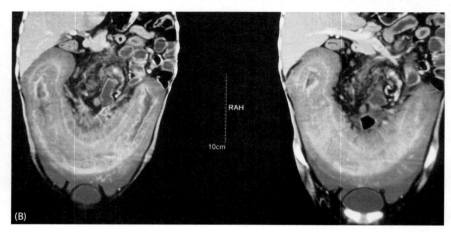

(A)

(B)

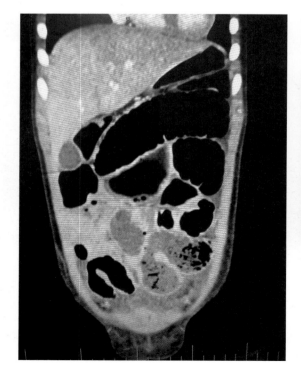

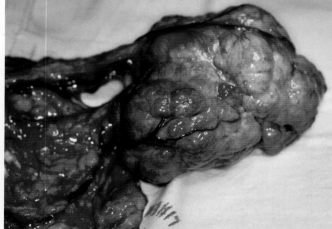

Fig. 5.42 Carcinoid tumour involving the greater omentum.

Fig. 5.41 Primary peritonitis on CT showing dilated bowel and thickening of the bowel wall.

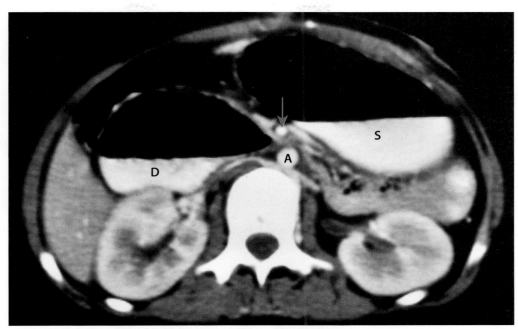

Fig. 5.43 Superior mesenteric artery compression of the duodenum in a 13-year-old girl, shown on CT with intravascular and intraluminal contrast. Note the fluid level in the distended stomach (S) and the proximal duodenum (D) with the third part of the duodenum compressed between the superior mesenteric artery (arrow) and the abdominal aorta (A).

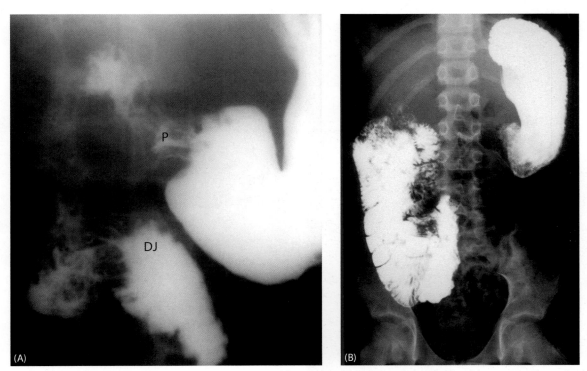

Figs. 5.44A, B (A) Sudden onset of bile-stained vomiting, with or without colicky abdominal pain, suggests intestinal malrotation with volvulus. The diagnosis is confirmed on an upper GI contrast study, which may show complete obstruction of the second part of the duodenum or will reveal that the duodenojejunal (DJ) flexure does not reach the level of the pylorus (P), as shown here. The normal C-shaped curve of the duodenum is lost, and it fails to cross the midline. (B) An upper GI contrast study in an older child with recurrent episodes of vomiting shows intestinal malrotation, with all the small bowel on the right side of the abdomen.

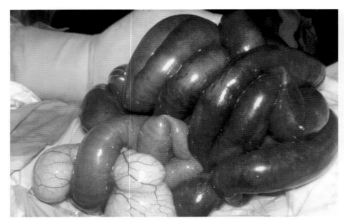

Fig. 5.45 Midgut volvulus complicating intestinal malrotation in older children may present with recurrent episodes of severe colicky abdominal pain, which may or may not be associated with bile-stained vomiting. If untreated, the blood supply to the midgut may be compromised.

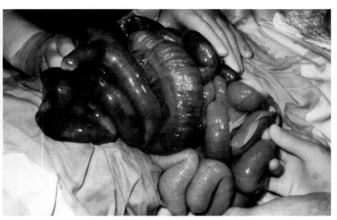

Fig. 5.46 If volvulus of the midgut obstructs the superior mesenteric vessels, gangrene of the small bowel will ensue.

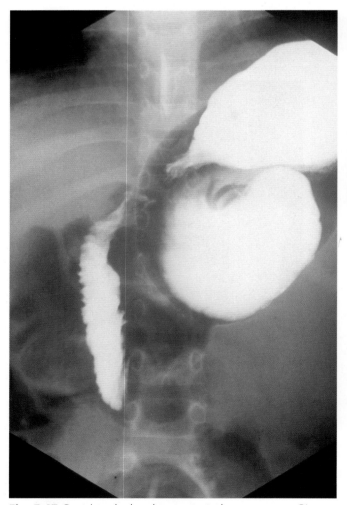

Fig. 5.47 Gastric volvulus demonstrated on an upper GI contrast study.

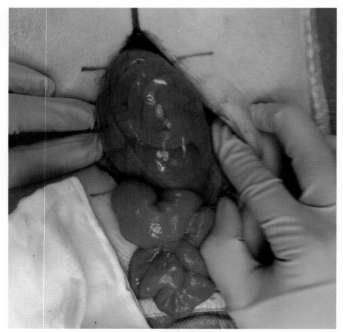

Fig. 5.48 Abdominal cocoon at laparotomy showing bowel encased in a membranous sac. This rare form of encapsulation of small bowel loops by a peritoneal membrane may be congenital or acquired (e.g. abdominal tuberculosis) and can cause a bowel obstruction.

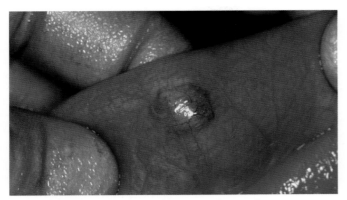

Fig. 5.49 Vascular anomaly of the small bowel.

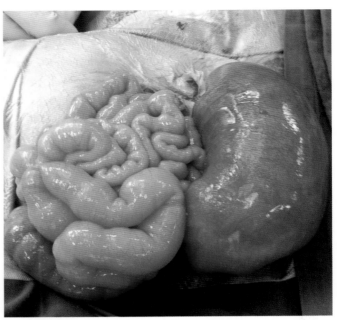

Fig. 5.50 Obstruction of the sigmoid colon in a neonate, showing the massive local dilatation at laparotomy. This could be caused by segmental dilatation of the colon in Hirschsprung disease or anorectal malformation and may lead to local volvulus.

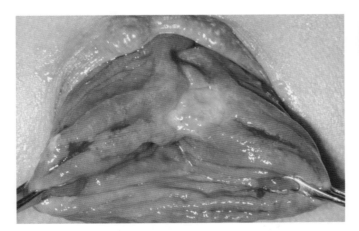

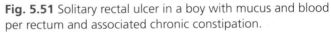

Fig. 5.51 Solitary rectal ulcer in a boy with mucus and blood per rectum and associated chronic constipation.

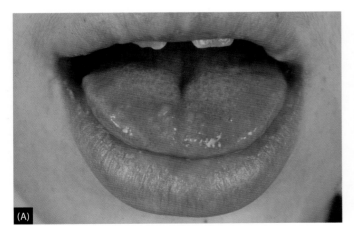

(A)

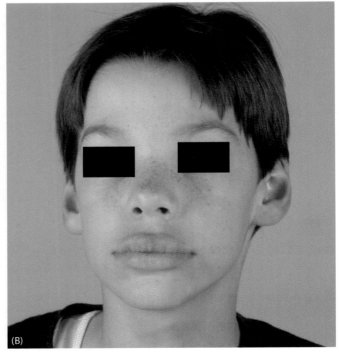

(B)

Figs. 5.52A, B (A) Mucosal neuromas on the tip of the tongue of this 5-year-old girl who presented with severe, chronic constipation. The nodules are pathognomonic for multiple endocrine neoplasia type 2B (MEN2B). (B) Patient with MEN2B and a history of chronic constipation, showing overgrowth of the lips from mucosal neuromas. In addition to colonic dysmotility, affected patients are at a high risk of developing medullary thyroid carcinoma and/or phaeochromocytoma.

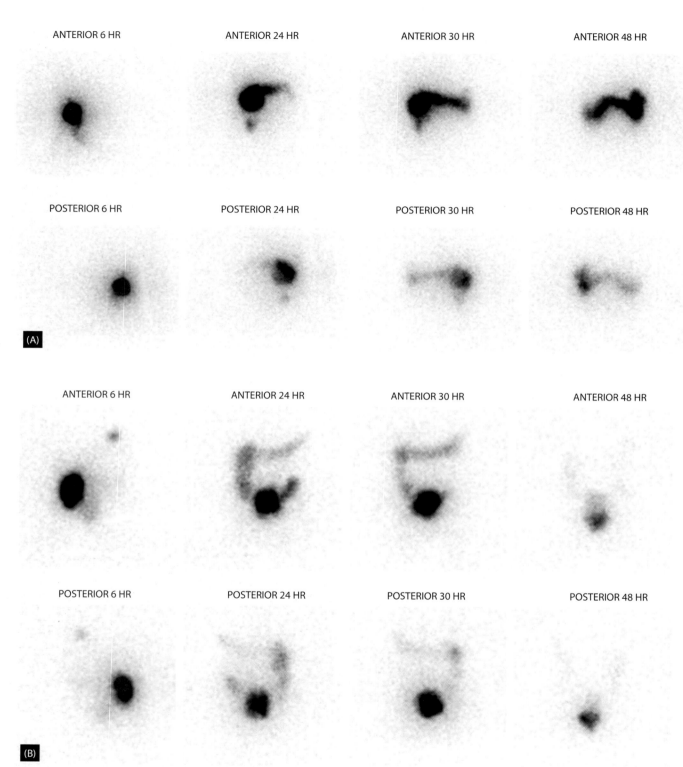

ANTERIOR 6 HR　ANTERIOR 24 HR　ANTERIOR 30 HR　ANTERIOR 48 HR

POSTERIOR 6 HR　POSTERIOR 24 HR　POSTERIOR 30 HR　POSTERIOR 48 HR

(A)

ANTERIOR 6 HR　ANTERIOR 24 HR　ANTERIOR 30 HR　ANTERIOR 48 HR

POSTERIOR 6 HR　POSTERIOR 24 HR　POSTERIOR 30 HR　POSTERIOR 48 HR

(B)

Figs. 5.53A, B (A) Nuclear transit study in a 9-year-old girl with severe, chronic constipation, showing anterior and posterior views at 6, 24, 30 and 48 hours. This study shows slow colonic transit, with tracer just reaching the splenic flexure at 48 hours. Children with this pattern of transit may respond to transcutaneous electrical stimulation. (B) Nuclear transit study in this 5-year-old girl shows paradoxically rapid colonic transit in the colon, with hold up in the rectosigmoid. This child was found to have sugar malabsorption, and responded to an exclusion diet with complete resolution of symptoms.

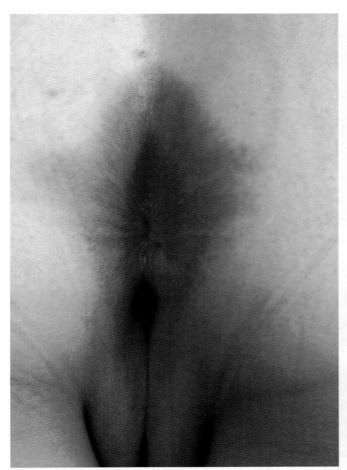

Fig. 5.54 Perianal excoriation secondary to spurious diarrhoea in chronic constipation. A differential diagnosis is perianal streptococcal dermatitis (see **Fig. 5.92**).

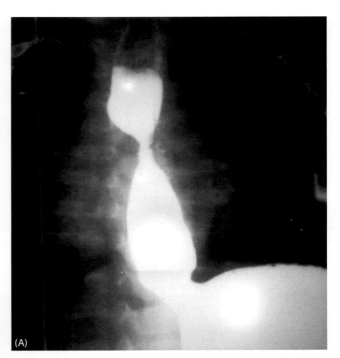

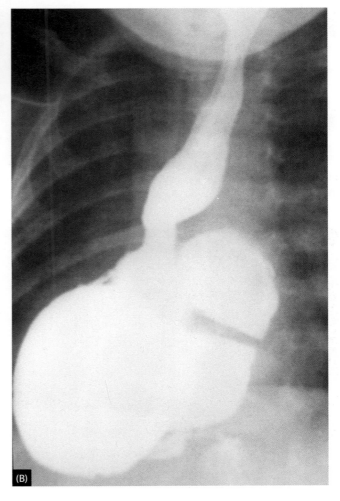

Figs. 5.55A, B (A) Oesophageal (peptic) stricture secondary to chronic reflux oesophagitis from gastro-oesophageal reflux into the lower oesophagus. (B) Congenital para-oesophageal hernia. When large, these are referred to as an intrathoracic stomach and may be associated with a short oesophagus. There is a risk of gastric volvulus.

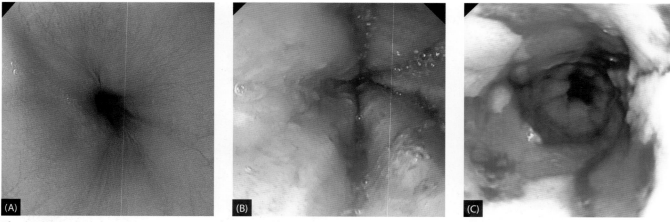

Figs. 5.56A–C Endoscopic appearance of normal distal oesophagus (A), mild reflux oesophagitis (B) and severe reflux oesophagitis with extensive ulceration (C).

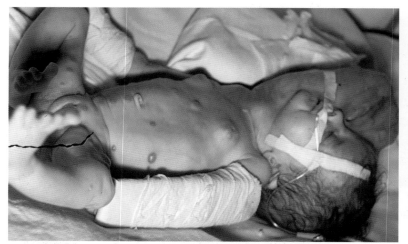

Fig. 5.57 A huge cervical neuroblastoma with multiple skin metastases in an infant.

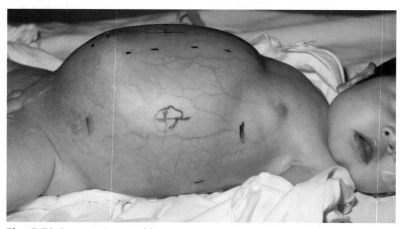

Fig. 5.59 Stage IVS neuroblastoma presenting with a rapidly enlarging abdominal mass.

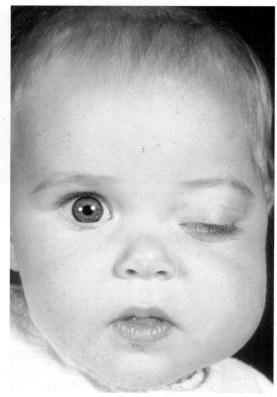

Fig. 5.58 Ptosis of left eyelid and proptosis of the left eye in an infant with an orbital metastasis of neuroblastoma. There is also a metastasis in the left maxilla. Sometimes this is the presentation of the abdominal tumour.

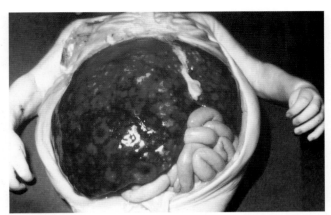

Fig. 5.60 Neuroblastoma metastases in the liver, causing gross hepatomegaly, shown at post-mortem.

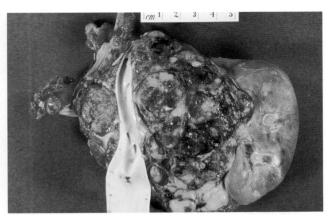

Fig. 5.61 Most neuroblastomas arise from the adrenal gland. In this post-mortem specimen, there is compression of the aorta and infiltration of the kidney from an adrenal neuroblastoma.

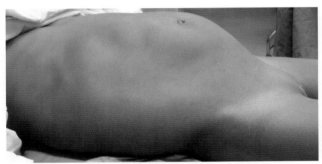

Fig. 5.62 Asymmetrical enlargement of the abdomen caused by a Wilms tumour.

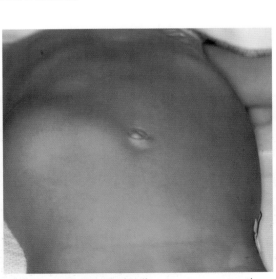

Fig. 5.63 A large right-sided Wilms tumour presenting as an abdominal mass. Clinically, tumours may extend from the costal margin to the iliac fossa. A Wilms tumour most commonly presents as a painless abdominal mass that reaches, but rarely crosses, the midline. Less common presentations include haematuria following minor trauma, hypertension, varicocele and abdominal pain.

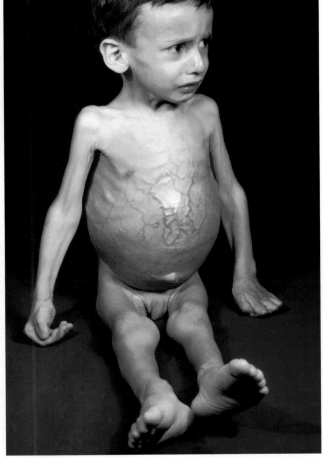

Fig. 5.64 Hepatoblastoma may present as an asymptomatic abdominal mass. This child has had surgery but has ongoing disease with features of weight loss and wasting, and increasing abdominal distension with pain. The prominent superficial abdominal wall veins reflect portosystemic shunting through collateral veins secondary to portal hypertension.

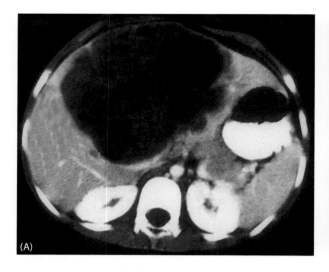

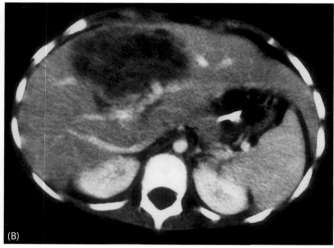

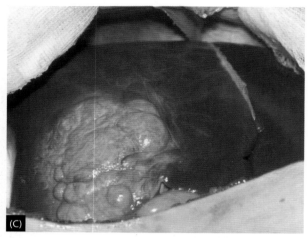

Figs. 5.65A–C (A, B) Abdominal CT scans of a 3-year-old girl with hepatoblastoma: (A) at presentation, (B) after four cycles of neoadjuvant chemotherapy. (C) Operative appearance of a hepatoblastoma in the right lobe of the liver.

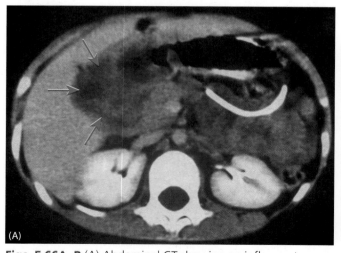

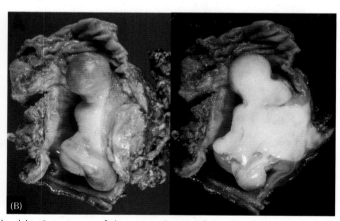

Figs. 5.66A, B (A) Abdominal CT showing an inflammatory myofibroblastic tumour of the second part of the duodenum (arrows). These tumours were previously known as inflammatory pseudotumours. (B, left) The excised duodenal tumour following Whipple pancreaticoduodenectomy. (B, right) The cut surface of the specimen demonstrates the dense fibrous nature of the tumour.

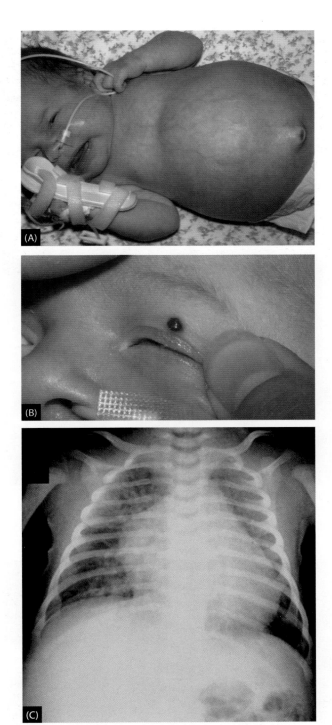

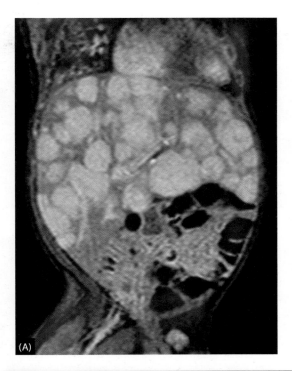

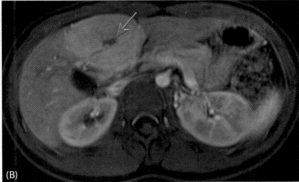

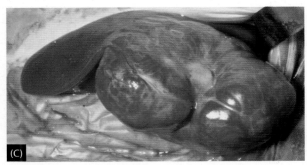

Figs. 5.67A–C (A) An infant with abdominal distension from a diffuse haemangioma of the liver (previously termed hepatic haemangioendothelioma). The lesion was also causing high-output cardiac failure from arteriovenous shunting. Thrombocytopaenia may be present. (B) Same patient: haemangiomas may be present at other sites outside the liver in such children (e.g. cutaneous, as shown, lung and brain). (C) A chest radiograph shows cardiomegaly and pulmonary oedema consistent with high-output cardiac failure. These tumours may respond to treatment with propranolol.

Figs. 5.68A–C (A) An MRI scan after gadolinium contrast showing a diffuse hepatic haemangioma. The hepatic artery is large in such cases because of the massive shunt though the liver. (B) Focal nodular hyperplasia of the liver. These tumours may be asymptomatic or present with pain (and rarely bleeding). They are more common in girls and in paediatric oncology patients. This MRI scan shows a typical central stellate 'scar' (arrow). (C) Operative appearance of focal nodular hyperplasia.

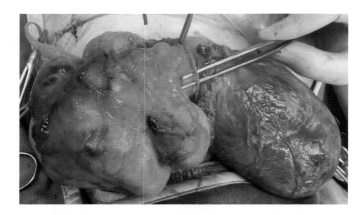

Fig. 5.69 Operative view of a retroperitoneal teratoma with the bile duct draped over the anterior surface of the tumour at surgery.

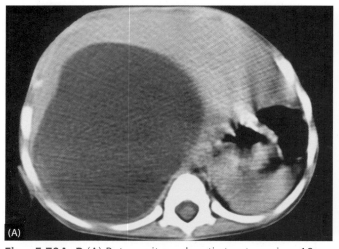

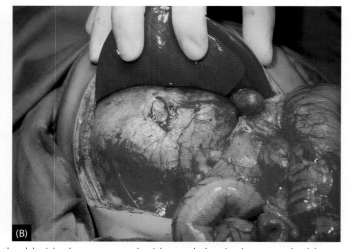

Figs. 5.70A, B (A) Retroperitoneal cystic teratoma in a 10-month-old girl who presented with an abdominal mass palpable below the liver. The large cystic mass was revealed on CT scan. (B) Same patient: at operation, a predominantly cystic retroperitoneal teratoma was identified. The benign lesion was well encapsulated.

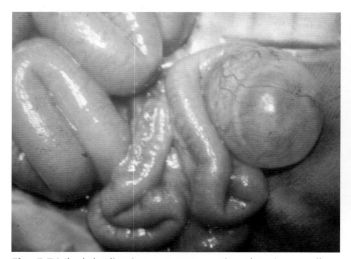

Fig. 5.71 Ileal duplication cyst at operation showing small bowel obstruction with dilated proximal bowel.

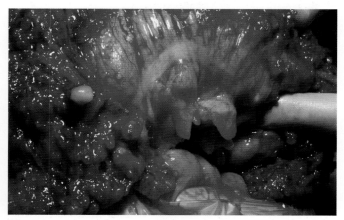

Fig. 5.72 Adenocarcinoma of the colon is extremely rare in childhood. It may be seen in long-standing inflammatory bowel disease and in adenomatous polyposis syndromes. This child presented with a large central abdominal mass and at operation was found to have a massive adenocarcinoma of the transverse colon infiltrating through the wall of the bowel. The prognosis is poor.

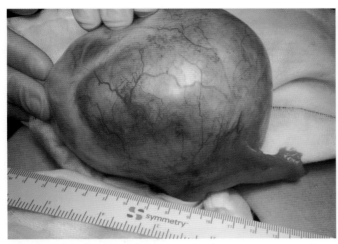

Fig. 5.73 Ovarian teratoma at removal.

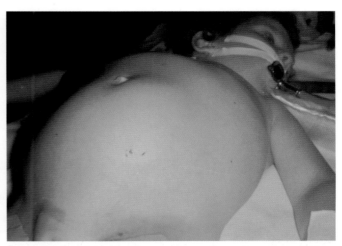

Fig. 5.74 A child with a large retroperitoneal sarcoma that extended from the costal margin to the pelvis.

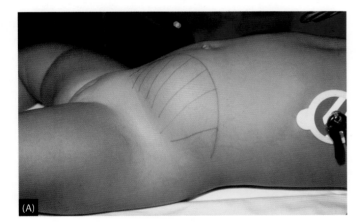

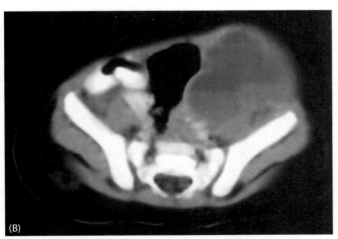

Figs. 5.75A, B (A) Multilocular lymphangioma in the retroperitoneum. This 9-month-old girl presented with a left iliac fossa mass, which was firm but yielding. (B) Same patient: CT scan demonstrating the multiloculated cystic mass in the retroperitoneum.

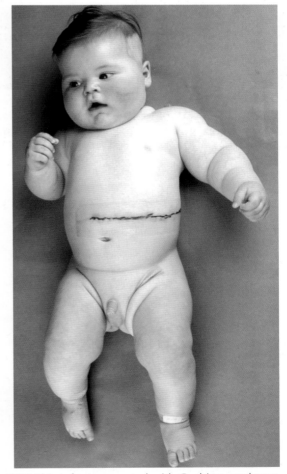

Fig. 5.76 This infant presented with Cushing syndrome (initially not appreciated) and hemihypertrophy of the left upper and lower limbs. Investigation of the hemihypertrophy revealed a left adrenal tumour, which was the cause of the Cushing syndrome.

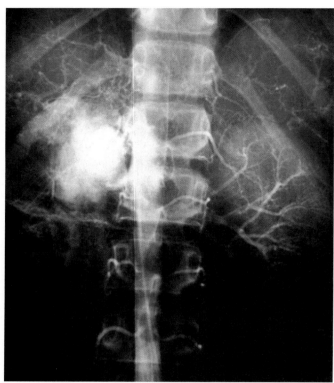

Fig. 5.77 Phaeochromocytoma in an 11-year-old girl who presented with a history of severe headaches and vomiting. She had tachycardia, hypertension, papilloedema and a renal bruit. The angiogram shows a lesion in the right adrenal.

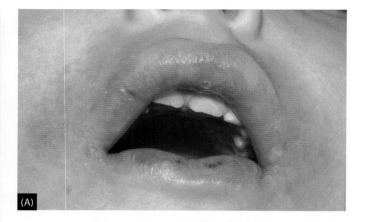

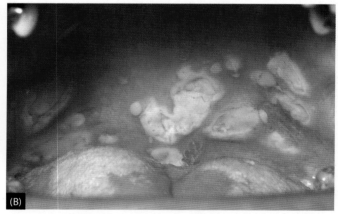

Figs. 5.78A, B (A) Perioral Crohn disease with erythema and oedema of the lips and mild angular cheilitis. (B) Intraoral Crohn disease with palatal and lingual ulceration.

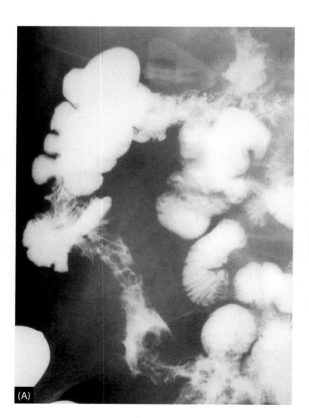

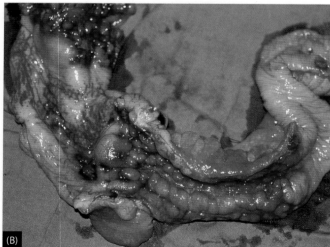

Figs. 5.79A, B (A) Contrast study demonstrating stricturing ileocaecal Crohn disease. (B) Operative specimen of the contrast study showing the pathological correlation. Note the thickened bowel wall and 'cobblestone' appearance of the mucosa, with linear ulceration in the terminal ileum.

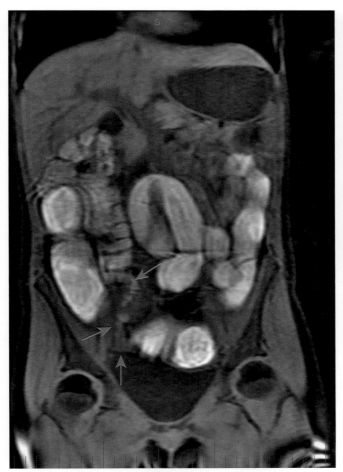

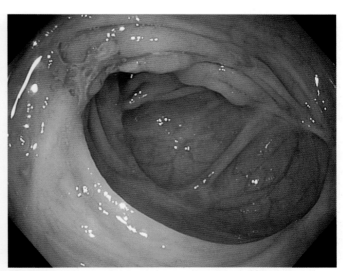

Fig. 5.81 Colonoscopic view of typical Crohn disease ulceration near the ileal papilla. Much of the caecal mucosa appears normal, emphasising the discontinuous nature of the disease.

Fig. 5.80 MR enterography showing a terminal ileal stricture (arrows) from Crohn disease.

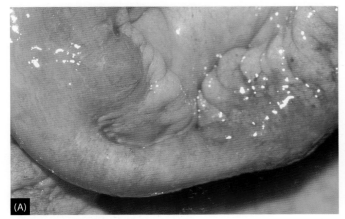

(A)

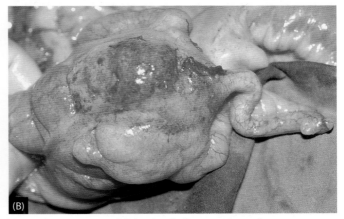

(B)

Figs. 5.82A, B Operative appearance of Crohn disease. (A) Small bowel stricture, and (B) caecal disease. Note the inflammation and creeping mesenteric fat.

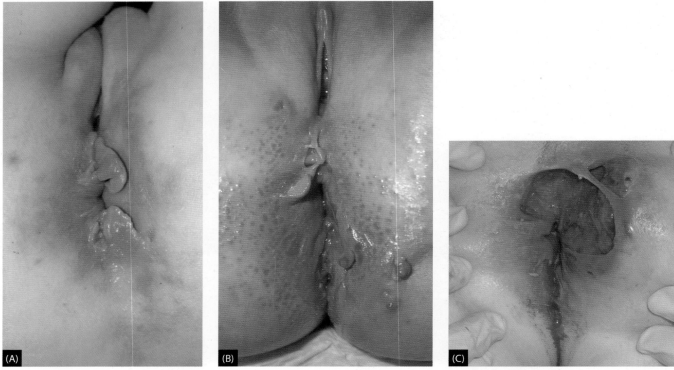

(A) (B) (C)

Figs. 5.83A–C The spectrum of perianal Crohn disease. Perianal disease may precede other manifestations of Crohn disease, but is usually a complication of pre-existing disease. Chronic perianal fissures may be relatively painless and frequently occur laterally as well as in the midline. Fleshy perianal skin tags, ulcers, abscesses and fistulae are other manifestations.

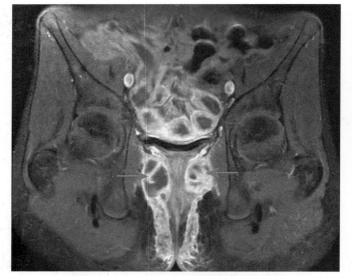

Fig. 5.84 Ischioanal abscess (arrows) in Crohn disease demonstrated on coronal MRI.

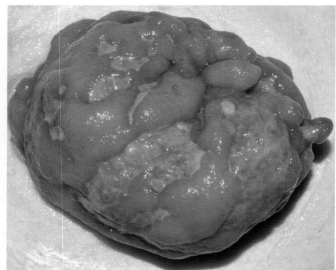

Fig. 5.85 Stomal Crohn disease in a child who had a partial colectomy with colostomy for colonic Crohn disease.

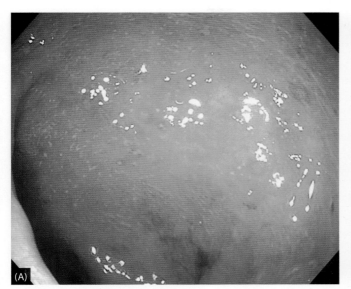 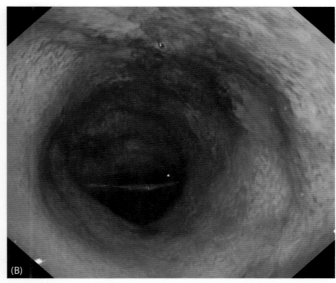

Figs. 5.86A, B Colonoscopic appearances of mild (A) and moderately severe (B) ulcerative colitis. Note the continuous nature of the mucosal disease with an erythematous, granular friable mucosa and loss of the normal mucosal vascular pattern.

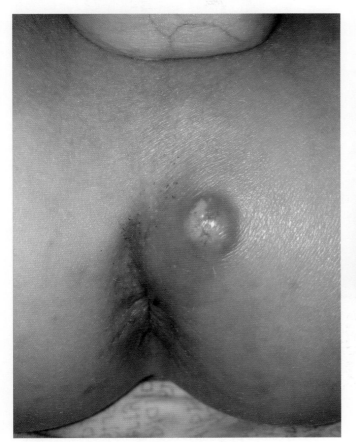

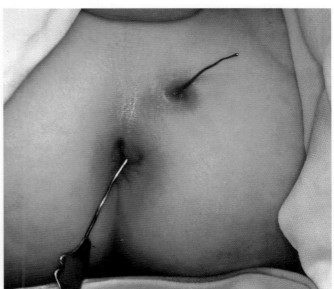

Fig. 5.88 Although a perianal abscess presents superficially, there is usually a fistulous tract connecting it with the anal canal, as shown by this probe.

Fig. 5.87 Perianal abscesses are common during infancy, especially in boys. They present with a small red and tender lump adjacent to the anus. They arise from infection of the anal glands, which open into the crypts of the anal valves.

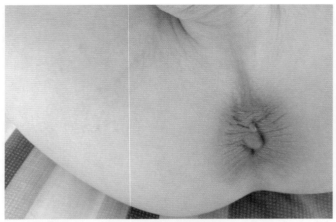

Fig. 5.89 External haemorrhoid with distension of the external haemorrhoidal plexus presenting as a painless blue perianal lump on straining.

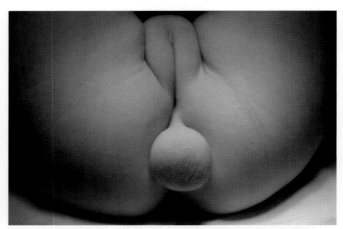

Fig. 5.90 Congenital lipomatous malformation presenting on a stalk arising from the perineal body. These lesions are commonly associated with anorectal malformations.

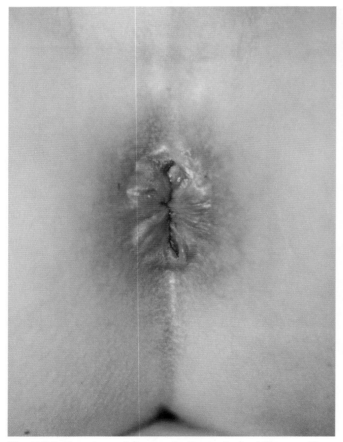

Fig. 5.91 Chronic anal fissures in the typical midline position.

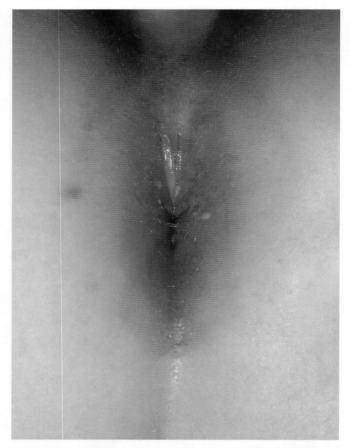

Fig. 5.92 Perianal streptococcal dermatitis is typically bright red and is caused by group A beta-haemolytic streptococci.

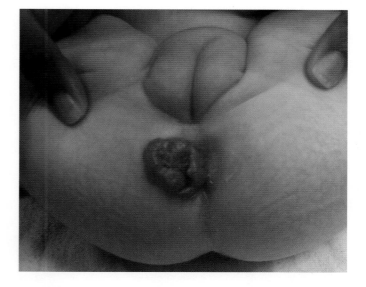

Fig. 5.93 Perianal infantile haemangioma with some secondary ulceration. These lesions should respond to propranolol promoting early regression to avoid bleeding and infection. Other causes of rectal bleeding (e.g. anal fissure, proctocolitis, Meckel diverticulum) are illustrated in other sections.

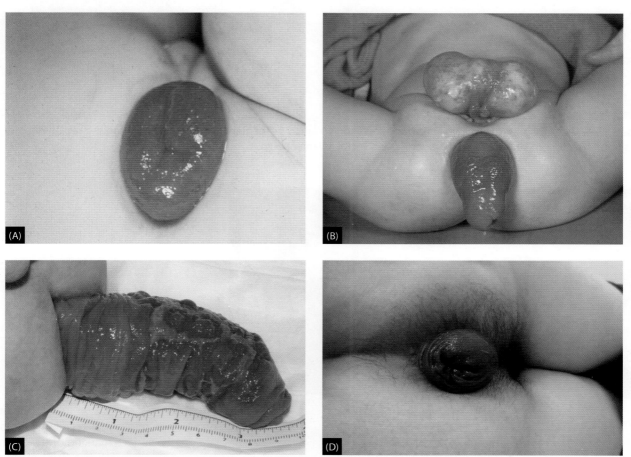

(A)

(B)

(C)

(D)

Figs. 5.94A–D (A) Rectal prolapse showing a doughnut shape when there is a circumferential mucosal prolapse. Rectal prolapse usually occurs in otherwise healthy toddlers. (B) A rectal prolapse is commonly seen in association with bladder exstrophy where it is due to disturbance of the structural support of the rectum. It is also seen in cloacal exstrophy. (C) A full-thickness rectal prolapse with some ulceration of the colon in an infant. A prolapsing intussusception must be considered if the child presents acutely. (D) Rectal prolapse in an older child. The differential diagnosis of the underlying cause includes cystic fibrosis, spina bifida, chronic constipation, post repair of an anorectal malformation or Hirschsprung disease after pull-though and disruption of the anal sphincter after sexual abuse.

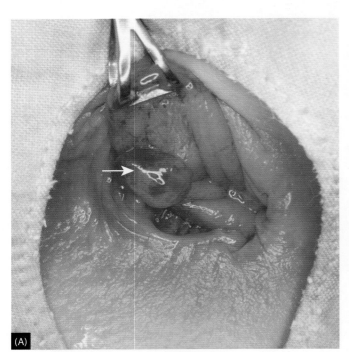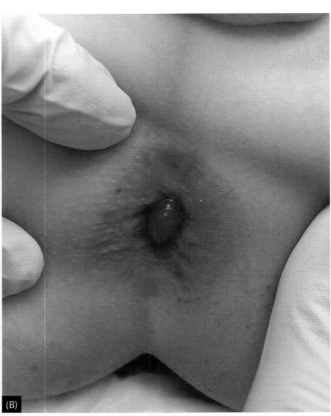

Figs. 5.95A, B (A) The operative appearance of a rectal polyp (arrow). The Babcock forceps delivering the rectal mucosa show the site of attachment of the polyp. (B) A prolapsing rectal juvenile polyp.

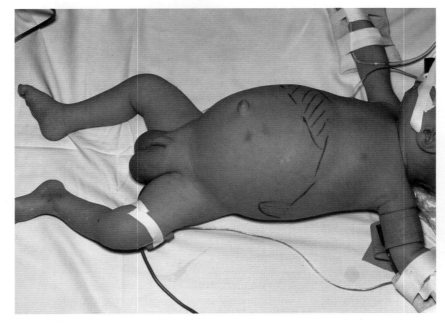

Fig. 5.96 Biliary atresia. In this preoperative photograph of a jaundiced infant with biliary atresia, the surface marking of the enlarged liver and spleen are shown. The enlarged scrotum is common, being secondary to ascitic fluid producing a hydrocele.

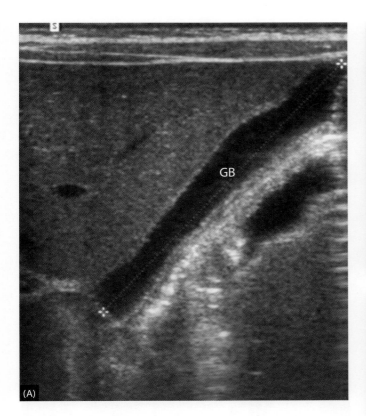

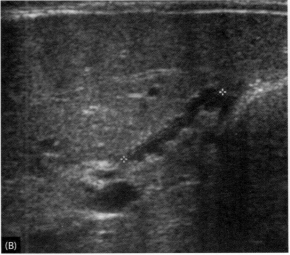

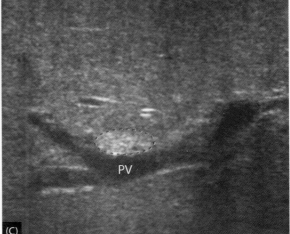

Figs. 5.97A–C Ultrasound features of biliary atresia. (A) Normal gallbladder (GB); (B) small irregular gallbladder in biliary atresia; (C) triangular cord sign at the porta hepatis (dotted oval) representing inflammatory tissue around occluded extrahepatic bile ducts between the bifurcation of the portal vein (PV).

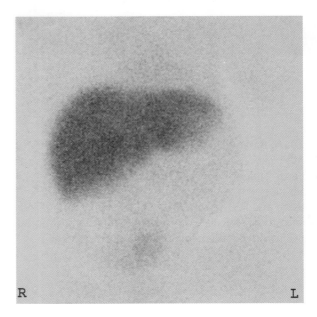

Fig. 5.98 Hepatobiliary iminodiacetic acid (HIDA) scan in biliary atresia. There is no isotope excretion from the liver into the extrahepatic bile ducts and gut.

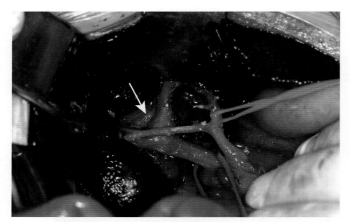

Fig. 5.99 Operative appearance of biliary atresia. The portal vein (blue sling) and hepatic artery (red sling) divide at the porta hepatis (arrow). Note the complete absence of the extrahepatic biliary structures and the dark cholestatic liver.

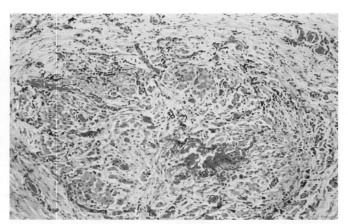

Fig. 5.100 The histological appearance in a cross-section of an atretic gallbladder in biliary atresia. There is evidence of inflammation, with lymphocytes in the wall of the gallbladder and obliteration of its lumen.

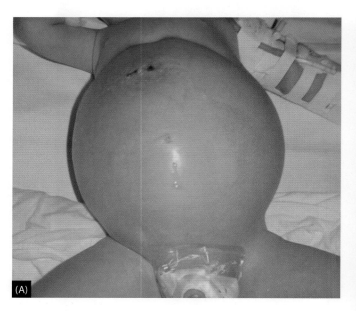

(A)

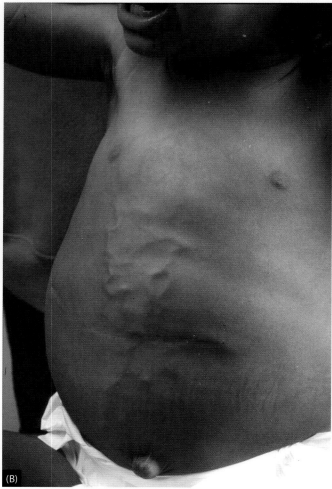

(B)

Figs. 5.101A, B (A) An 11-month-old deeply jaundiced infant with biliary atresia. Massive hepatosplenomegaly and ascites is evident. This child had an unsuccessful Kasai operation. Progressive cirrhosis causes portal hypertension and liver failure. (B) An older child with a failed portoenterostomy for biliary atresia, exhibiting signs of portal hypertension with cutaneous varices and portosystemic shunting.

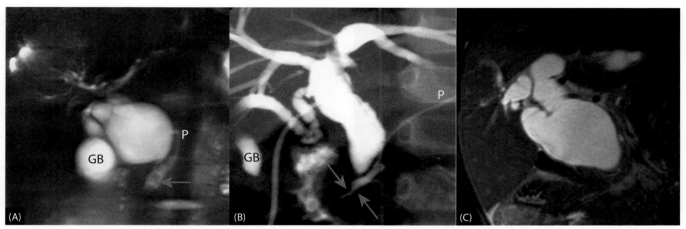

Figs. 5.102A–C Common types of choledochal cyst. (A) MRCP showing type I cyst with a common pancreaticobiliary channel containing debris (arrow). (B) Intraoperative cholangiogram showing type I fusiform cyst with pancreaticobiliary malunion (arrows). (C) MRCP showing a type IVa cyst with segmental extra- and intrahepatic duct dilatations. GB, gallbladder; P, pancreatic duct.

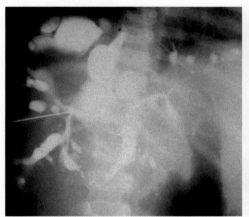

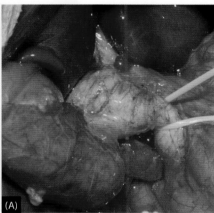

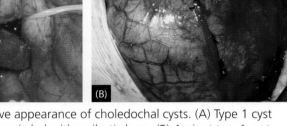

Fig. 5.103 Caroli disease shown on a percutaneous transhepatic cholangiogram. There are multiple saccular dilatations of the intrahepatic bile ducts. When combined with renal anomalies and hepatic fibrosis this is known as Caroli syndrome.

Figs. 5.104A, B Operative appearance of choledochal cysts. (A) Type 1 cyst with the distal segment encircled with a silastic loop. (B) A giant type1 cyst with secondary liver fibrosis.

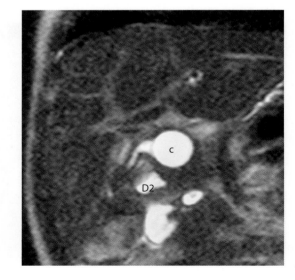

Fig. 5.105 MRCP of an infant with biliary atresia and an extrahepatic biliary cyst (c). There are no dilated intrahepatic ducts. This must not be mistaken for a choledochal cyst or the opportunity of a successful portoenterostomy may be missed. D2, second part of duodenum.

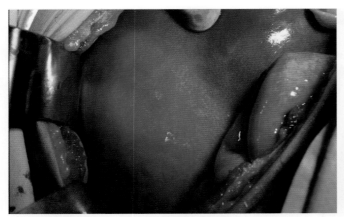

Fig. 5.106 Hydatid cyst in the right lobe of the liver. The operative photograph shows normal liver parenchyma becoming attenuated over the large cyst. The thick white capsule of the hydatid cyst is visible through the parenchyma.

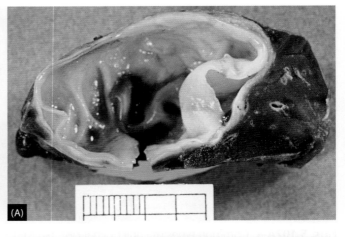

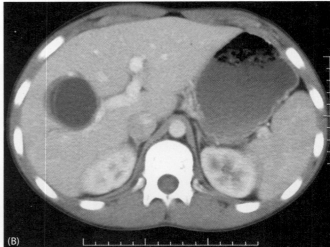

Figs. 5.107A–C (A) Operative specimen of a hydatid cyst within a segment of excised liver. Note the white laminated membrane that surrounds the germinal membrane of the cyst. External to these is the adventitia, which is the secondary fibrous cover that represents the host reaction to the cyst. (B) CT scan of a hydatid cyst in the liver of a 14-year-old boy. (C) The same child had a pulmonary hydatid cyst shown on chest CT.

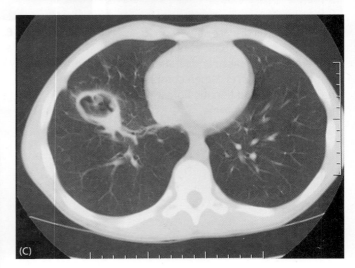

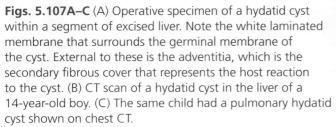

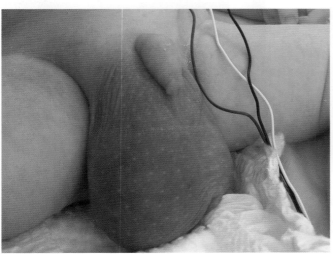

Fig. 5.108 Bile-stained fluid in a hydrocele of an infant with spontaneous biliary perforation.

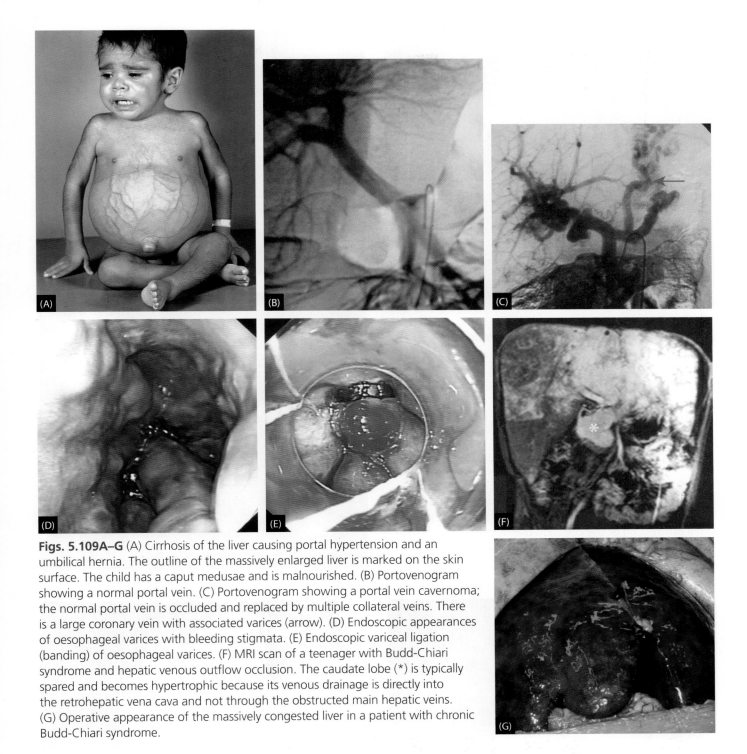

Figs. 5.109A–G (A) Cirrhosis of the liver causing portal hypertension and an umbilical hernia. The outline of the massively enlarged liver is marked on the skin surface. The child has a caput medusae and is malnourished. (B) Portovenogram showing a normal portal vein. (C) Portovenogram showing a portal vein cavernoma; the normal portal vein is occluded and replaced by multiple collateral veins. There is a large coronary vein with associated varices (arrow). (D) Endoscopic appearances of oesophageal varices with bleeding stigmata. (E) Endoscopic variceal ligation (banding) of oesophageal varices. (F) MRI scan of a teenager with Budd-Chiari syndrome and hepatic venous outflow occlusion. The caudate lobe (*) is typically spared and becomes hypertrophic because its venous drainage is directly into the retrohepatic vena cava and not through the obstructed main hepatic veins. (G) Operative appearance of the massively congested liver in a patient with chronic Budd-Chiari syndrome.

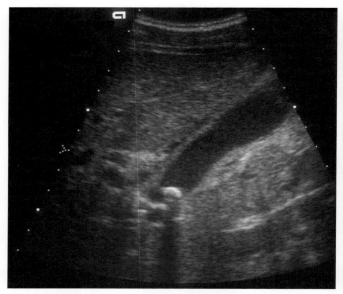

Fig. 5.110 Ultrasound scan showing a gallstone within the gallbladder; the stone casts an acoustic shadow.

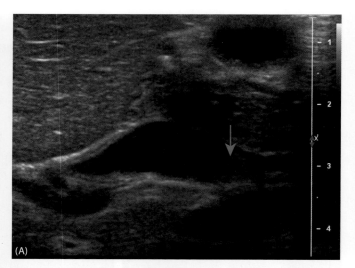

(A)

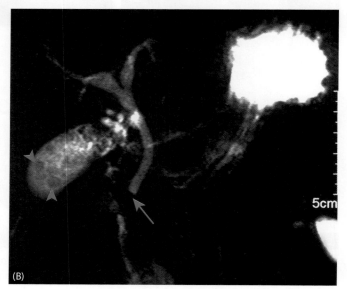

(B)

Figs. 5.111A, B (A) Ultrasound scan showing a sludge ball (arrow) obstructing the common bile duct. (B) MRCP showing multiple gallbladder stones (arrowheads) and distal obstruction of the common bile duct from a gallstone (arrow). This 13-year-old girl presented with gallstone pancreatitis.

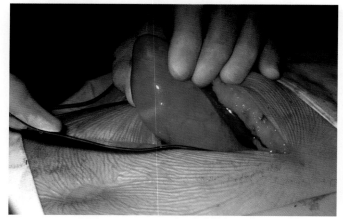

Fig. 5.112 Mucocele of the gallbladder secondary to a cholesterol stone in the cystic duct.

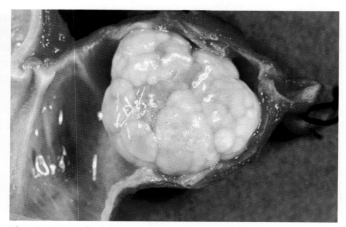

Fig. 5.113 A cholesterol stone in the neck of the gallbladder.

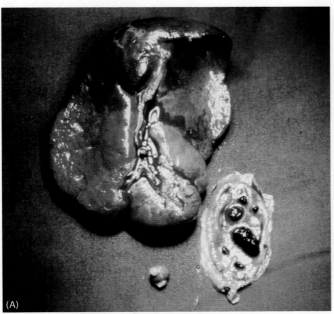

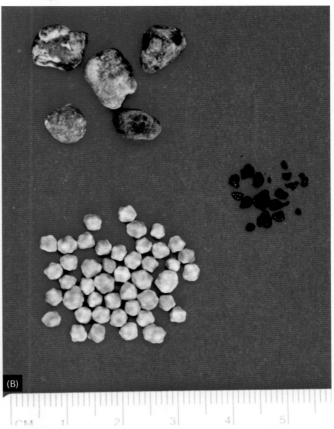

Figs. 5.114A, B (A) Black pigment calculi (calcium bilirubinate) are seen in haemolytic anaemias such as spherocytosis and thalassaemia. This child with splenomegaly and cholelithiasis had pigmented stones within the gallbladder at the time of splenectomy. (B) Common types of gallstones: mixed cholesterol (above), pure cholesterol (below) and black pigment stones.

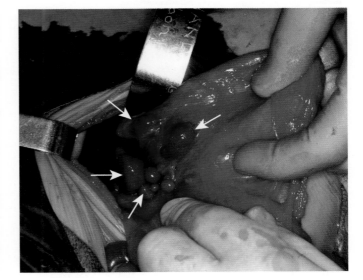

Fig. 5.115 Polysplenia may be associated with cardiac abnormalities, interruption of the inferior vena cava, situs inversus and biliary atresia. Asplenia may be seen in conjunction with complex cardiac abnormalities and situs anomalies or can be isolated; some cases are familial.

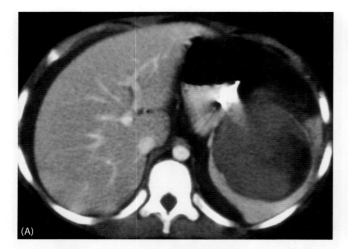

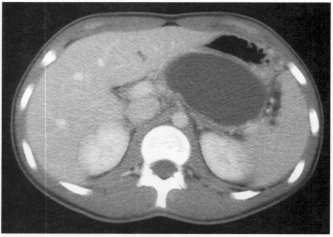

Fig. 5.117 Pancreatic pseudocyst (after traumatic pancreatitis) shown on CT scan. Note that the cyst lies immediately posterior to the stomach.

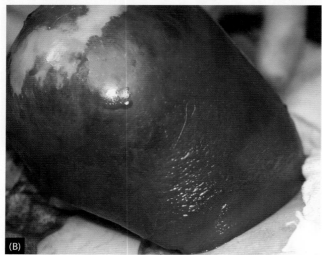

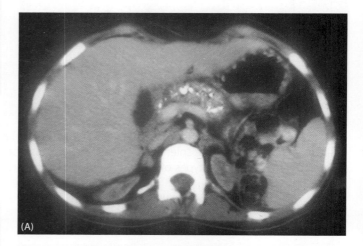

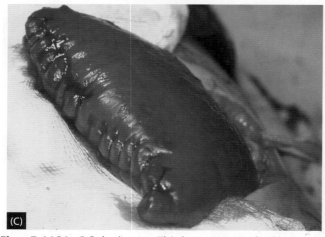

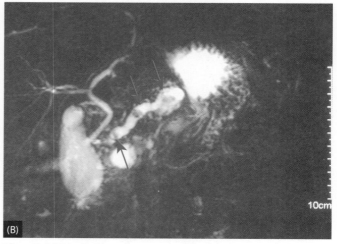

Figs. 5.116A–C Splenic cyst. This boy presented with left upper quadrant pain and a mass. A splenic cyst was identified on ultrasound scan and showed evidence of partial rupture on CT (A). At operation a large splenic cyst was confirmed (B), and completely excised with a partial splenectomy (C). Histology showed a congenital epidermoid cyst. Splenic cysts may be parasitic, congenital or neoplastic.

Figs. 5.118A, B Chronic pancreatitis. (A) CT scan showing pancreatic calcification. (B) MRCP in another patient showing a dilated, irregular pancreatic duct containing calculi (arrows).

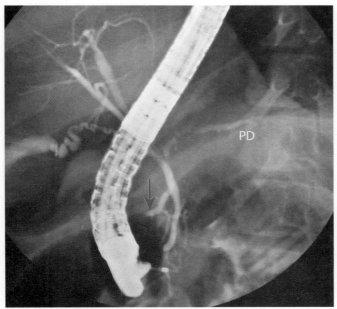

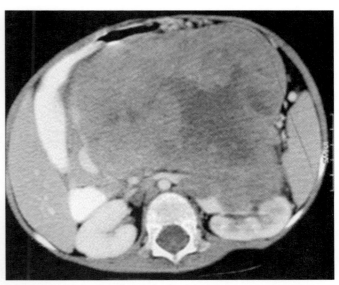

Fig. 5.120 CT scan of a patient with a large pancreatic tumour displacing the stomach. The tumour was a pancreatoblastoma.

Fig. 5.119 Pancreas divisum shown on ERCP. There is a dominant dorsal pancreatic duct (PD) opening into the minor duodenal papilla (arrow).

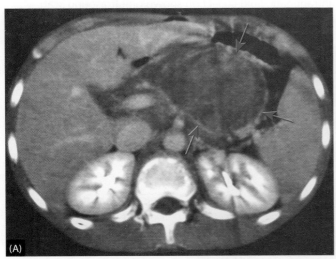

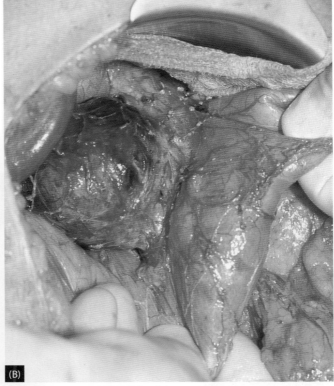

Figs. 5.121A, B Papillary cystic tumour of the pancreas. (A) CT scan of a tumour in the tail of the pancreas (arrows) of a 12-year-old boy presenting with abdominal pain and a mass. (B) Operative appearance of a papillary cystic tumour in the head of the pancreas in a 13-year-old girl; the duodenum has been Kocherised and elevated medially off the tumour.

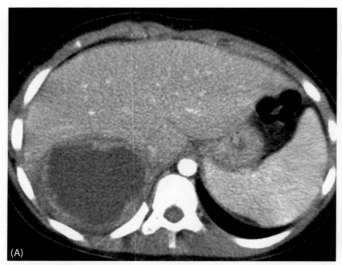 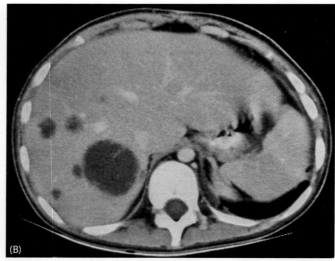

Figs. 5.122A, B Pyogenic liver abscess. (A) CT scan of a primary liver abscess in an 8-year-old boy (*Strep. intermedius*). (B) Multiple pyogenic abscesses in a 9-year-old girl with acute appendicitis complicated by portal pyaemia.

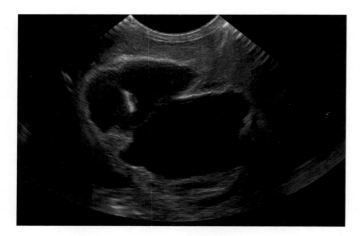

Fig. 5.123 Neonatal total parenteral nutrition (TPN) intrahepatic fluid collection shown on ultrasound scan.

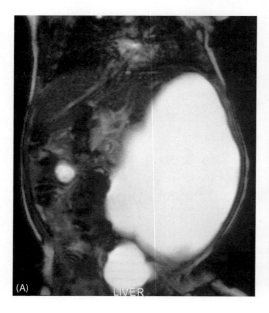 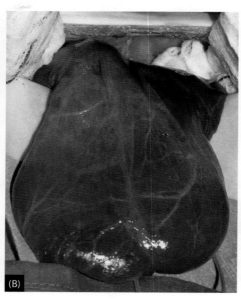

Figs. 5.124A, B 'Simple' liver cyst in an infant with abdominal distension and associated respiratory and gastrointestinal symptoms. (A) MRI scan. (B) Operative appearance at resection (after partial decompression).

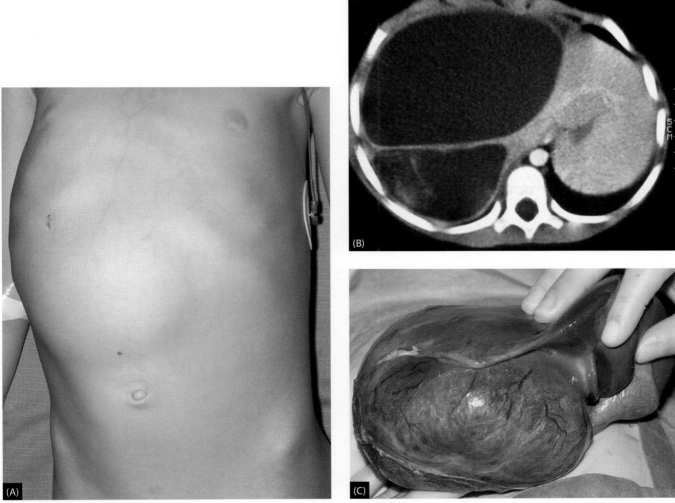

Figs. 5.125A–C Mesenchymal hamartoma of the liver. (A) This girl presented with an abdominal mass. (B) CT of same patient. (C) Operative appearance of the tumour in another child. Mesenchymal hamartomas typically present as a large multicystic liver mass.

The abdominal wall and inguinoscrotal conditions | CHAPTER 6

THE UMBILICUS

Before birth, the umbilical ring is a normal opening in the ventral abdominal wall at the site of attachment of the umbilical cord to the fetus. Early in development, the midgut communicates with the yolk sac via the vitelline duct (yolk stalk) but this normally involutes by birth. Persistence of part or all of the vitelline duct produces a variety of conditions, including Meckel diverticulum, ectopic mucosa at the umbilicus and patency of the vitello-intestinal duct. The urachus connects the bladder to the allantois in the umbilical cord. Failure of the urachus to obliterate results in urinary discharge from the umbilicus or a urachal sinus or cyst. At the time of birth, the main structures passing through the umbilical ring are the two umbilical arteries and the umbilical vein. After birth, the umbilical stump desiccates and separates from the umbilicus, leaving a dry corrugated dimple. Failure of contraction of the umbilical ring in the first few weeks after birth may lead to an umbilical hernia, in which peritoneum protrudes into the skin-covered defect. Some degree of umbilical herniation is present in about 20% of newborn babies, and is even more common in the premature. When the infant lies quietly, the umbilical skin looks redundant, but on crying or straining, bowel fills the hernia, giving the umbilicus a tense and slightly blue appearance beneath the shiny skin; however, it is non-tender and reduces easily. The vast majority of umbilical hernias close spontaneously in the first few years of life. The skin overlying the hernia never ruptures and strangulation of the contents is exceptionally rare.

The umbilicus should be dry within days of separation of the umbilical cord stump. If it remains moist and there is an ongoing weeping discharge from granulation tissue at its base, an umbilical granuloma should be suspected. A diagnosis of umbilical granuloma should be made only after careful examination has shown no evidence of a sinus or fistula opening and if no urine, air or faecal discharge has been observed issuing from it. An umbilical granuloma becomes apparent in the first month or two of life, whereas sinuses and cysts of urachal or vitelline origin may present at a later date. Clinically, an umbilical granuloma can be difficult to distinguish from a sequestered island of intestinal mucosa, which discharges mucus. The ectopic tissue appears as a small, red, shiny moist lesion at the base of the umbilical cicatrix.

Faeces and air discharging from the umbilicus is diagnostic of a patent vitello-intestinal duct (omphalomesenteric duct).

There is a small opening in the umbilicus, into which a fine feeding tube may be passed to demonstrate the communication with the ileum. A broader vitello-intestinal duct may allow prolapse of ileum, producing a double-horned protrusion, unless there is an associated atresia, in which case the protrusion will be single-horned.

Urine may drain from the umbilicus through a patent urachus. If the urine is infected, it may be difficult to distinguish from faecal fluid. Again, a sinus opening will be evident. Patency of the urachus may occur in association with obstruction of urinary outflow from the bladder (e.g. posterior urethral valve) or an anorectal malformation. Injection of contrast material into the opening and/or an ultrasound scan will delineate the anatomy.

THE PENIS

The penis and its foreskin are common causes of trouble and concern in boys. The normal foreskin protrudes beyond the glans penis, and its inner surface is adherent to the glans for a variable period in childhood. Beneath this adherence, particularly in the region of the coronal groove, secretions and desquamation of keratin can accumulate as deposits of smegma. These deposits have a creamy or bright yellow appearance through the skin and, until separation of the adherent foreskin provides a communication with the outside, they remain sterile and cause no inflammation. Smegma itself requires no treatment, but is often mistaken for pathology.

The penis may become red, swollen and painful, secondary to balanoposthitis (often simply called 'balanitis'). This is a superficial infection of the foreskin, and is often due to infected pooled urine or partially expelled smegma between the glans and foreskin. The infection can produce rapid swelling. Occasionally, painless penile swelling may be part of idiopathic scrotal oedema.

Phimosis

Phimosis is stenosis of the preputial orifice. Mild phimosis causes no symptoms, but in severe phimosis it is impossible to retract the foreskin behind the glans penis. There may be a history of marked ballooning of the foreskin, which persists after micturition has ceased, and scarring of the foreskin may reduce the opening to a pin-hole. The scar appears as pale, unyielding tissue, which may split and fissure on attempted retraction. Phimosis occurs from tearing of the foreskin during overzealous retraction, ammoniacal dermatitis producing recurrent or chronic inflammation, or from infection under the foreskin (balanoposthitis).

Paraphimosis

Paraphimosis occurs in older children who have a mild degree of phimosis. The foreskin has been retracted proximal to the coronal groove and cannot be returned to its former position. Compression of the shaft of the penis at the coronal groove causes venous obstruction of the glans penis and leads to engorgement and oedema of both the glans and foreskin. The foreskin appears as a pale and eccentric 'tyre'. Prompt diagnosis is important, since delay allows progression of the oedema and makes subsequent reduction more difficult.

Hypospadias

Hypospadias is caused by incomplete formation of the urethra and its adjacent structures in the male. The urethral orifice is proximal to its normal position and may be situated anywhere on the ventral surface of the penis in the midline, as far proximal as the scrotum. Chordee, or ventral bending of the shaft of the penis, is present in almost all boys with hypospadias; the deficient periurethral tissue effectively shortens its ventral length. Chordee can be demonstrated either by pulling the dorsal hood upwards or by pulling the side of the skin of the shaft downwards. The degree of chordee, which is best assessed from the side, tends to become worse with growth of the penis. The foreskin is deficient ventrally, producing a dorsal 'hood', and the median raphe is often deviated or abnormal in its formation. In the most common variant of hypospadias, the urethral orifice is near the corona. Often there are several pit-like openings distal to the ventral urethral meatus, which itself can be demonstrated by pulling the meatal skin away from the shaft, thus opening up the meatus. Immediately proximal to the orifice the skin is thin and the adjacent tissues deficient. Where there is severe hypospadias with marked chordee and a urethral meatus on the scrotum or at the penoscrotal junction, the possibility of other urinary tract abnormalities and defective sexual differentiation must be considered. Similarly, the presence and location of testes in patients with severe hypospadias must be determined, so that disorders of sex development, particularly congenital adrenal hyperplasia, can be excluded.

Chordee can occur in the absence of a proximal urethral orifice, a condition sometimes called 'hypospadie sans hypospadie'. In epispadias, the urethral meatus opens on the dorsal surface of the penis. In many ways this condition is best considered a minor form of bladder exstrophy.

Miscellaneous conditions of the penis

A wide variety of rare abnormalities of the penis may occur.

THE 'ACUTELY PAINFUL SCROTUM'

An 'acutely painful scrotum' is where the contents of the scrotum are acutely painful and swollen or there are other signs of inflammation. Torsion of a testicular appendage and torsion of the testis itself account for the majority of cases in children. Idiopathic scrotal oedema and epididymo-orchitis are seen only occasionally (*Table 6.1*).

The incidence of testicular torsion peaks at two ages: first, in the perinatal period, when the whole tunica and its contents twist ('extravaginal torsion'); and secondly, shortly before or at puberty, when the enlarging testis can twist on its long mesorchium ('intravaginal torsion'). Torsion of the testis needs to be recognised early, so that immediate operative intervention can salvage the testis before it becomes infarcted. Perinatal torsion with infarction is one cause of a vanishing testis.

Torsion of an appendage (e.g. 'hydatid of Morgagni') in the 10–12-year-old prepubertal boy is more common than torsion of the testis. The boy complains of severe pain in the scrotum or the ipsilateral iliac fossa. In its early stages, a testicular appendage may be visible as a blue–black spot beneath the skin of the scrotum near the upper pole of the testis. It is extremely painful, whereas the testis itself is non-tender. The epididymis feels normal and is not enlarged. Subsequently, a reactive hydrocele develops and the whole scrotum becomes tender to palpation, oedematous and red. When this occurs, it may be difficult to distinguish it clinically from torsion of the testis. In the latter, the testis and epididymis are both exquisitely tender, but may be partially obscured by the overlying scrotal oedema and the reactive hydrocele. Once the scrotal tissues become indurated, complete infarction of the testis has almost certainly occurred. The testis that has undergone torsion may assume a location high in the scrotum, secondary to the shortening effect of torsion on the intravaginal length of the spermatic cord.

Epididymitis or epididymo-orchitis in the paediatric age group usually occurs secondary to an abnormality of the urinary tract (especially in the first 6 months of life) or after urethral instrumentation, trauma or surgery. In some patients, no cause is found and a viral aetiology is presumed. In adolescent boys a sexually transmitted infection may be the cause. Epididymo-orchitis occurring in infancy suggests a urinary tract abnormality, for which a micturating cystourethrogram and renal ultrasound scan should be performed after the

TABLE 6.1 Causes of the acute scrotum in children	
Condition	**Frequency**
Torsion of a testicular appendage	>60%
Torsion of the testis	<30%
Idiopathic scrotal oedema	<10%
Epididymitis	<10%

epididymitis has subsided and any co-existing urinary tract infection treated. Mumps orchitis is extremely rare prior to puberty. Infiltration of the testis is also uncommon, but may be seen in leukaemia or with a primary neoplasm (e.g. germ cell tumour) or a benign tumour of the interstitial cells of Leydig. Paratesticular rhabdomyosarcoma is an important differential diagnosis.

Idiopathic scrotal oedema produces a scrotum that rapidly becomes puffy with oedema that spreads into the inguinal region, the penis (including the foreskin) and on to the perineum. The swelling often involves both halves of the scrotum. The discomfort is slight and on palpation there is no tenderness of the testes. There may be localised erythema and a pale pink discolouration of the inguinal region on one side. The condition most often affects boys under 10 years of age.

HERNIAS AND HYDROCELES

During the seventh month *in utero,* the testis descends into the scrotum along with a tube of peritoneum, the processus vaginalis. Shortly before birth the latter begins to obliterate, leaving only the tunica vaginalis surrounding the testis. Hernia, hydrocele and encysted hydrocele of the cord result from failure of complete obliteration of the processus vaginalis.

An indirect inguinal hernia occurs when there is wide patency of the processus vaginalis in continuity with the abdominal cavity. A hydrocele occurs where the processus remains narrowly patent, such that only peritoneal fluid can trickle through the communication and collect in the tunica vaginalis. An encysted hydrocele of the cord develops when the peritoneal fluid drains into a loculus of expanded processus vaginalis at some point along its course in the spermatic cord. Combined abnormalities of the three may occur also. These abnormalities are seen more frequently on the right side, perhaps because the right testis descends later than the left. The higher incidence in premature babies is caused by delivery either very soon after the testes have descended or even before descent. The higher post-partum intra-abdominal pressures make it more difficult for spontaneous closure of the processus vaginalis to occur.

An inguinal hernia becomes noticeable when it contains bowel (or in the female, an ovary). The parent may report an intermittent swelling overlying the child's external ring, often during crying or straining. The groin lump disappears spontaneously as the hernial contents return to the peritoneal cavity. There is little pain or discomfort, except when the bowel becomes stuck in the sac (incarceration). Strangulation of an inguinal hernia is a complication that is seen frequently in infancy, but is somewhat less common in older children. The infant cries in pain and a tense, tender swelling over the external inguinal ring is evident. If unrecognised and untreated, generalised colicky abdominal pain with vomiting and abdominal distension will develop. Rarely, there may be redness and induration overlying the lump or signs of peritonitis, both of which are suggestive of ischaemia of the entrapped bowel (strangulation). A strangulated inguinal hernia needs to be distinguished from an encysted hydrocele of the cord (which may also appear suddenly) and an undescended testis. An encysted hydrocele is non-tender and the cyst moves readily in line with the spermatic cord. Abdominal features are absent. A strangulated hernia may occur in conjunction with an undescended testis. Inguinal lymphadenitis and a local inguinal abscess can be distinguished by their exact location in most cases, but occasionally an ultrasound scan and/or surgical exploration may be warranted to clarify the diagnosis.

Several features of a hydrocele distinguish it from a hernia: the swelling involves the scrotum alone and the normal narrow spermatic cord can be identified above the swelling ('you can get above it').

UNDESCENDED TESTIS

An undescended testis is one that cannot be made to reach the bottom of the scrotum. Most undescended testes have no primary abnormality, but may become secondarily dysplastic if they are allowed to remain outside the scrotum. In the vast majority, the cause of maldescent is unknown.

A true undescended testis has to be distinguished from a retractile testis. A retractile testis is one that can be manipulated to the bottom of the scrotum and remains in the scrotum after manipulation. The retractile testis resides spontaneously in the scrotum, at least some of the time, and should be normal in size. All prepubertal boys have some degree of retractility of their testes. The position of their testes is controlled by the cremaster muscle, which is capable of retracting the testis out of the scrotum. Cremasteric retraction is not seen in the first few months of life, and is maximal at between 2 and 8 years.

Examination of a child with suspected undescended testes is performed with the child lying supine and comfortable. If the testes are not seen in the region of the scrotum, their location can be determined by first placing the flat of the hand over the inguinal pouch. The testis is felt as a mobile, ovoid structure between the subcutaneous fat and the abdominal wall muscles. Once the testis is located, it is manipulated towards the scrotum. The fingers of one hand are pressed firmly against the abdominal wall lateral to the known position of the testis, and the testis is 'milked' towards the scrotum where the fingers of the opposite hand can snare it through the thin scrotal skin. The testis can then be pulled down towards the normal scrotal position and an estimate made of the degree of descent achieved. A child with cryptorchidism may have a testis that is small, ill-formed and relatively immobile on a short spermatic cord, which prevents it from reaching the bottom of the scrotum. Most undescended testes are located near the external inguinal ring, although others may reside at a higher level in the inguinal canal. Some of these can be manipulated through the external ring, but when palpation ceases they return to an impalpable position. The testis may remain completely impalpable despite manipulation if it is residing at a higher level within the inguinal canal or is intra-abdominal. Less commonly, a testis may be absent or ectopic.

VARICOCELE

A varicocele is enlargement of the veins of the pampiniform plexus in the spermatic cord, and almost always involves the left side and develops around the time of puberty. There may be little abnormality to observe when the adolescent is supine apart from an asymmetrical scrotum (with the left side redundant), but on standing the veins fill and become visible, and feel like 'a bag of worms'. A small secondary hydrocele may be observed. Varicoceles are usually symptomless, although some boys complain of a dragging ache or discomfort in the groin. If untreated, the left testis may not grow as much as the right testis at puberty, a reflection of the effect on spermatogenesis of unilateral warming of the testis by the surrounding veins. Uncommonly, a varicocele may develop from obstruction of one of the renal veins by a renal or perirenal tumour, of which Wilms tumour and neuroblastoma are the most common. Because the left testicular vein drains directly into the left renal vein, this sign is seen almost always on the left side. Consequently, an underlying cause must be suspected in a boy under 6 years of age who develops a varicocele; the tumour will usually be palpable as an abdominal mass.

SACROCOCCYGEAL TERATOMA

Most sacrococcygeal teratomas are strikingly obvious at birth. A few, however, are less obvious, particularly if they are largely intrapelvic and have few manifestations: these tend to present later in childhood.

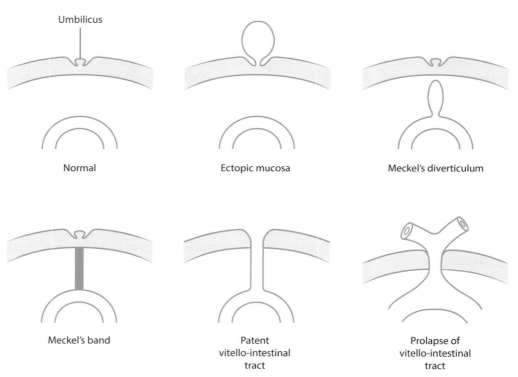

Fig. 6.1 A schematic representation of a variety of abnormalities produced by persistence of part or all of the vitello-intestinal duct.

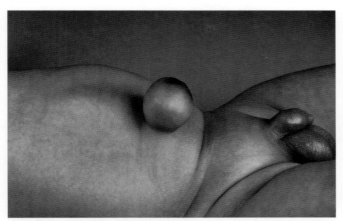

Fig. 6.2 An umbilical hernia in an infant appears after the umbilical cord has separated. It results from persistence of the defect in the umbilical cicatrix following obliteration of the umbilical vessels. It is completely covered by skin. The natural history is for spontaneous closure of the umbilical ring. In addition to the umbilical hernia, this infant has divarication of the rectus abdominis muscles.

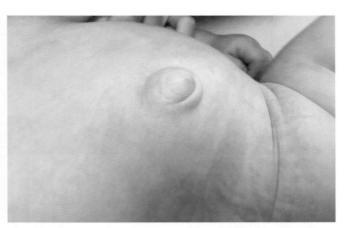

Fig. 6.3 The typical appearance of an umbilical hernia. The swelling is more obvious when the child is straining.

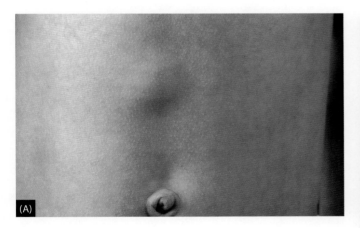

(A)

Figs. 6.4A, B (A) Epigastric hernias usually appear in the midline midway between the xiphisternum and the umbilicus. Occasionally they may be multiple. There is a minor defect in the linea alba, which allows protrusion of extraperitoneal fat. There is no hernial sac as such. They cause discomfort following meals in some children and may present with 'recurrent abdominal pain'. They are not usually reducible. (B) Epigastric hernia in an infant who also has an umbilical hernia.

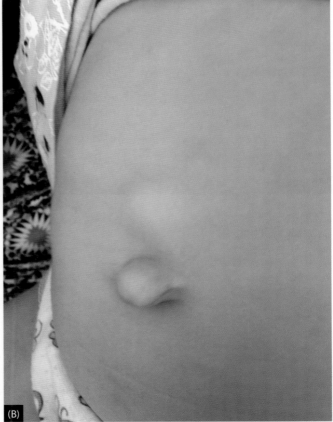

(B)

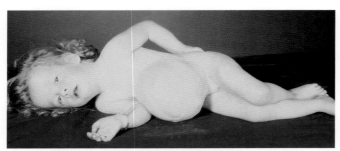

Fig. 6.5 This infant had a large exomphalos, which was allowed to heal by epithelialisation after painting with antiseptic. Ultimately the child was left with a large ventral hernia.

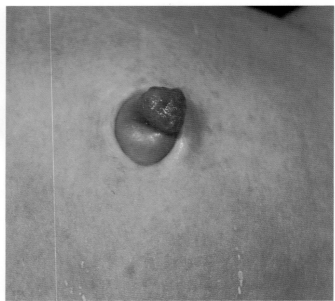

Fig. 6.6 An umbilical granuloma presents with ongoing weeping discharge from granulation tissue at the base of the umbilicus following separation of the umbilical cord stump.

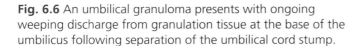

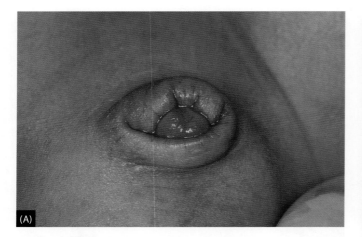

(A)

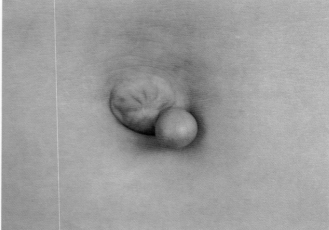

Fig. 6.8 An inclusion dermoid cyst of the umbilicus. Skin epithelium has become sequestered during separation of the umbilical cord.

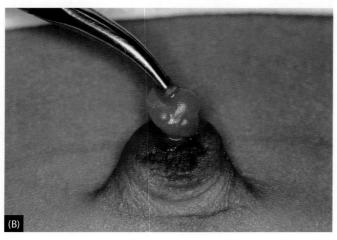

(B)

Figs. 6.7A, B (A) Examination of an umbilical granuloma reveals no evidence of a sinus or fistula opening, and there is no urine, air or faecal discharge from it. An umbilical granuloma may be difficult to distinguish clinically from ectopic bowel mucosa, which may become sequestered in the base of the umbilicus. (B) Same patient: even an umbilical granuloma within the umbilicus may be pedunculated.

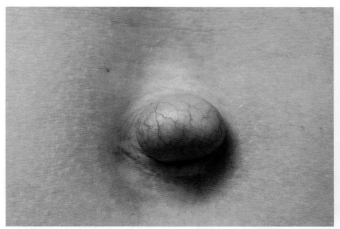

Fig. 6.9 Iatrogenic inclusion dermoid cyst of the umbilicus. This lesion enlarged slowly over several years following an umbilical hernia repair.

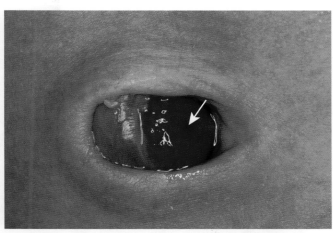

Fig. 6.10 Patent vitello-intestinal duct (omphalomesenteric duct). The umbilicus is moist and there is fluid discharging from the opening of the vitello-intestinal duct (arrow).

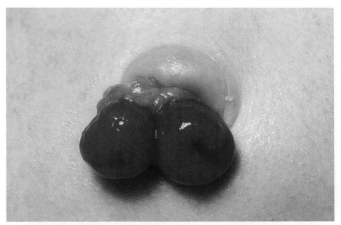

Fig. 6.11 Double-horned patent vitello-intestinal duct after prolapse of both proximal and distal ends of adjacent ileum. The mucosa of the ileum is exposed.

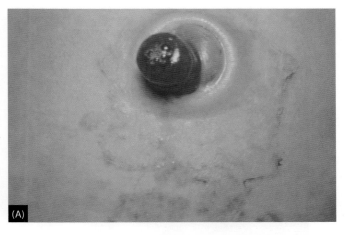

(A)

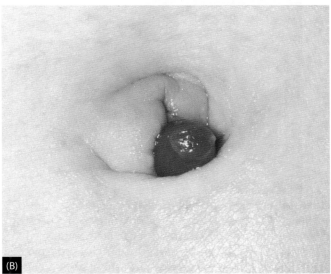

(B)

Figs. 6.12A, B (A) Intestinal fluid can be seen discharging from the patent vitello-intestinal duct. Note the surrounding skin excoriation from irritation by the ileal fluid. (B) Ectopic mucosa, often gastric, which may represent a remnant of a vitello-intestinal duct. This needs to be distinguished from an umbilical granuloma.

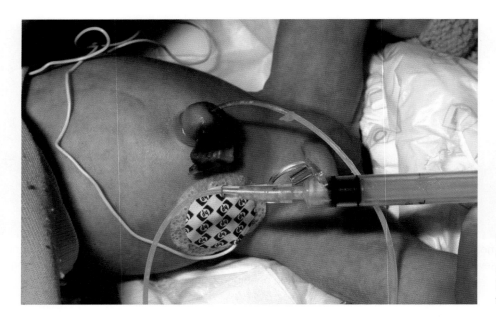

Fig. 6.13 The communication of a patent vitello-intestinal duct can be demonstrated by inserting a fine catheter and withdrawing ileal fluid.

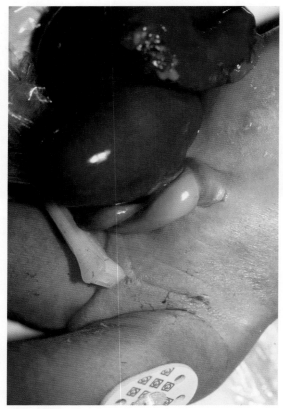

Fig. 6.14 A single-horned protrusion of a prolapsed vitello-intestinal duct. The reason there is only one horn is because there is an associated ileal atresia. It can be distinguished from gastroschisis by the fact that the mucosal surface of the bowel is exposed (rather than the serosal surface) and an opening can be seen at its end.

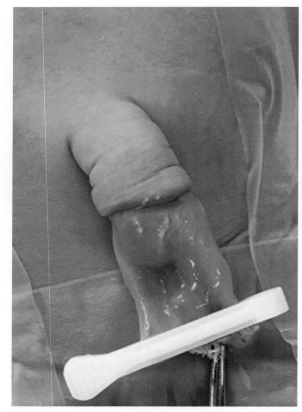

Fig. 6.15 Urachal remnant visible through the amnionic membrane of the umbilical cord.

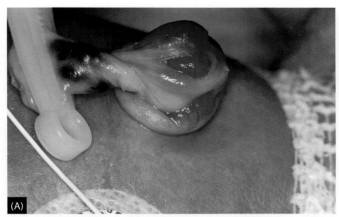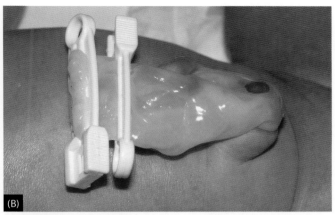

Figs. 6.16A, B (A) A patent urachus. Fluid drained freely through the opening. Without the observation of urine discharge, the appearance is similar to that of exomphalos minor with an incomplete sac. Distal urinary tract obstruction should be excluded, but is uncommon as the urachus normally obliterates soon after urine is first produced at 10 weeks' gestation. (B) In this newborn neonate with a patent urachus, mucosa is exposed on the side of the umbilical cord, through which urine discharges.

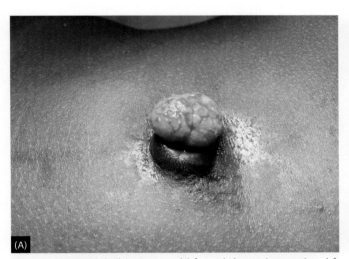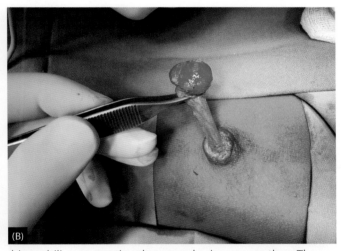

Figs. 6.17A, B (A) This 6 year old found that urine squirted from his umbilicus every time he passed urine per urethra. The umbilicus was dry between attempts at micturition. (B) Operative view of the patent urachal fistula as it was followed down towards the bladder prior to excision.

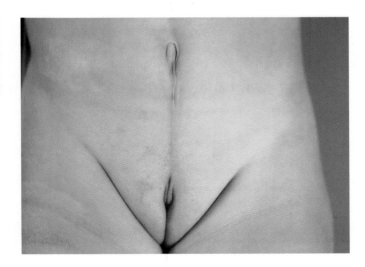

Fig. 6.18 A median cleft extending from the umbilicus to the clitoris, which is likely to be a variant of the exstrophy-epispadias complex.

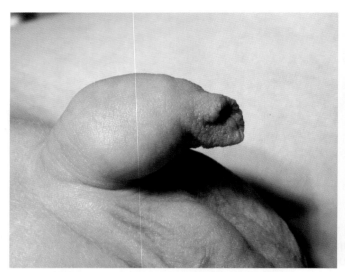

Fig. 6.19 The normal appearance of the foreskin in an uncircumcised boy. The foreskin protrudes beyond the glans penis and causes no obstruction to micturition.

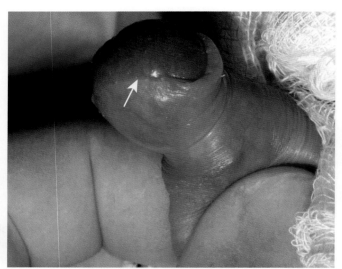

Fig. 6.20 Retraction of the normal foreskin in a young child will reveal congenital adherence of the inner surface of the foreskin to the glans penis (arrow). With growth, this adherence separates unevenly around the circumference of the glans penis until, by puberty, the foreskin should be fully retractable as far as the coronal groove.

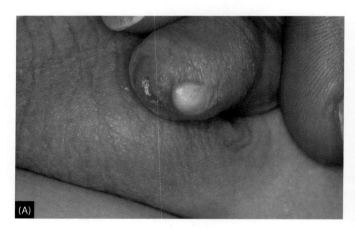

(A)

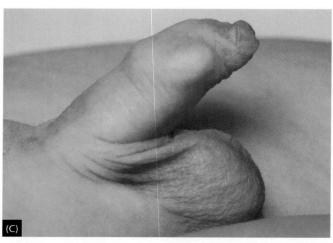

(C)

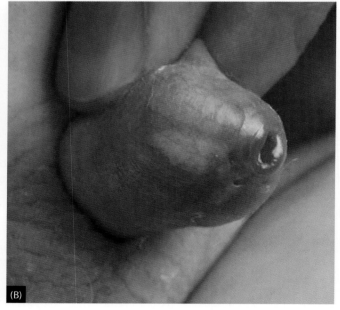

(B)

Figs. 6.21A–C (A) Smegma is a collection of secretions and desquamated epithelium that accumulates under the foreskin, which is still adherent to the glans penis. These deposits are a normal finding in small children. Ultimately, the adhesions separate and the smegma will be discharged as cheesy white material. (B) In this toddler there is accumulated smegma during the normal phase of separation of the foreskin. (C) Multiple nodules of smegma around the coronal groove.

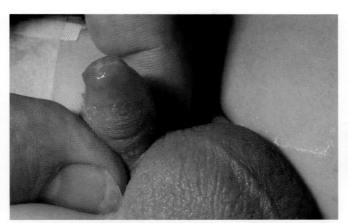

Fig. 6.22 Balanoposthitis. The foreskin is red and swollen and pus can be seen issuing from the end of the foreskin. This boy complained of pain on micturition.

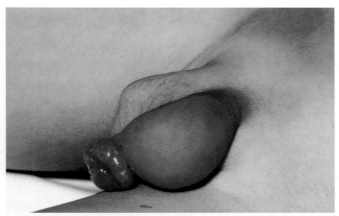

Fig. 6.23 Balanoposthitis, where the inflammation and oedema has extended beyond the foreskin to involve the penile shaft. The penile swelling in this boy was relatively painless. Note the erythema extending to the right inguinal region. During the previous day there was some scrotal oedema as well.

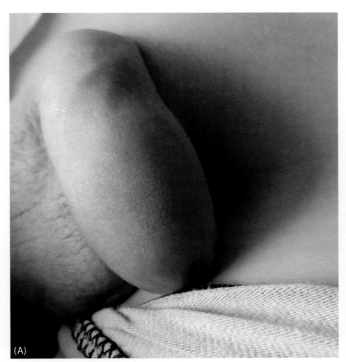

(A)

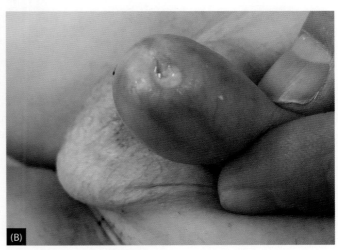

(B)

Figs. 6.24A, B (A) Balanitis xerotica obliterans causing ballooning of the foreskin and urinary retention, which may require urgent surgical correction. (B) Another picture of the same patient showing drops of urine and the phimosis.

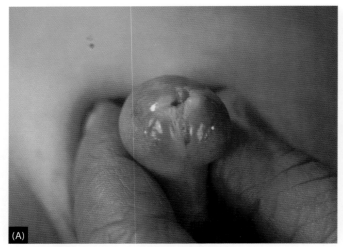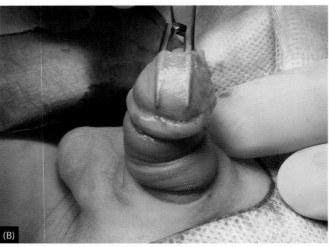

Figs. 6.25A, B (A) Severe phimosis and balanitis xerotica obliterans. Note the circumferential white scar around the opening of the foreskin, and skin splitting. There is chronic inflammation of the inner surface of the foreskin and glans. (B) Balanitis xerotica obliterans. Following retraction of the foreskin under anaesthetic there is commonly an inflammatory pseudomembrane between the glans and the foreskin, as demonstrated here by the forceps under it.

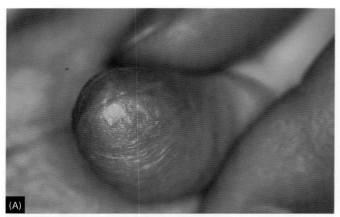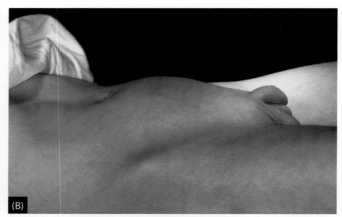

Figs. 6.26A, B (A) Severe phimosis in which there is only a pinhole opening. This patient went into acute urinary retention. (B) Acute urinary retention secondary to severe phimosis in the same patient. The grossly distended bladder is evident.

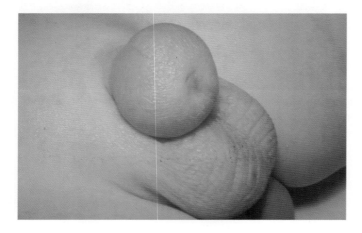

Fig. 6.27 Ballooning of the foreskin during and following micturition. The urinary obstruction created by phimosis causes urine to collect under pressure between the inner surface of the foreskin and glans.

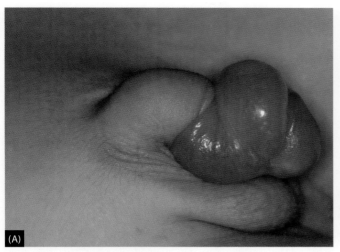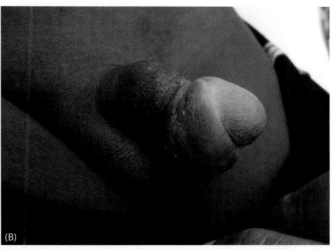

Figs. 6.28A, B (A) Paraphimosis, in which the foreskin has been left retracted proximal to the coronal groove and later is unable to return to its former position. The constriction has resulted in gross oedema and engorgement of the glans and foreskin. This often presents to the emergency department in the middle of the night after the boy goes to sleep with the foreskin still retracted and later is woken by the pain. (B) Chronic paraphimosis (present for 2 weeks) in a 5-year-old boy.

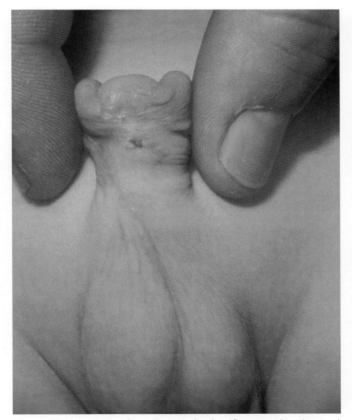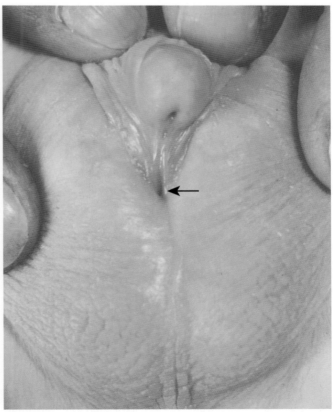

Fig. 6.29 In hypospadias, the urethral orifice may be situated anywhere on the ventral surface of the penis in the midline from the glans to the scrotum. In this child, the urethral meatus can be seen mid-shaft.

Fig. 6.30 A more severe degree of hypospadias with marked chordee or ventral bending and shortening of the shaft of the penis. The urethral meatus opens at the level of the scrotum (arrow). In the absence of testes in the scrotum, a disorder of sex development should be suspected.

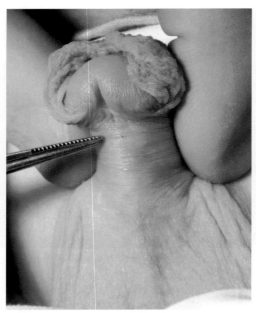

Fig. 6.31 The degree of chordee is variable in hypospadias. In this infant, the chordee is predominantly distal, such that the glans is tilted ventrally, but there is a reasonable length of ventral shaft of the penis. Note that there is failure of fusion of the foreskin on the ventral side.

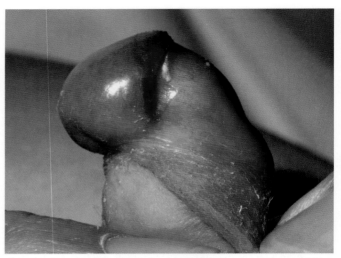

Fig. 6.32 Retraction downwards on either side of the shaft will demonstrate the degree of distal chordee. The glans penis is rotated about 60 degrees ventral to its correct orientation.

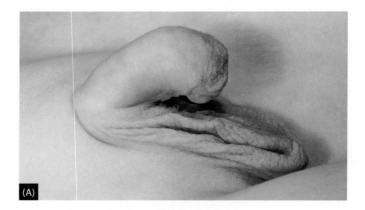

(A)

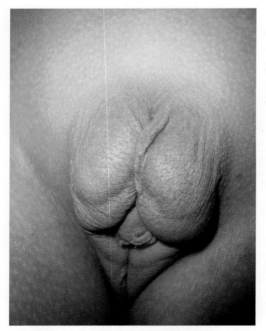

Fig. 6.33 Penoscrotal transposition associated with proximal hypospadias and chordee in a child who needs investigation for disorders of sex development.

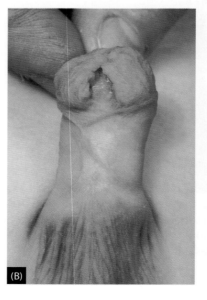

(B)

Figs. 6.34A, B (A) Beware the square-looking foreskin. This infant has hypospadias. (B) In this same infant, the hypospadias with dorsal hood, distal chordee and marked deviation of the median raphe is not obvious until the ventral aspect of the penis is examined.

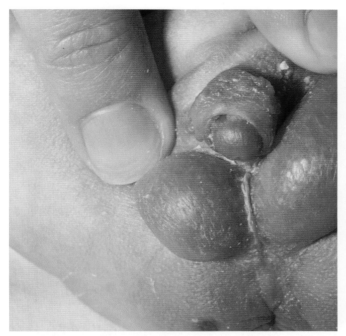

Fig. 6.35 Severe hypospadias with marked chordee and a penoscrotal urethral meatus may occur in association with other urinary tract abnormalities and defective sexual differentiation (disorders of sex development).

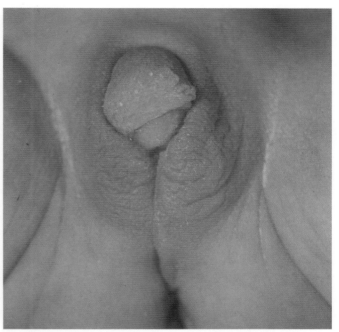

Fig. 6.36 The presence and location of testes in patients with severe hypospadias must be determined so that disorders of sex development can be excluded. This infant has congenital adrenal hyperplasia and is a genetic female, accounting for the absence of testes in the labioscrotal folds.

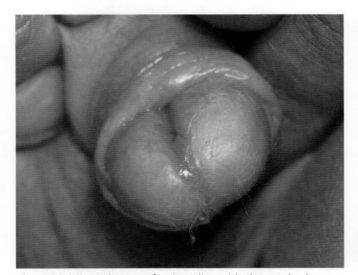

Fig. 6.37 Minor degree of epispadias with the urethral meatus on the dorsal surface of the glans penis.

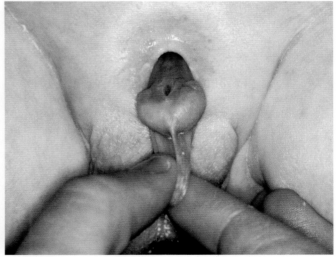

Fig. 6.38 Severe epispadias with the urethral meatus on the dorsal surface of the penile shaft at its base. The urethral plate extends along the dorsal shaft as far as the glans. The verumontanum is just within the opening, hidden from view. This is a less severe variant of the bladder exstrophy spectrum, and there is diastasis of the pubic bones.

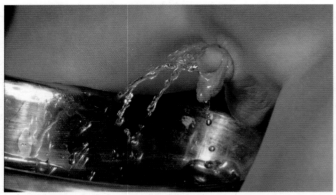

Fig. 6.39 Photograph taken during micturition in a child with epispadias, demonstrating the urine emanating from the dorsal surface of the penis.

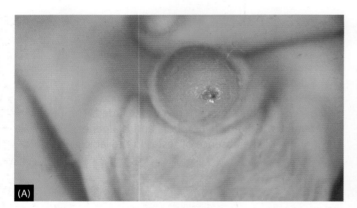

(A)

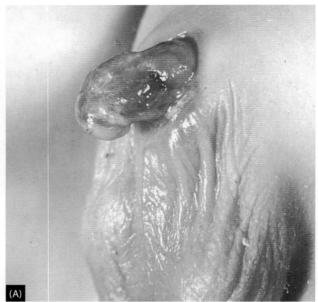

(A)

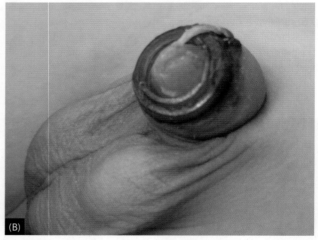

(B)

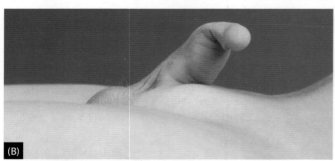

(B)

Figs. 6.40A, B (A) Meatal stenosis is a complication of circumcision in which meatal ulceration has occurred. Contraction of the scar following meatal ulceration leads to meatal stenosis. Meatal stenosis may also be caused by balanitis xerotica obliterans. (B) Dermoid cyst involving the distal part of the foreskin in an uncircumcised boy.

Figs. 6.41A–C (A) Diathermy injury during circumcision has led to major destruction of the skin and corpora cavernosa. (B) Retained Plastibell ring with secondary infection after elective circumcision. (C) Retained Plastibell ring with swelling of the penile shaft consistent with significant haemorrhage.

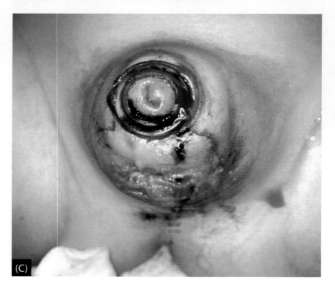

(C)

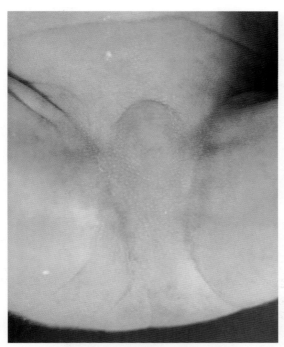

Fig. 6.42 Absence of both external genitalia and anus is an extremely rare abnormality, and is part of the spectrum of caudal regression.

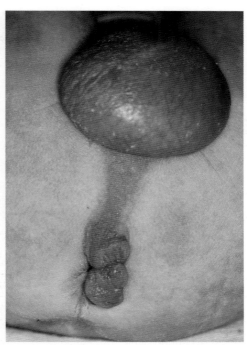

Fig. 6.43 Posterior ectopia of the penis presenting as apparent penile agenesis. There was no phallus cranial to the scrotum. A small pedunculated spongy lesion at the anterior rim of the anus extended deeply as corpus cavernosum, which on post-mortem was clearly the shaft of the penis buried in the perineal body. Absence of the scrotal raphe, as in this patient, is usually associated with severe renal dysplasia.

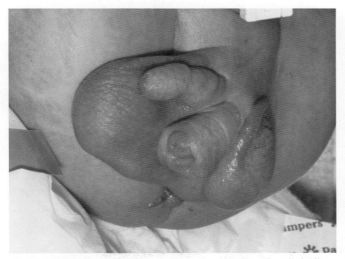

Fig. 6.44 Duplication of the external genitalia. The diphallus was associated with double bladders, multiple urethrae and rectourethral and rectocutaneous fistulae. Infants born with diphallus often have diastasis of the pubic bones and lumbosacral spinal abnormalities.

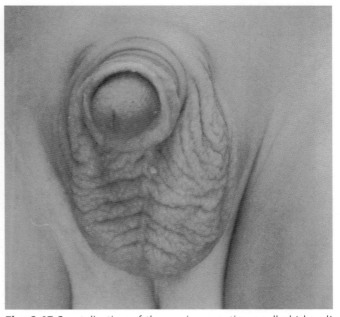

Fig. 6.45 Scrotalisation of the penis, sometimes called 'shawl' scrotum. Both the penis and scrotum are normal, but the wrinkled skin of the scrotum extends around the base of the penis.

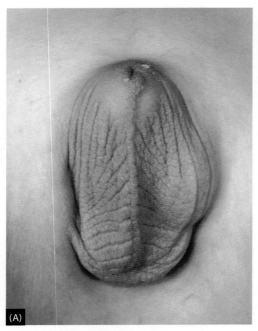

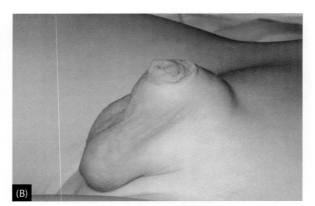

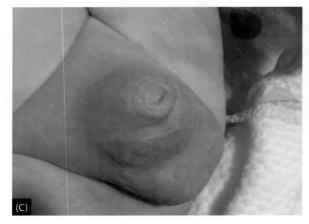

Figs. 6.46A–C (A) Buried penis. The penile shaft is normal but there is minimal skin of the shaft. (B) Buried penis where there is likely to be a megaprepuce, which is filling with urine. (C) Congenital megaprepuce.

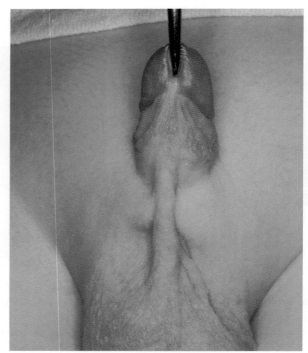

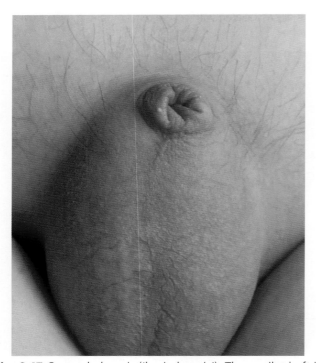

Fig. 6.47 Concealed penis ('buried penis'). The penile shaft is concealed by skin. Beware of the possibility of epispadias in these patients.

Fig. 6.48 Penoscrotal web, best seen when the penis is pulled upwards.

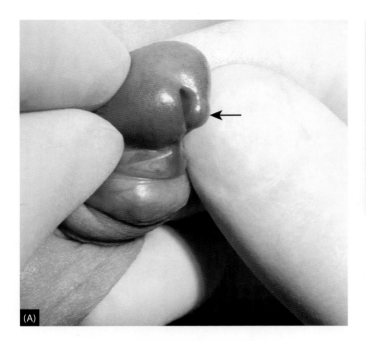

(A)

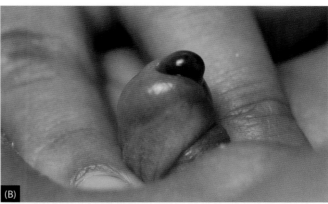

(B)

Figs. 6.49A, B (A) Partial collateral urethral duplication with obstruction. This child presented with a cyst adjacent to his normally situated external urethral meatus. The cyst (arrow) was lined by transitional epithelium but ended blindly. (B) The twin brother of the child in (A). A similar collateral urethral duplication into which bleeding has occurred produced a 'blood blister' adjacent to the urethral meatus.

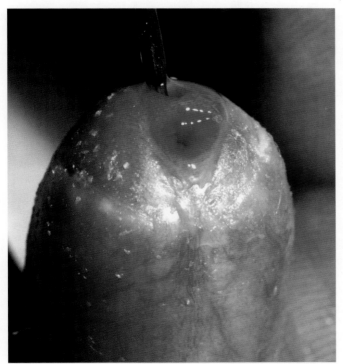

Fig. 6.50 Dorsal duplication of the urethra. The dorsal urethral tract (probed) extended to the base of the penis but had no demonstrable communication with the ventral urethra or bladder. Dorsal duplications are more common than collateral duplications of the urethra.

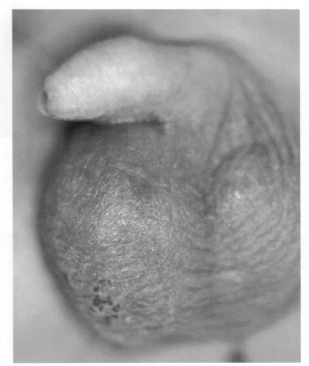

Fig. 6.51 Torsion of the testis in the perinatal period. The hemiscrotum is enlarged and may be indurated. It does not appear to be tender. The torsion is of the extravaginal type and the testis is nearly always dead by the time the scrotum is explored. Extravaginal torsion occurs just after the testis has descended into the scrotum, as there is an enzymatically-created plane around the gubernaculum allowing it to migrate through the tissues. Torsion can occur before the plane is obliterated by new collagen formation.

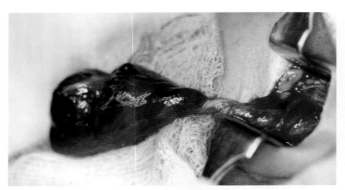

Fig. 6.52 Operative appearance of neonatal torsion of the testis, revealing that the whole cord has twisted (i.e. 'extravaginal torsion').

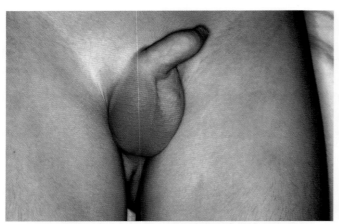

Fig. 6.53 Acute torsion in a pre-adolescent boy. The right hemiscrotum is swollen and red and the right testis is extremely painful. The inflammation is localised by the tunica vaginalis.

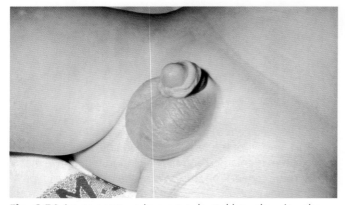

Fig. 6.54 Acute scrotum in a prepubertal boy showing the inflammation confined to the hemiscrotum. This means that the pathology is arising from within the tunica vaginalis, making the differential diagnosis testicular torsion or torsion of an appendage. Epididymitis also can occur but is very uncommon between 6 months and 13–14 years of age.

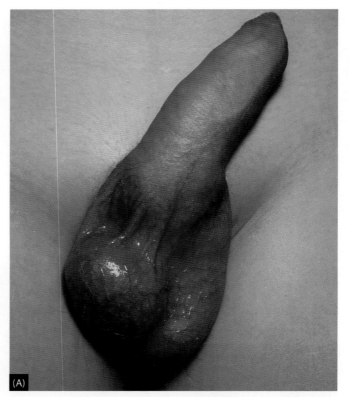

(A)

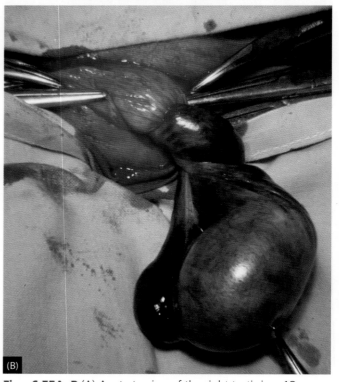

(B)

Figs. 6.55A, B (A) Acute torsion of the right testis in a 13-year-old boy. The testis is extremely tender to palpation and is riding high in the scrotum. (B) Same patient: surgical exploration shows the testis and epididymis infarcted secondary to torsion of the long mesorchium ('intravaginal torsion').

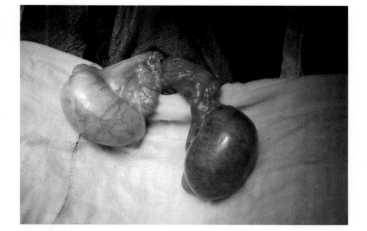

Fig. 6.56 Scrotal exploration showing the bilateral bell-clapper anomaly of the mesorchium, which has predisposed to left-sided torsion. The bell-clapper anatomical variant is usually bilateral, hence the need for bilateral fixation.

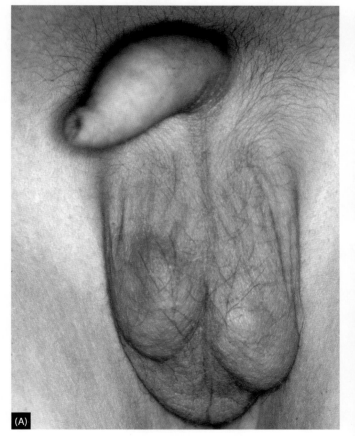

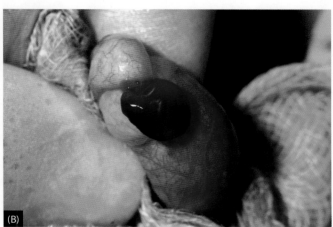

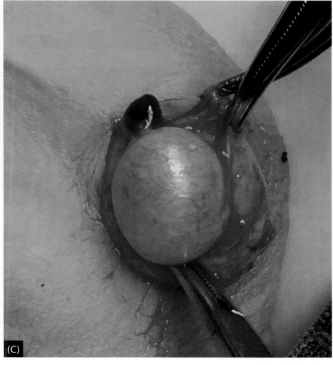

Figs. 6.57A–C (A) Torsion of a testicular appendage (e.g. hydatid of Morgagni) may be visible in the early stages as a blue–black spot in the scrotum near the upper pole of the testis. Subsequently, a reactive hydrocele will develop and it may be difficult to distinguish this clinically from torsion of a testis. (B) Operative appearance of torsion of an appendix testis. The appendix testis is gangrenous. Note the reactive inflammatory change of the epididymis. (C) Appendix testis (hydatid of Morgagni) showing haemorrhagic infarction at scrotal exploration.

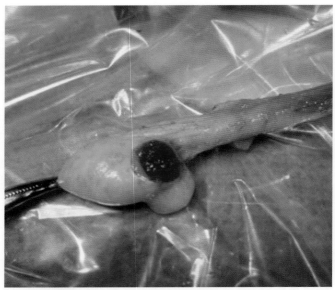

Fig. 6.58 Splenogonadal fusion shown at operation. This is a rare cause of the blue-dot sign, which is seen in an infarcted, haemorrhagic appendix testis.

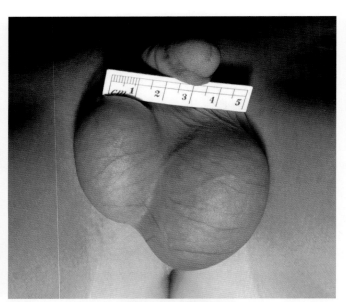

Fig. 6.59 Leukaemic infiltration of the testis.

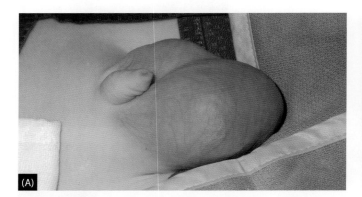

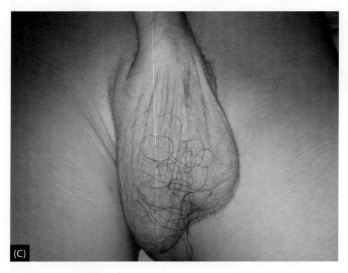

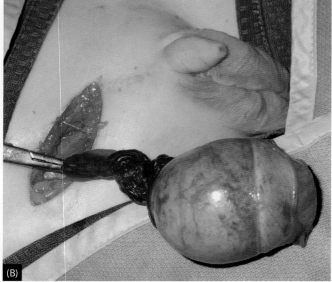

Figs. 6.60A–C (A) Yolk sac tumour showing massive enlargement of the hemiscrotum before surgery. (B) Operative treatment of a testicular tumour (here a yolk sac tumour) with an inguinal approach and clamping the spermatic cord before delivering the testis. (C) Leydig cell tumour causing some virilisation with production of hair.

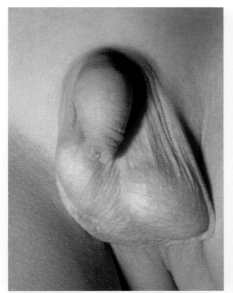

Fig. 6.61 A benign tumour of the interstitial cells of Leydig. Other neoplasms that occur in the testis include embryonal carcinoma, teratoma and seminoma.

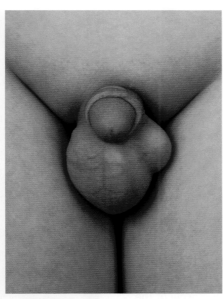

Fig. 6.62 Paratesticular rhabdomyosarcoma.

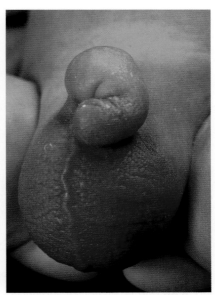

Fig. 6.63 Idiopathic scrotal oedema. This scrotum is oedematous and 'puffy'. The erythema and oedema extend into the inguinal region (here on the left side). The penis and foreskin are also oedematous. There is no tenderness of either testis.

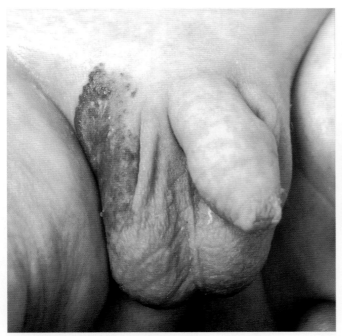

Fig. 6.64 Capillary haemangioma of the scrotum. This lesion developed in the first few weeks after birth and is now involuting.

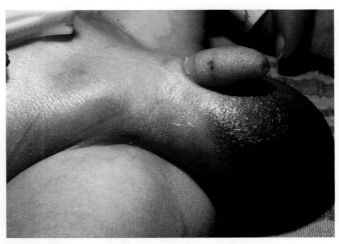

Fig. 6.65 Birth trauma to the scrotum causing bleeding into the processus vaginalis. Examination of the abdomen was unremarkable. Occasionally, neonatal peritonitis and haemoperitoneum (or adrenal haemorrhage) may present with a scrotal swelling similar in appearance to this from peritoneal fluid or blood tracking down a patent processus vaginalis.

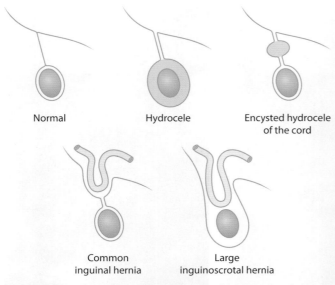

Normal   Hydrocele   Encysted hydrocele of the cord

Common inguinal hernia   Large inguinoscrotal hernia

Fig. 6.66 Hernia, hydrocele and encysted hydrocele of the cord result from failure of complete obliteration of the processus vaginalis after testicular descent is complete in boys, and as a less common anomaly in girls.

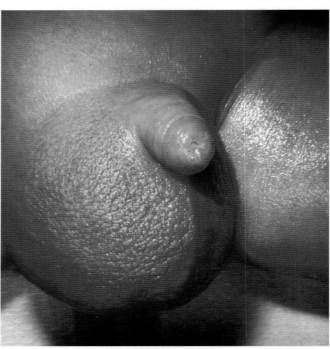

Fig. 6.67 Right indirect inguinal hernia, appearing on the first day of life as a swelling in the groin and contiguous with the right hemiscrotum. It is readily reducible.

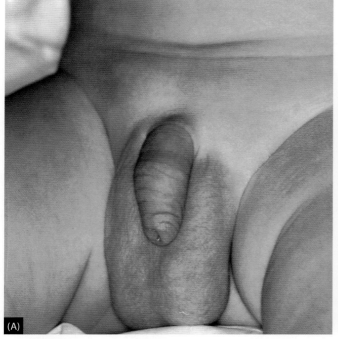

(A)

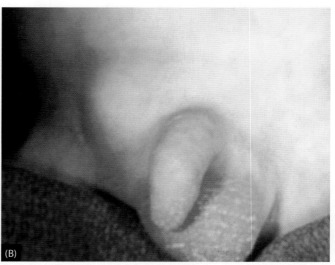

(B)

Figs. 6.68A, B (A) The typical appearance of a right inguinal hernia in an infant. A lump intermittently appears in the region of the external inguinal ring, particularly on crying or straining. The testis is palpable in the scrotum, distinct from the hernia. (B) Strangulated inguinal hernia presenting as an obvious mass in the groin.

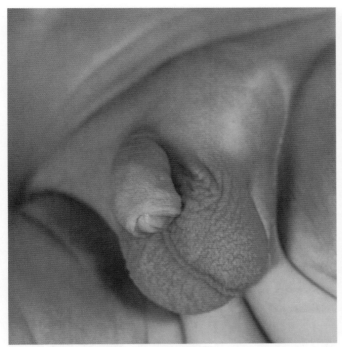

Fig. 6.69 A left indirect inguinal hernia, which is tense to feel but can be reduced by manipulation ('taxis'). The majority of inguinal hernias in infants and children are confined to the groin and do not extend to the scrotum clinically.

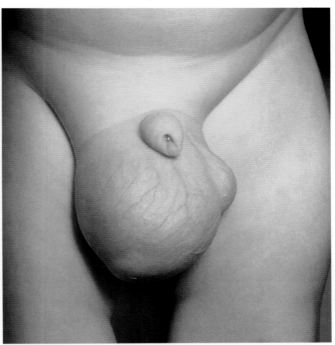

Fig. 6.70 Right inguinoscrotal hernia in which the large sac extends into the scrotum. This tends to be seen in long-standing cases that have not been treated.

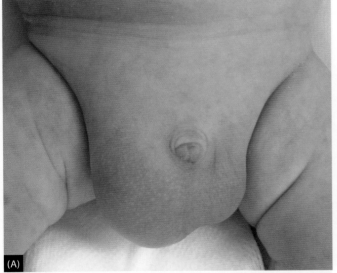

(A)

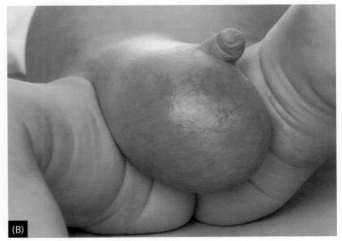

(B)

Figs. 6.71A, B (A) Bilateral inguinal hernias. (B) A large inguinoscrotal hernia containing multiple loops of bowel. This type of hernia is common in extremely premature infants and is best repaired before discharge from the neonatal ward.

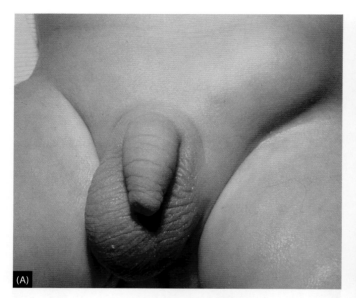

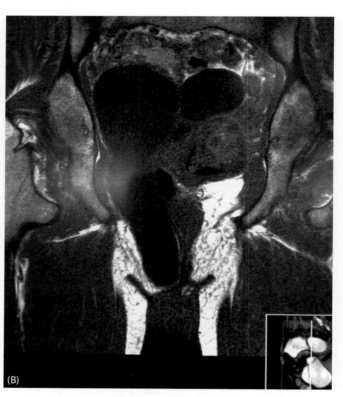

Figs. 6.72A, B (A) Strangulated left inguinal hernia. There is a tender irreducible lump overlying the inguinal canal. Note there is a hydrocele on the contralateral side. This boy has a large hernia in association with a left undescended testis. (B) MRI of incarcerated inguinal hernia, showing dilated, fluid-filled loops in the hernial sac. MRI is not normally indicated for a strangulated hernia.

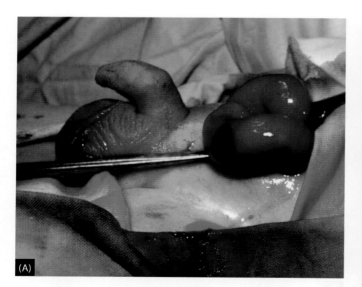

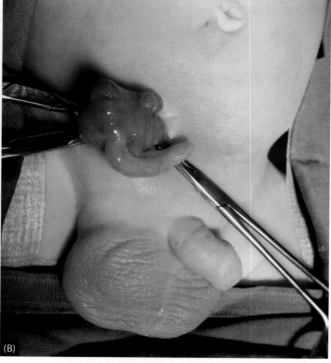

Figs. 6.73A, B (A) Operative appearance of a strangulated inguinal hernia that was irreducible on external manipulation. The bowel within the hernial sac was congested and oedematous, and there was a small area of bowel necrosis at the level of the neck of the sac. (B) Amyand's hernia containing appendix.

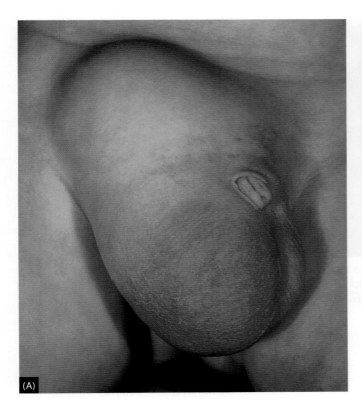

(A)

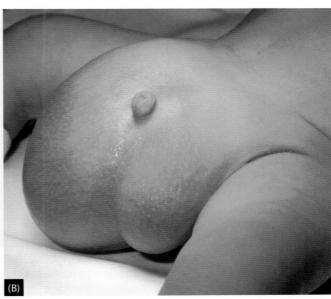

(B)

Figs. 6.74A, B (A) Large inguinoscrotal hernia accentuating a 'buried penis'. (B) Very large bilateral inguinoscrotal hernia in a baby. The large size of the hernias is responsible for the apparent burying of the penis.

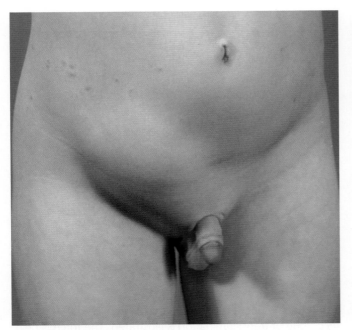

Fig. 6.75 Large direct inguinal hernia. These are rare except in association with: (1) previous extreme prematurity, (2) collagen disorders (3) cystic fibrosis, (4) direct inguinal trauma (e.g. a handlebar injury) or (5) a previously difficult inguinal herniotomy.

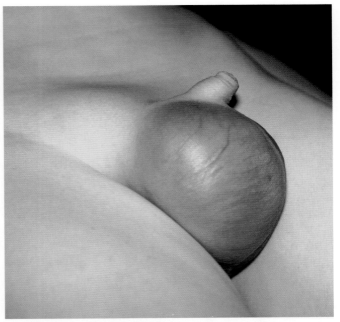

Fig. 6.76 Paratesticular rhabdomyosarcoma, which masqueraded as an irreducible inguinoscrotal hernia.

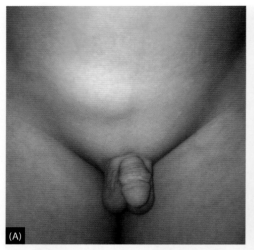 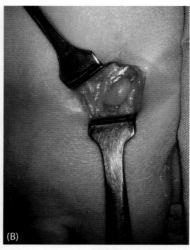 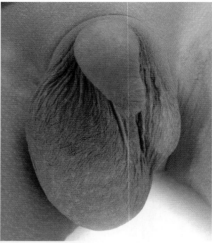

Figs. 6.77A, B (A) Preoperative view of a direct inguinal hernia showing an obvious bulge above the pubic tubercle and no extension down the spermatic cord to the scrotum. (B) A view of the sac during herniotomy in a patient with a direct inguinal hernia.

Fig. 6.78 Indirect inguinal hernia extending to the scrotum and sac containing fluid similar to a hydrocele. This occurs commonly when the omentum is in the neck of the sac and the transudate of the omentum is preferentially filling the sac. External compression of the scrotum usually identifies this as a hernia if it is easily emptied.

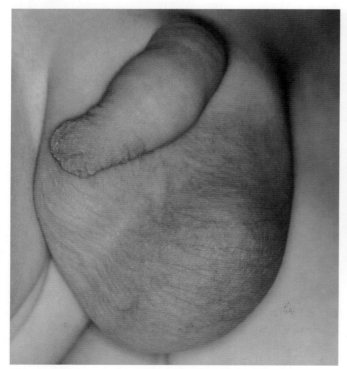

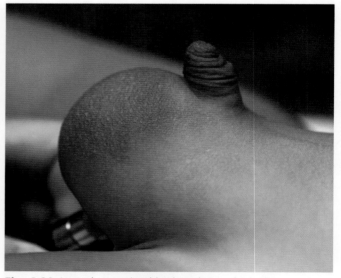

Fig. 6.80 A moderate-sized hydrocele in which the technique of transillumination is illustrated. The torch is held behind the scrotum.

Fig. 6.79 The typical appearance of a small hydrocele in an infant. There is a slight bluish hue to the hydrocele beneath the scrotal tissues. The testis is non-tender and the swelling is irreducible. Hydroceles rarely cause discomfort.

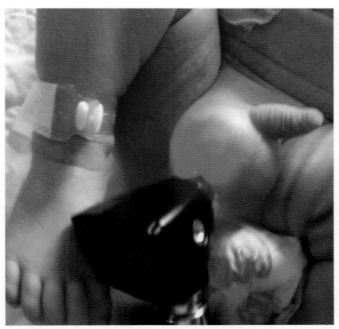

Fig. 6.81 Transillumination of the scrotum in a hydrocele.

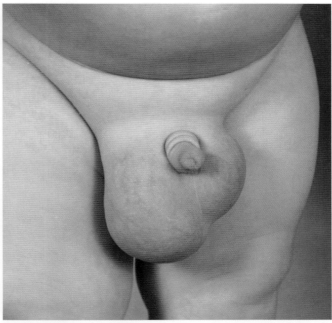

Fig. 6.82 Bilateral hydroceles with the right hydrocele the larger. Both sides of the scrotum transilluminated brilliantly. There is no extension of the swelling into the groin and it does not reduce. These features distinguish it from an inguinoscrotal hernia.

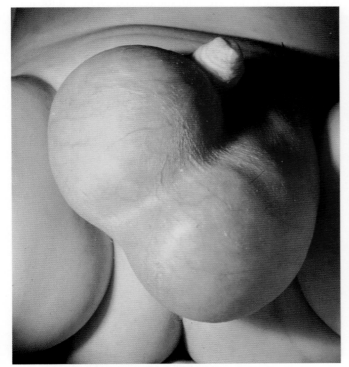

Fig. 6.83 Bilateral symmetrical hydroceles. The dumb-bell appearance when viewed from below suggests that the fluid is contained within the tunica vaginalis on each side of the scrotum (cf. **Fig. 6.85**).

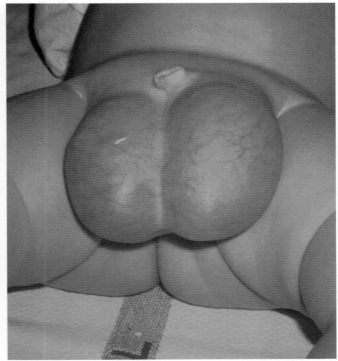

Fig. 6.84 This child with bilateral large hydroceles has a secondary 'buried' penis.

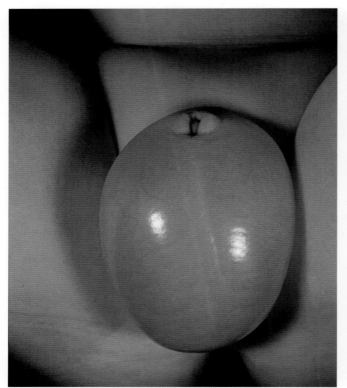

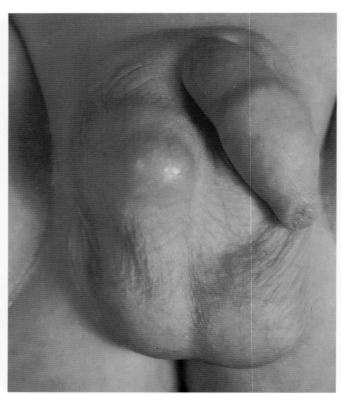

Fig. 6.85 Nephrotic syndrome with scrotal oedema, masquerading as hydroceles. The fluid in the scrotum is not confined to the tunica (and hence the spherical rather than dumb-bell shape), a feature that distinguishes it from bilateral hydroceles.

Fig. 6.86 Encysted hydrocele of the right spermatic cord. A cystic swelling discrete from the testis is evident. It moves in line with the spermatic cord and is irreducible and non-tender.

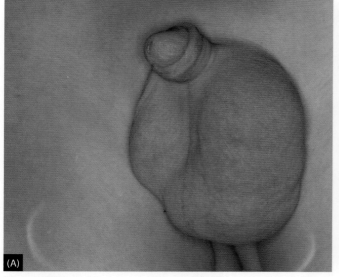

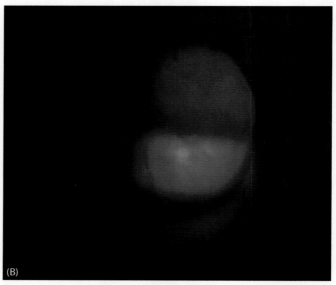

Figs. 6.87A, B (A) A larger encysted hydrocele of the left spermatic cord. It can be distinguished from a scrotal hydrocele when the testis is clearly palpable separate from and below the cystic swelling. An encysted hydrocele situated higher in the spermatic cord may be distinguished from an irreducible inguinal hernia by its mobility and absence of pain or tenderness. (B) Same patient: transillumination of the encysted hydrocele.

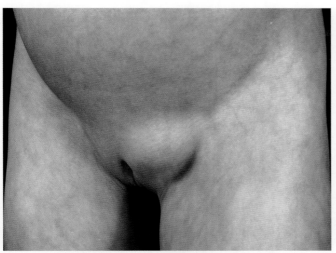

Fig. 6.88 Encysted hydrocele of the canal of Nuck is the female equivalent of an encysted hydrocele of the spermatic cord. Clinically, it needs to be distinguished from an inguinal hernia containing an ovary.

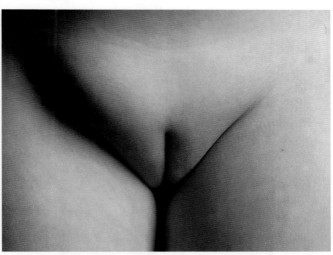

Fig. 6.89 The differential diagnosis of an inguinal hernia in a girl includes both an encysted hydrocele of the canal of Nuck and inguinal lymphadenitis (shown here).

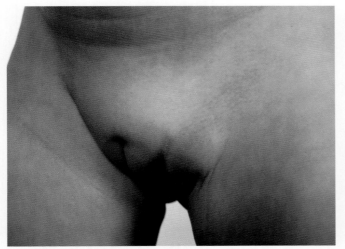

Fig. 6.90 Lymphatic malformation presenting as a mass in the upper thigh.

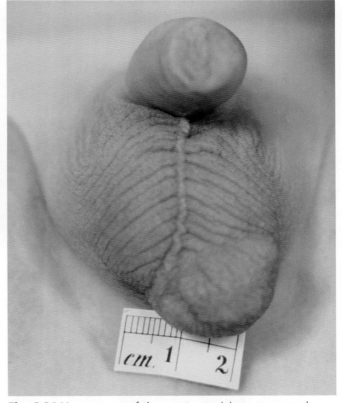

Fig. 6.91 Hamartoma of the scrotum, giving an unusual appearance of the scrotal skin.

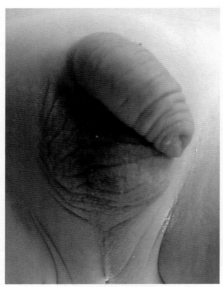

Fig. 6.92 Empty right hemiscrotum and slightly enlarged left hemiscrotum. If the left testis is larger than normal (i.e. normally, it should be similar to the volume of the glans), then there may have been a vanishing testis on the right, and the remaining testis has undergone enlargement by compensatory hypertrophy.

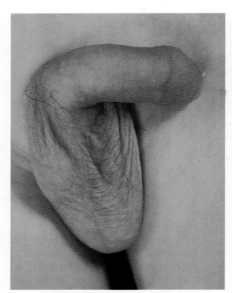

Fig. 6.93 An older child with a right undescended testis. The scrotum is not as obviously empty on the right and cord coverings (spermatic fascia) can be felt within it.

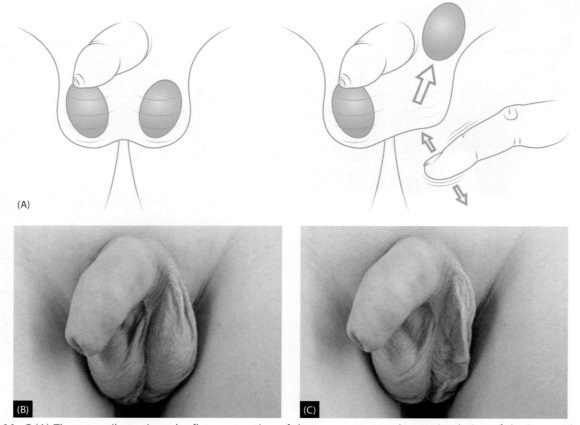

(A)

(B)

(C)

Figs. 6.94A–C (A) The retractile testis and reflex contraction of the cremaster muscle on stimulation of the inner side of the thigh. (B) The appearance of the scrotum before eliciting the cremasteric reflex. (C) The appearance after the reflex.

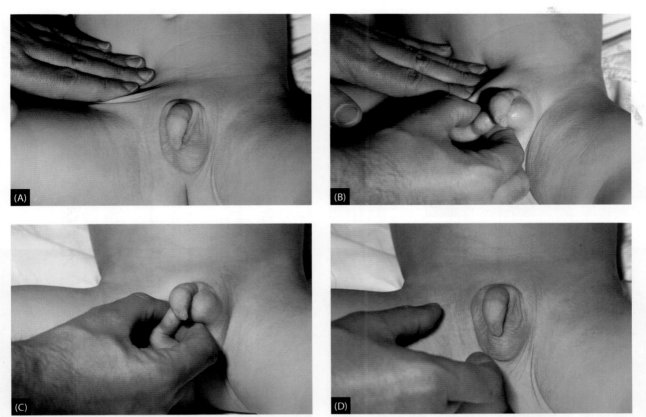

Figs. 6.95A–D (A) Examination of a child with suspected undescended testis. The left hand 'milks' the testis along the line of the inguinal canal towards the scrotum. (B) The left hand prevents retraction of the testis as the right hand grasps it within the scrotum. (C) The left hand is removed while the right hand holds the testis in the scrotum in its most distal position. (D) On release of the right hand the testis, if it is undescended, will immediately disappear back into the inguinal region. In contrast, a retractile testis will stay in the scrotum for a period.

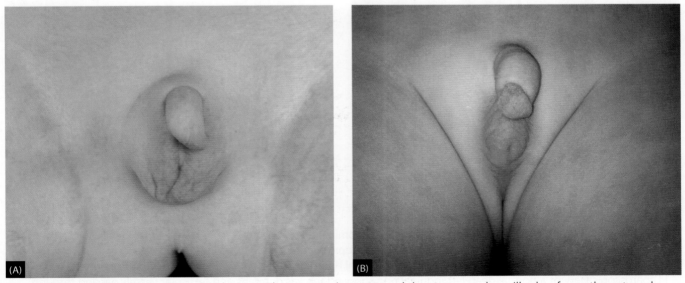

Figs. 6.96A, B (A) Bilateral undescended testes. The scrotum is empty and the testes can be milked as far as the external inguinal ring only. (B) Bilateral undescended testes with empty scrotum. The right testis is inguinal and there is a subtle bulge to the right of the penis, while the left testis is impalpable.

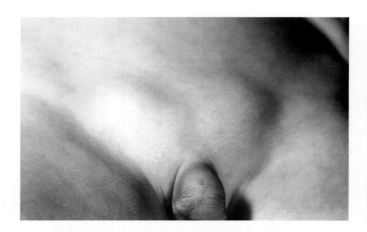

Fig. 6.97 Bilateral undescended testes residing in the 'superficial inguinal pouch', overlying the pubis on each side.

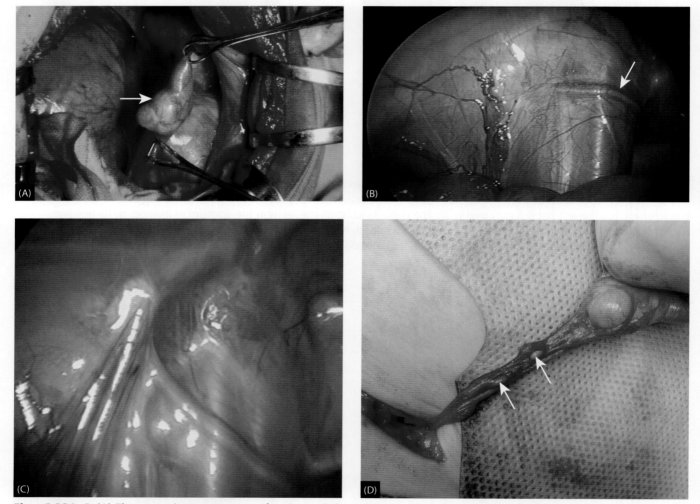

Figs. 6.98A–D (A) The operative appearance of an intra-abdominal testis (arrow). Such a testis is impalpable on clinical examination and difficult to locate radiologically. (B) Laparoscopic picture showing a blind-ending vas deferens (arrow) and no gonadal vessels passing through a closed left deep inguinal ring. This is seen in a vanishing testis after perinatal torsion. (C) Laparoscopic view of a normal deep left inguinal ring showing the vas deferens and testicular vessels passing through the ring and with no patency of the processus vaginalis. In this circumstance the testis should be located beyond the deep inguinal ring. (D) Operative appearance of adrenal rests in the spermatic cord (arrows). These are quite common and need no treatment.

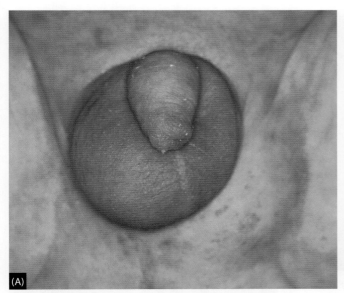

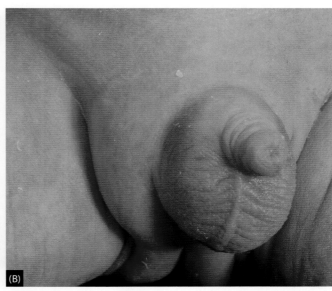

Figs. 6.99A, B (A) Perineal ectopic testis. The left testis is seen as a swelling behind the left hemiscrotum and anterior to the anus. (B) Ectopic testis in the perineum.

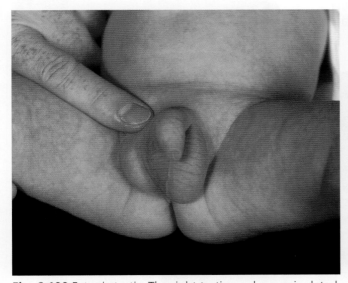

Fig. 6.100 Ectopic testis. The right testis can be manipulated lateral to, rather than into, the right hemiscrotum.

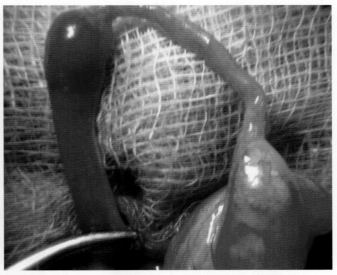

Fig. 6.101 Splenogonadal fusion, in which the testis is attached by a fibrous cord to splenic tissue. (See also **Fig. 6.58**.)

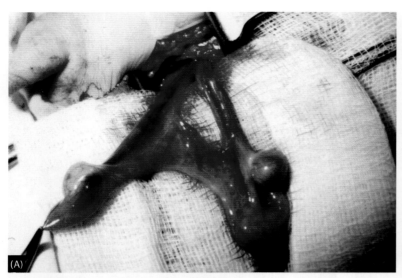

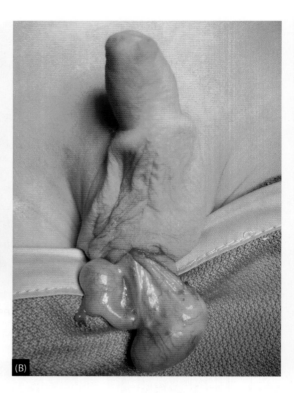

Figs. 6.102A, B (A) Transverse testicular ectopia (crossed testicular ectopia) is where both testes descend down the same inguinal canal. There is no testis in the canal on the contralateral side. It should be distinguished from polyorchidism. One or both testes will be undescended and there is usually a hernial sac associated with the lesion. (B) Polyorchidism caused by likely duplication of the gonad in early embryogenesis. This boy has three testes.

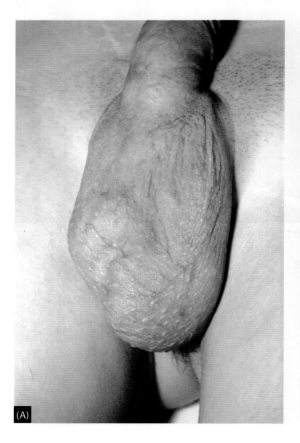

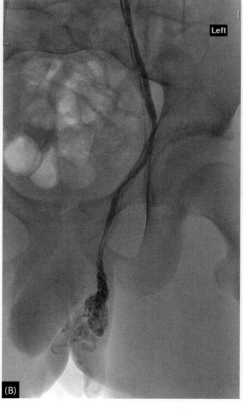

Figs. 6.103A, B (A) A varicocele almost always involves the left side and usually develops around the time of puberty. In this photo the scrotal asymmetry is obvious (despite the patient lying supine), but the 'bag of worms' will be more obvious once the boy is stood up. (B) Venogram in a boy with a varicocele showing the dilated pampiniform plexus (prior to embolisation).

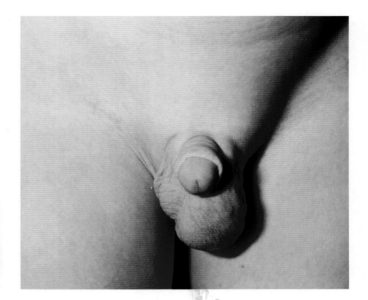

Fig. 6.104 A varicocele in association with a Wilms tumour or neuroblastoma is seen occasionally. This occurs because the left testicular vein drains directly into the left renal vein, which may be obstructed by the tumour.

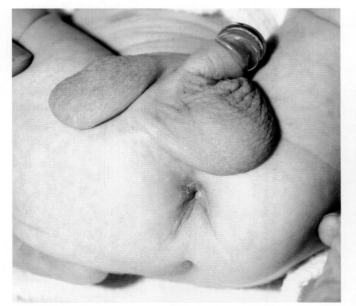

Fig. 6.105 Ectopic right hemiscrotum in an infant who has had a Plastibell circumcision. The cause of this anomaly is commonly external pressure on the genital fold by the heel of one of the feet of the fetus during early development. This deformity is rarely genetic but usually secondary to abnormal fetal position. The ectopic hemiscrotum is quite likely to contain the testis, which has migrated into it despite the anomalous location. Associated ipsilateral renal abnormalities are likely.

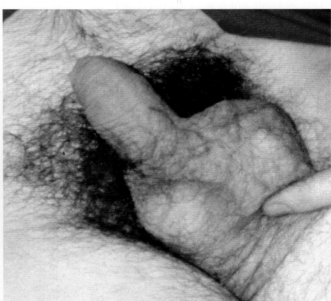

Fig. 6.106 Testicular teratoma in the left testis in a young man.

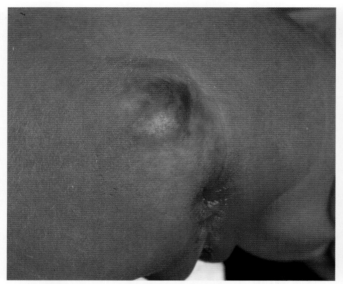

Fig. 6.107 A sacrococcygeal teratoma presenting at birth, masquerading as a haemangioma. There was a significant intrapelvic component.

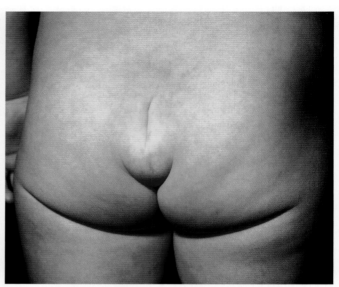

Fig. 6.108 A predominantly intrapelvic sacrococcygeal teratoma showing relatively minor swelling in the region of the coccyx. The more obscure sacrococcygeal teratomas tend to present beyond the neonatal period and are more likely to become malignant.

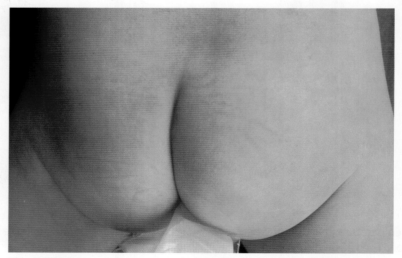

Fig. 6.109 Intrapelvic sacrococcygeal teratoma with subtle fullness of the right buttock being its only external manifestation. A large presacral mass was palpable on rectal examination.

The urinary tract | CHAPTER 7

Urinary tract disorders are often diagnosed on antenatal ultrasonography (see Chapter 1). Postnatally they present with either vague generalised features related to infection or specific symptoms such as dysuria, loin pain, wetting or haematuria. Small infants with urinary tract infections display non-specific features of infection, such as vomiting, lethargy, poor feeding, failure to thrive and fever. Consequently, if an infant develops these non-specific signs of sepsis, the urinary tract should be excluded as their cause; this is done by looking for white cells and bacteria in the urine. Suprapubic aspiration of urine is more reliable than a bag specimen in infants, whereas a mid-stream specimen of urine should be collected under aseptic technique in the older child.

Pyelonephritis and upper urinary tract obstruction (e.g. pelviureteric junction obstruction) may cause continuous or colicky loin pain radiating to the ipsilateral iliac fossa or genitalia. The renal parenchyma and collecting system become inflamed (or may even form an abscess) in pyelonephritis, often producing severe systemic signs of sepsis and toxicity. Children with pyelonephritis may have a fullness in the renal angle, local tenderness and compensatory scoliosis. In chronic pelviureteric junction obstruction with hydronephrosis there may be a large ballotable mass in the flank. The underlying pathology is determined by a renal ultrasound scan and nuclear renal scan.

Hypertension is rare in children but is present in a significant number who have urinary tract abnormalities. The blood pressure should always be measured in children who present with urinary tract infections, known congenital renal abnormalities or Wilms tumour. It is important to select a blood pressure cuff that is appropriate to the size of the child. The blood pressure should be correlated with normal values for the child's age. Hypertension is seen most often in association with scarring of the renal parenchyma secondary to chronic glomerulonephritis, pyelonephritis or vesicoureteric reflux. Occasionally, renal artery stenosis or compression by Wilms tumour may be responsible.

Urinary incontinence or wetting is normal in infants and even some school-age children when they are asleep (i.e. nocturnal enuresis). The cause of wetting usually can be determined from the history. Acute causes of wetting (e.g. psychological or infective) should be distinguished from long-standing abnormalities such as neurogenic bladder and ectopic ureter.

Haematuria is another important urinary tract sign, and the diagnosis can be made on the basis of the history and clinical findings. Most medical causes of haematuria, including glomerulonephritis and other renal disorders, produce evenly blood-stained urine throughout micturition. By contrast, spots of blood passed at the end of micturition suggest a lower urinary tract abnormality, such as meatal ulcer, urethral diverticulum or a minor tear in the foreskin. It is important to remember that Wilms tumour or congenital abnormalities of the urinary tract may produce haematuria, and trivial trauma may cause haematuria when there is a hydronephrotic kidney. Occasionally, bleeding from the vagina and ingestion of coloured dyes or vegetables containing red pigment can be mistaken for haematuria.

INVESTIGATIONS

Children presenting with urinary signs or symptoms should have an initial renal ultrasound scan and sometimes a micturating cystourethrogram. These are good screening tests and will detect most significant abnormalities. Should an abnormality be found, further investigation of the anatomy and function of the urinary tract may be required (e.g. nuclear isotopic scan [and occasionally antegrade or retrograde pyelograms]). A number of rare congenital defects may be found on investigation, including retrocaval ureter, crossed renal ectopia or a patent urachus (although urachal remnants are now recognised to be more common since the advent of ultrasonography). Anomalies not directly related to the urinary tract may cause secondary urinary symptoms (e.g. bladder and urethral compression in pelvic tumours).

WILMS TUMOUR

A Wilms tumour is an embryonal tumour of the kidney. Most commonly, it presents as an abdominal mass that is discovered incidentally during infancy or early childhood. Sometimes a trivial injury causes haematuria, while hypertension and varicocele are rare presentations. Wilms tumour may be unilateral or bilateral.

PELVIURETERIC OBSTRUCTION

Obstruction by stenosis or kinking at the pelviureteric junction causes dilatation of the pelvicalyceal system, known as hydronephrosis. The obstruction may be persistent or intermittent. It can be identified on an antenatal ultrasound scan or postnatally because of infection, loin pain and vomiting or haematuria. Pelviureteric junction obstruction diagnosed prenatally needs careful assessment after birth, since the blockage may be a transient feature that resolves spontaneously with growth. An ultrasound scan and micturating cystourethrogram are performed immediately after birth, followed by a renal mercaptoacetyltriglycine 3 (MAG3) scan when the baby is 6 weeks old. If renal function is preserved and the degree of dilatation is not progressive, surgery may not be needed. The aim of surgery is to prevent ongoing destruction of renal parenchyma. Pelviureteric junction obstruction may occur in association with other urinary tract anomalies (e.g. horseshoe kidney) or vesicoureteric obstruction.

VESICOURETERIC OBSTRUCTION

Blockage at the lower end of the ureter is caused by stenosis or a mucosal flap creating a valve. Ureteric dilatation is often dramatic and leads to urinary stasis and infection. However, the back pressure on the kidney is less than is seen in pelviureteric junction obstruction and the kidney may be undamaged. A MAG3 or diethylenetriamine pentaacetic acid (DTPA) scan identifies the level of obstruction: antegrade and retrograde pyelography can define the anatomical problem more precisely.

VESICOURETERIC REFLUX

The commonest cause of urinary tract infection is vesicoureteric reflux. Bacteria in the lower urinary tract are not expelled during micturition, and can ascend up the refluxing ureter to the kidney. The child is at risk of developing pyelonephritis with renal scarring, and subsequent renal failure and hypertension. An inadequate length of intravesical ureter ('submucosal tunnel') is the cause of reflux, and is a frequent finding in infants. As the child grows the submucosal tunnel lengthens, frequently leading to spontaneous resolution of reflux.

Reflux is commonly diagnosed after an antenatal ultrasound scan has shown dilatation of the urinary tract. These infants often have severe reflux with associated dysplastic kidneys and other congenital malformations of the urinary tract. Other children present later with a urinary tract infection. Reflux is diagnosed on micturating cystourethrography, and the presence of scarring and renal dysplasia is documented with ultrasonography or a dimercaptosuccinic acid (DMSA) nuclear scan.

URETEROCELE

A ureterocele is a cystic dilatation of the intravesical end of the ureter. There is often a congenital stenosis of the ureteric opening in association with deficiency of the muscular wall of the distal ureter, allowing dilatation within the bladder to form a mucosa-covered cyst. Ureteroceles occur in children with duplex ureters and, occasionally, with a single ureter. A subservient renal segment will have little or no function if it is obstructed by the ureterocele. Reflux or obstruction of the adjacent orthotopic ureter is a frequent finding. If the ureteric opening is ectopic, the ureterocele may open in the urethra. Some ureteroceles are large and redundant, allowing prolapse down the urethra like a polyp. Ureteroceles need to be distinguished from bladder diverticula.

DOUBLE KIDNEYS AND URETERS

Where two ureteric buds develop instead of one, a double or duplex kidney will be formed. This may be associated with other abnormalities, such as stenosis of one of the ureters producing a ureterocele, or an opening of one of the ureters in an ectopic position, such as the bladder neck or vagina. An ectopic ureter opening distal to the bladder sphincter in a girl may present with continuous wetting. Occasionally, the only radiological evidence of a duplex kidney is lateral displacement of the functioning lower pole by the non-functional upper pole.

URINARY TRACT STONES

The incidence and composition of urinary stones in children varies between geographical regions. Metabolic disorders such as cystinuria or oxalosis are rare causes, whereas hypercalcuria is more common. Urinary tract infection and structural abnormalities are important predisposing factors in many cases. One notable cause of stone formation in children is in association with various forms of urinary diversion in a neurogenic bladder (e.g. spina bifida). Attempts to produce urinary continence in a neurogenic bladder by augmentation with a segment of ileum or colon may cause stones to develop within the augmented bladder. The stones form on epithelial debris or mucus.

POSTERIOR URETHRAL VALVE

Posterior urethral valves affect the male urethra and cause obstruction to urinary outflow.

Persistence of mucosal folds attached to the verumontanum block the posterior urethra (type I valve). Rarely, there may be persistence of the urogenital part of the cloacal membrane, producing a more distal obstruction (type III valve). Boys with a posterior urethral valve present with a poor urinary stream, sepsis from urinary tract infection or renal failure. The urinary obstruction has been present throughout the formation of the urinary tract: if the obstruction is severe, renal dysplasia may ensue. On occasion, this is so severe the child has intrauterine renal failure and dies shortly after birth with Potter syndrome. A micturating cystourethrogram confirms the diagnosis postnatally and a renal nuclear scan allows assessment of renal function and upper tract obstruction. Severe vesicoureteric reflux is often coexistent.

RARE URETHRAL ANOMALIES

Apart from posterior urethral valve, anomalies of the urethra are rare. In males, congenital, post-traumatic or postoperative diverticula of the anterior urethra may cause obstruction. Rarely, urethral polyps and prolapsing ureteroceles may obstruct the posterior or bulbar urethra. Bright bleeding at the end of micturition may be caused by ulceration of the fossa navicularis within the glans penis.

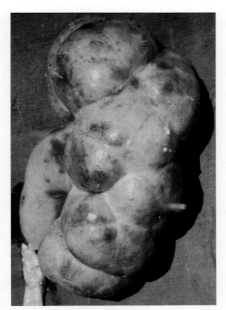

Fig. 7.1 Large tuberculous pyonephrosis. There were two strictures in the ureter.

Figs. 7.2A, B (A) Magnetic resonance urogram (MRU) in a 2-year-old infant who presented with antenatal hydronephrosis and suspected duplex systems. Further imaging after birth showed a horseshoe kidney, which can be seen here on the MRU. (B) In these T2 images from another patient it can be seen that the infant does have duplex systems and that the dilated, upper pole ureter on the left is ectopic and enters the urethra just below the bladder neck.

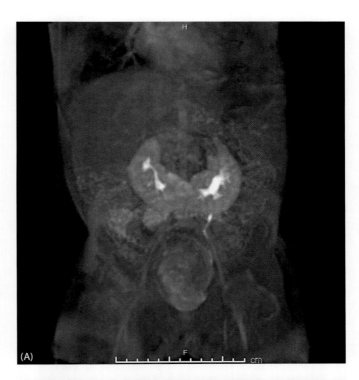

(A)

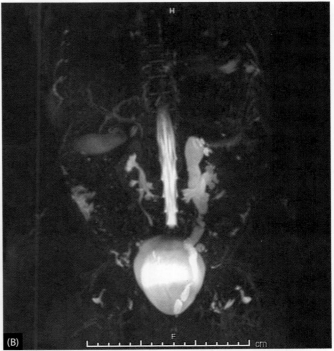

(B)

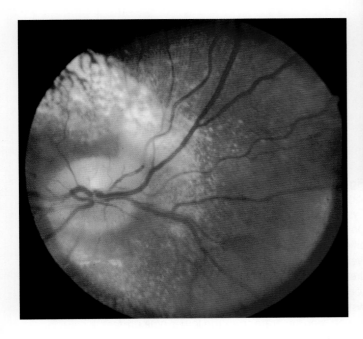

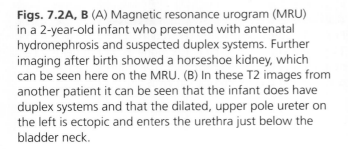

Fig. 7.3 Hypertension may occur in association with renal abnormalities. This child with a Wilms tumour presented with hypertension and examination of the retina revealed papilloedema.

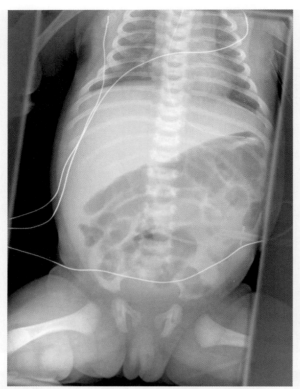

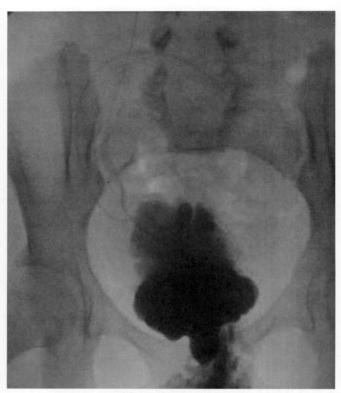

Fig. 7.4 Plain abdominal radiograph in a baby who presented with a urinary tract infection a few weeks after birth; this radiograph was taken to exclude necrotising enterocolitis. The sacral agenesis was missed until the baby came to urology outpatients at 3 months of age.

Fig. 7.5 Fluoroscopic image taken during urodynamics in this 11-year-old girl with spina bifida, done as part of her regular neurogenic bladder management. The trabeculated bladder is visible and the vertebral anomaly is also seen.

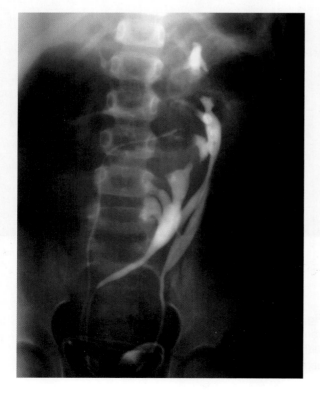

Fig. 7.6 Crossed renal ectopia. This 6-year-old child presented for investigation after a documented urinary tract infection. Cystoscopy revealed three ureteric openings within the bladder. On the left side there was a single opening, which led to a bifid upper ureter and calyceal system. On the right side there were two openings, catheterisation of which revealed that both ureters crossed the midline to the left side. This film shows contrast in the lower pole ureter of the right crossed ectopic system. The upper pole catheter has no contrast within it but can be seen separate from the lower pole ureter.

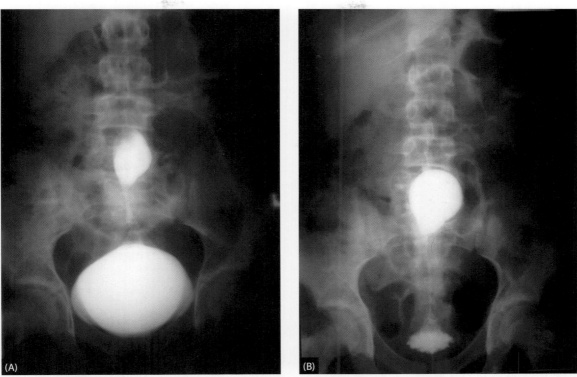

Figs. 7.7A, B (A) Urachal cyst in an 11-year-old girl who developed a urinary tract infection. The bladder communicates with the urachal cyst. On the lateral view (not shown) the cyst could be seen in the anterior abdominal wall. (B) Same patient: contrast remains in the urachal cyst following micturition and emptying of the bladder.

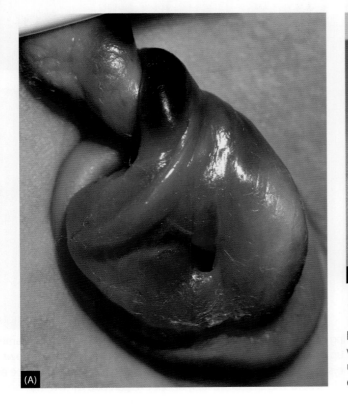

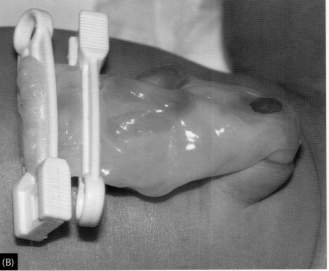

Figs. 7.8A, B (A) A patent urachus is evident from birth when urine is observed passing through an opening at the umbilicus. (B) Another baby with a patent urachus obvious even before separation of the cord.

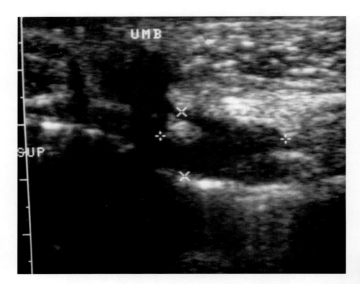

Fig. 7.9 Infected urachal remnant in an 11-year-old boy who presented with a short history of a painful tender lump at the umbilicus, which was discharging pus. He had marked localised tenderness below the umbilicus, and ultrasound demonstrated a cavity located within the anterior abdominal wall immediately below the umbilicus. The appearance was consistent with an infected urachal cyst.

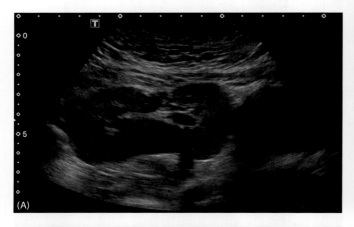

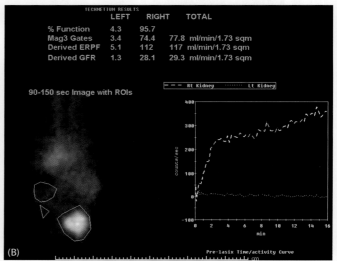

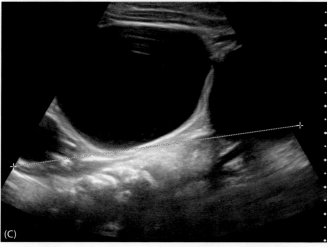

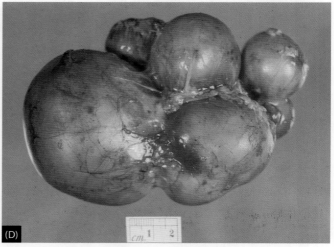

Figs. 7.10A–D (A) Ultrasound scan of a single pelvic kidney, showing its abnormal orientation in the pelvis. (B) MAG3 scan of the same 2-year-old boy with a single pelvic kidney showing tracer taken up on one side of the pelvis. (C) Five-month-old girl with a known renal abnormality on antenatal ultrasonography showing a multicystic dysplastic kidney (MCDK) that was originally thought to be a hydronephrosis, but which was found on nuclear scan to have no function. There is controversy about excision of a MCDK, but here the parents requested surgery as the mass was compressing the duodenum and she was failing to thrive. Surgery corrected the failure to thrive. (D) Pathological specimen of a MCDK showing loss of the renal outline and cysts of variable size.

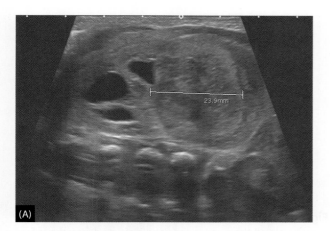

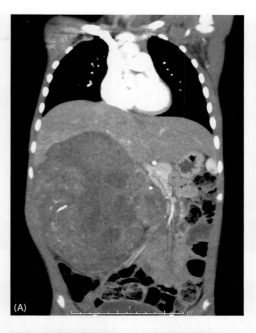

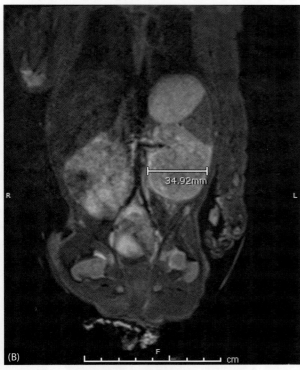

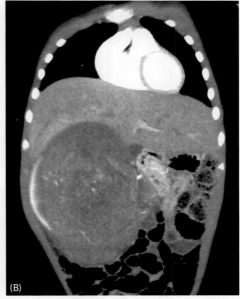

Figs. 7.11A, B (A) An expanding lesion in the lower pole of the left kidney in a 1-week-old baby seen on ultrasound scan. This was confirmed on nephrectomy to be a mesoblastic nephroma. (B) Same patient: MR image showing a relatively homogeneous lesion replacing the lower pole.

Figs. 7.12A–C (A) CT of the abdomen showing a massive tumour arising in the right flank and extending beyond the midline and distorting the great vessels. Biopsy confirmed this to be a Wilms tumour, and this 6-year-old boy was immediately commenced on chemotherapy. (B) Another CT section showing a thin crescent of functioning renal tissue draped across and distorted by the tumour arising from the right kidney. (C) Same patient after 6 weeks of chemotherapy, showing significant shrinkage of the tumour.

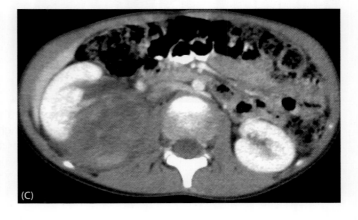

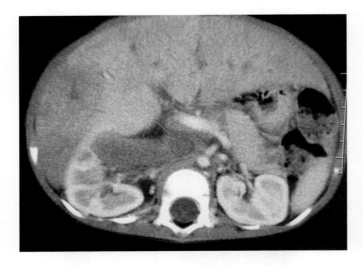

Fig. 7.13 CT with contrast showing extension of Wilms tumour along the right renal venal vein and into the inferior vena cava (arrow).

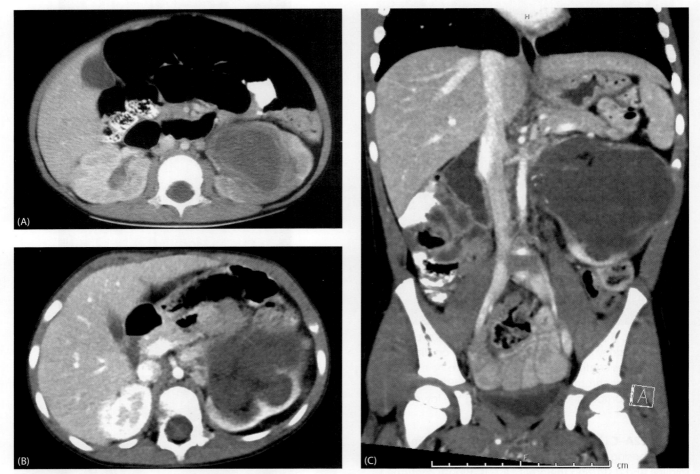

Figs. 7.14A–C (A) CT scan showing bilateral Wilms tumours after chemotherapy. (B) CT of the abdomen in a 3-year-old boy with a left kidney containing a Wilms tumour and a normal right kidney. (C) Another view of the same patient showing the rim of functional renal parenchyma stretched over the inferior margin of the tumour.

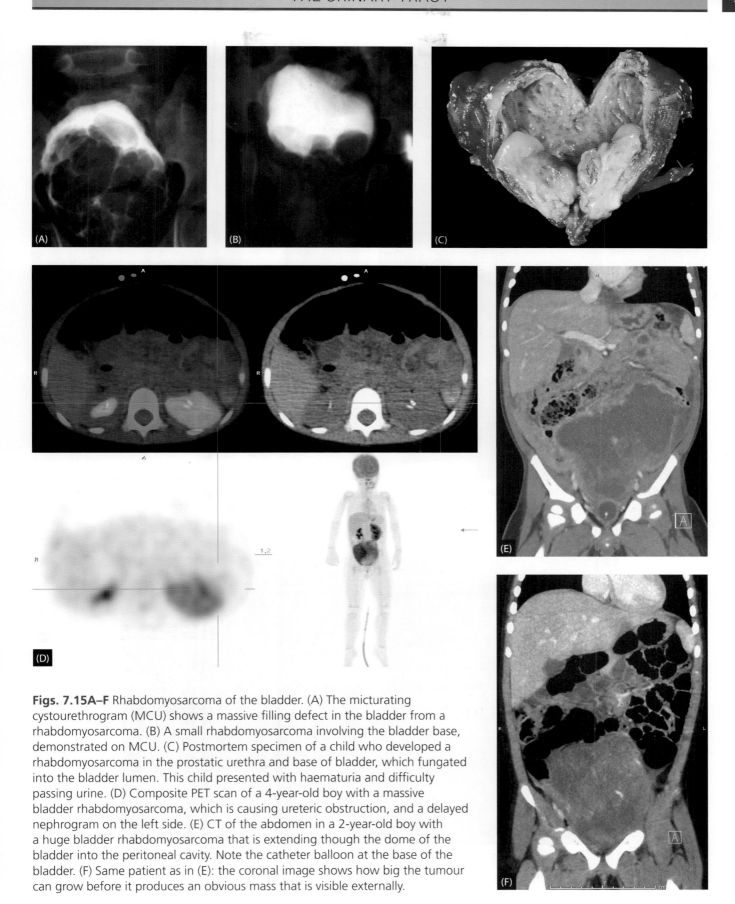

Figs. 7.15A–F Rhabdomyosarcoma of the bladder. (A) The micturating cystourethrogram (MCU) shows a massive filling defect in the bladder from a rhabdomyosarcoma. (B) A small rhabdomyosarcoma involving the bladder base, demonstrated on MCU. (C) Postmortem specimen of a child who developed a rhabdomyosarcoma in the prostatic urethra and base of bladder, which fungated into the bladder lumen. This child presented with haematuria and difficulty passing urine. (D) Composite PET scan of a 4-year-old boy with a massive bladder rhabdomyosarcoma, which is causing ureteric obstruction, and a delayed nephrogram on the left side. (E) CT of the abdomen in a 2-year-old boy with a huge bladder rhabdomyosarcoma that is extending though the dome of the bladder into the peritoneal cavity. Note the catheter balloon at the base of the bladder. (F) Same patient as in (E): the coronal image shows how big the tumour can grow before it produces an obvious mass that is visible externally.

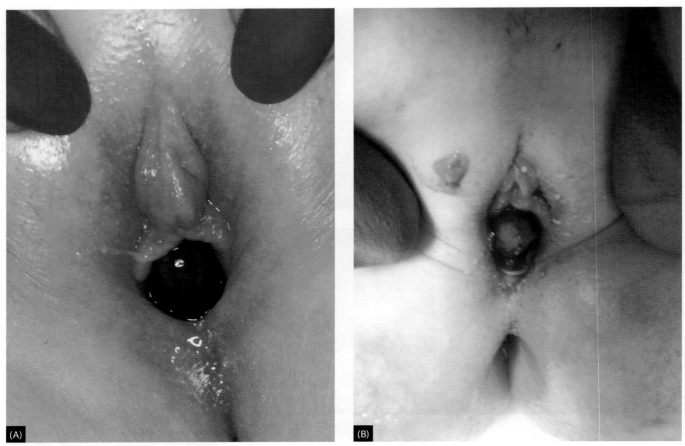

Figs. 7.16A, B (A) Vaginal rhabdomyosarcoma. This 2-year-old girl presented with a mass protruding from the vagina, which was shown to be a rhabdomyosarcoma arising from the vault of the vagina. (B) Rhabdomyosarcoma presenting as sarcoma botryoides.

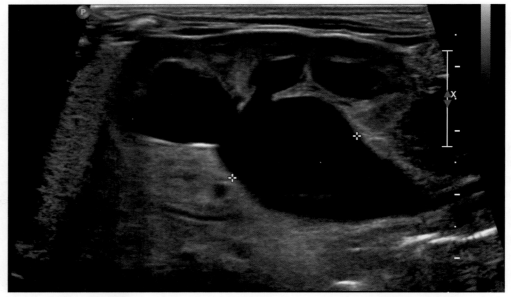

Fig. 7.17 Dilated renal pelvis and calyces in a 1-year-old girl who had antenatal hydronephrosis documented on ultrasonography.

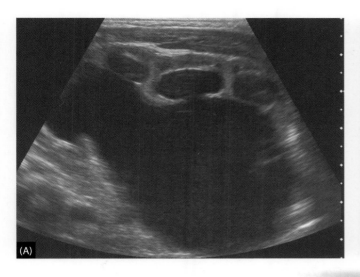
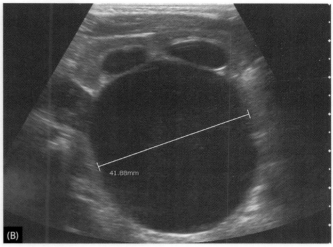

90–150 sec image with ROIs

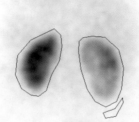

Height = 136 cm
Weight = 40 kg
Age = 7 yrs
BSA = 1.21 sq m

TECHNETIUM RESULTS

	LEFT	RIGHT	TOTAL
MAG3 Gates	174.1	122	296.1
Derived ERPF	328.5	230.1	558.7
Derived GFR	65.7	46	111.7
% Function	58.8	41.2	

LASIX ADMIN @ 15 MINS

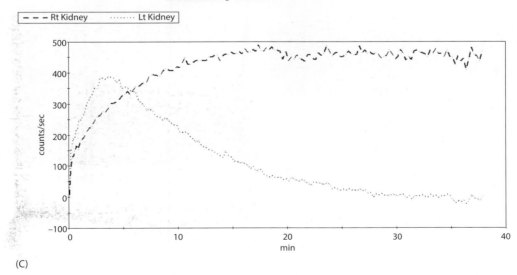

(C)

Figs. 7.18A–C (A) A 6-day-old infant with severe hydronephrosis caused by pelviureteric junction obstruction. The degree of distension seen on this ultrasound scan suggests that the function may be compromised (and that pyeloplasty is needed), which would be determined by nuclear scan. (B) Another view on ultrasound showing an almost spherical pelvis, consistent with significant obstruction. (C) Same patient showing the reduced function in the obstructed right kidney on nuclear scan, suggesting that pyeloplasty would be helpful.

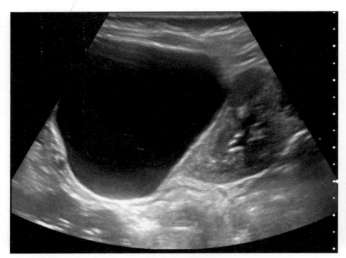

Fig. 7.19 Massive hydronephrosis of the upper pole in a duplex kidney seen on ultrasound scan; the lower pole is relatively unaffected.

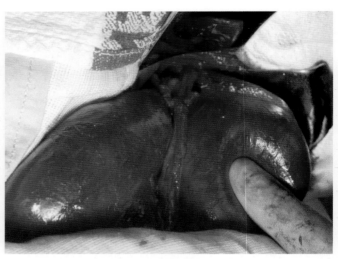

Fig. 7.20 Operative photograph of a horseshoe kidney with a bridge of kidney joining the two sides. The surgeon's finger is pressed against the dilated renal pelvis. Hydronephrosis in a horseshoe kidney is common because the ureter tends to be compressed as it courses across the front of the kidney.

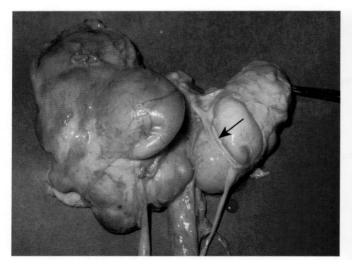

Fig. 7.21 Hydronephrosis in a horseshoe kidney in a postmortem specimen. The dilated pelvicalyceal systems on both sides are evident with the left renal vessels causing pelviureteric junction obstruction (arrow). The small calibre ureter distal to the obstruction is seen.

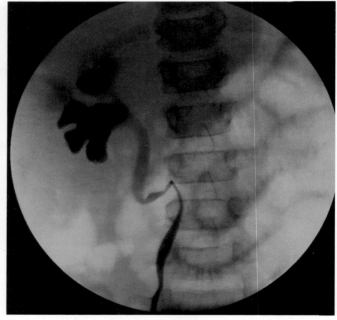

Fig. 7.22 A 7-year-old boy presented with intermittent right-sided abdominal pain and was found to have right hydronephrosis. On a MAG3 scan there was delayed drainage from the right kidney, with an obstruction in the upper ureter, but below the pelviureteric junction. This retrograde pyelogram shows the ureter passing behind the inferior vena cava.

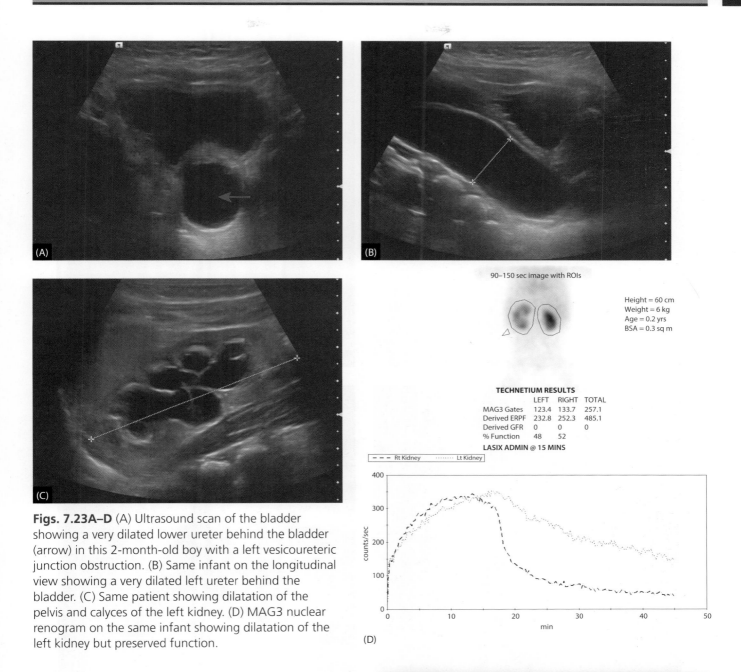

90–150 sec image with ROIs

Height = 60 cm
Weight = 6 kg
Age = 0.2 yrs
BSA = 0.3 sq m

TECHNETIUM RESULTS

	LEFT	RIGHT	TOTAL
MAG3 Gates	123.4	133.7	257.1
Derived ERPF	232.8	252.3	485.1
Derived GFR	0	0	0
% Function	48	52	

LASIX ADMIN @ 15 MINS

--- Rt Kidney .... Lt Kidney

Figs. 7.23A–D (A) Ultrasound scan of the bladder showing a very dilated lower ureter behind the bladder (arrow) in this 2-month-old boy with a left vesicoureteric junction obstruction. (B) Same infant on the longitudinal view showing a very dilated left ureter behind the bladder. (C) Same patient showing dilatation of the pelvis and calyces of the left kidney. (D) MAG3 nuclear renogram on the same infant showing dilatation of the left kidney but preserved function.

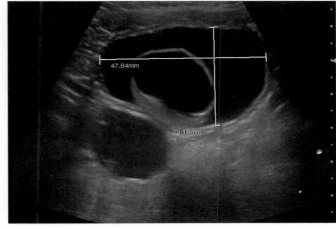

Fig. 7.24 A large ureterocele is seen on this transverse view of the bladder. A dilated ureter is seen behind the bladder on the right side. A ureterocele as large as this is at risk of prolapse into the urethra and causing bladder outlet obstruction.

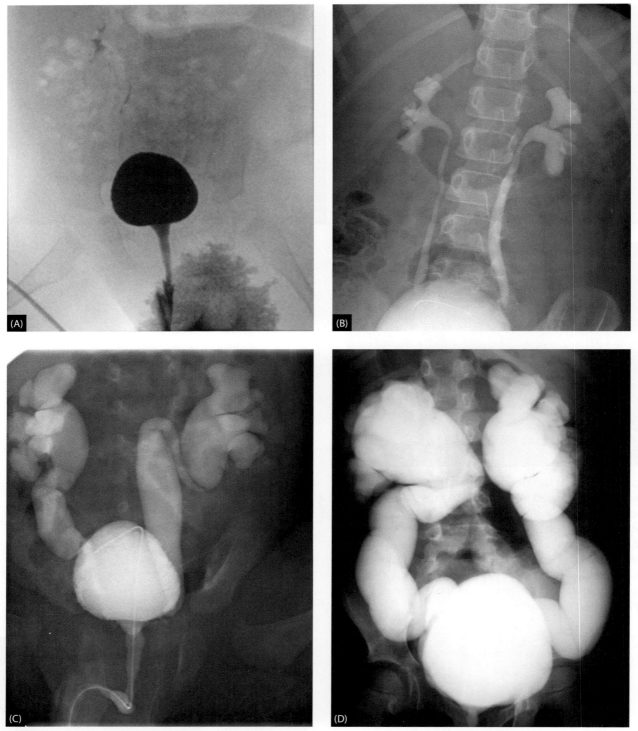

Figs. 7.25A–D (A) Micturating cystourethrogram (MCU) in a 6-month-old girl with grade 2/5 vesicoureteric reflux (VUR), showing a trace of contrast reaching the non-dilated pelvis on the right side. (B) MCU in a 6-year-old girl showing grade 3/5 VUR with contrast reaching the dilated pelvis and calyces. (C) VUR grade 4/5 on MCU. (D) Grade 5 bilateral VUR. This infant has dysplastic kidneys and ureters with severe reflux. Note the tortuous ureters.

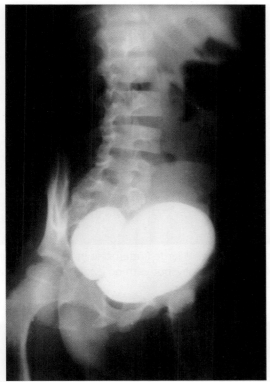

Fig. 7.26 Posterior bladder diverticulum as it appears on a lateral view during micturating cystourethrography.

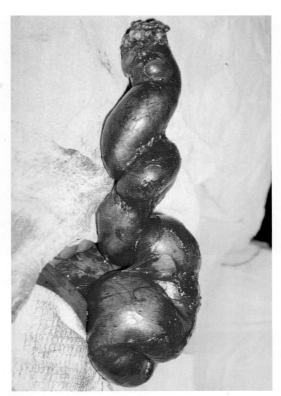

Fig. 7.27 Giant megaureter crowned by a small non-functioning dysplastic left kidney.

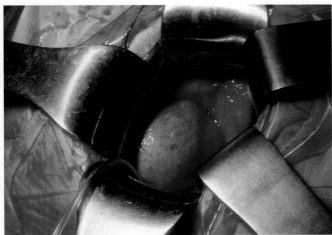

Fig. 7.28 Operative appearance of a moderately large ureterocele in the bladder.

Fig. 7.29 Massive ureterocele in an infant with duplex kidneys, shown at postmortem. The ureterocele opening is not visible, but may be in the bladder neck. The orthotopic left ureteric orifice is visible (arrow).

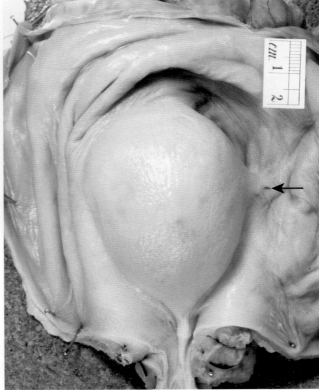
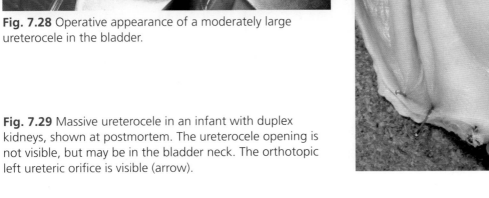

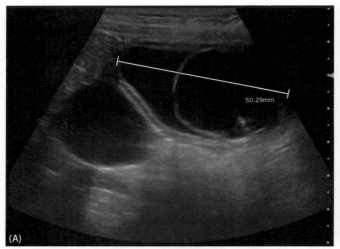

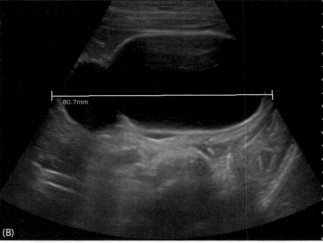

Figs. 7.30A, B (A) Longitudinal view on ultrasound scan of the bladder in a boy with a large ureterocele in the bladder and a dilated ureter behind the bladder. (B) Same infant showing dilatation of the right kidney, but with no evidence on this scan of a duplex.

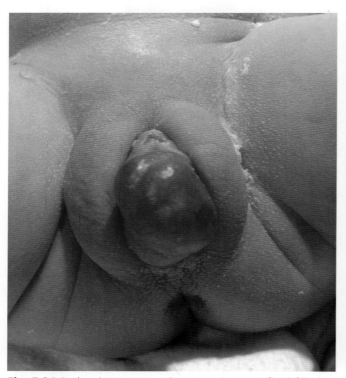

Fig. 7.31 Prolapsing ureterocele presenting as a fluid-filled mucosal swelling in the introitus.

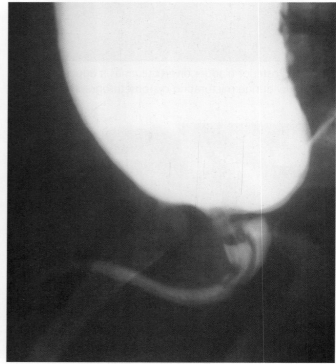

Fig. 7.32 Lateral view of a prolapsing ureterocele causing a filling defect in the proximal urethra. The contrast was introduced through a catheter, which can be seen still in the urethra.

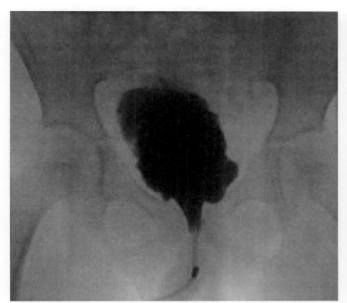

Fig. 7.33 Fluoroscopic image during urodynamics of a 9-year-old boy with a neurogenic bladder, showing a partially open bladder neck and a small volume, trabeculated bladder.

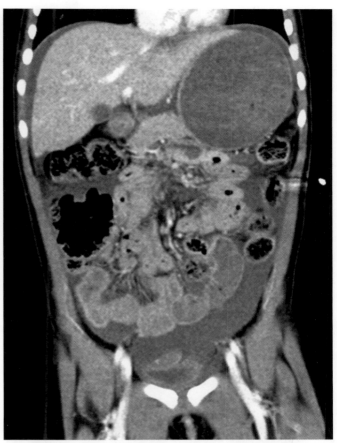

Fig. 7.34 Urinary ascites on CT scan in a child with a perforated neurogenic bladder, which is one of the complications of clean intermittent catheterisation.

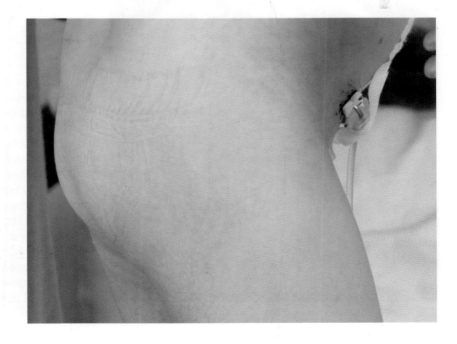

Fig. 7.35 Lateral view of the buttocks in a boy with sacral agenesis and a neurogenic bladder, showing a very flattened natal cleft. The natal cleft has been replaced by fat between the atrophic gluteal muscles. Note the presence of a Chait caecostomy button in a recently created appendix stoma for antegrade enemas to manage his chronic constipation.

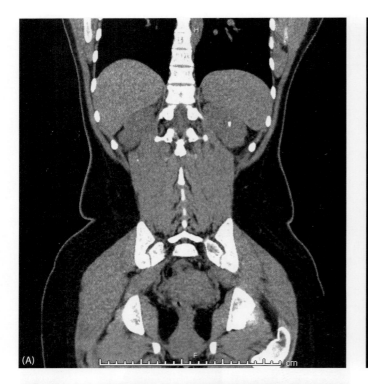

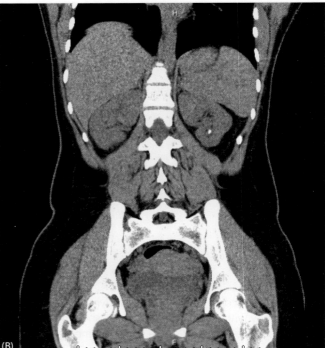

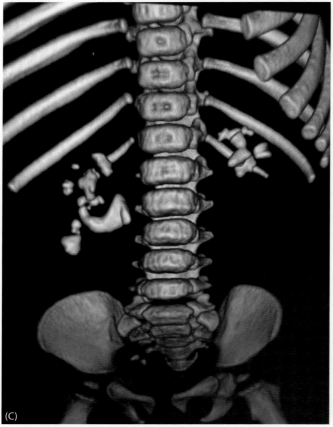

Figs. 7.36A–G (A) CT showing a stone in the left kidney in a 17-year-old girl. (B) Another image of the same patient demonstrating another stone in the lower pole calyx. (C) CT reconstruction without contrast showing multiple stones in the left kidney but also a few small fragments in the right kidney, in a 17-year-old girl with a stone-forming diathesis. (D) Her 15-year-old sibling also had a stone, probably in the pelvis or upper ureter. (E) CT scan of the same sibling showing the stone in the renal pelvis or upper ureter. (F) Renal ultrasound scan showing a stone in the right kidney in a 12-year-old boy. Improvement in ultrasound imaging means that a stone no longer always casts an acoustic shadow. (G) CT without contrast showing a stone in the left renal pelvis in a 15-year-old boy.

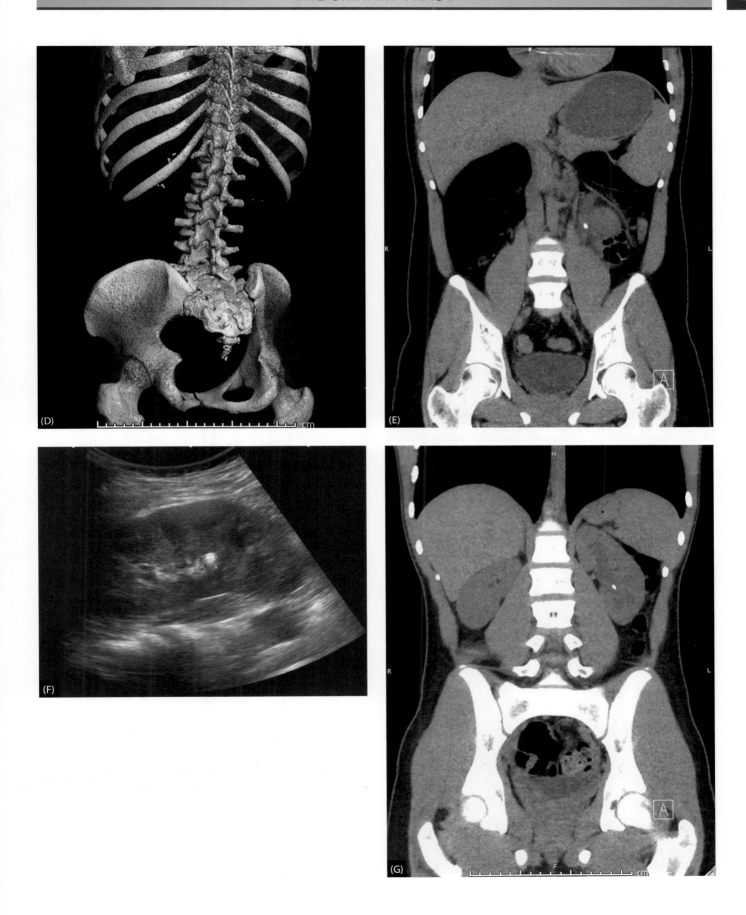

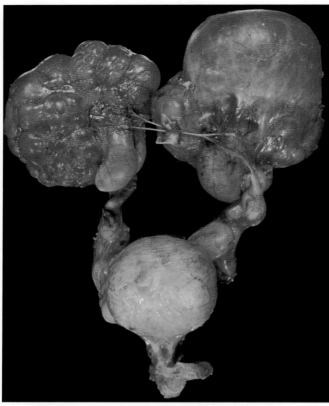

Fig. 7.37 Postmortem specimen of the renal tract in posterior urethral valve. The urethral obstruction has caused bilateral ureteric diverticula, bilateral vesicoureteric reflux, hydronephrosis and renal failure. This infant with Potter syndrome, secondary to the urethral obstruction, died shortly after birth from respiratory insufficiency.

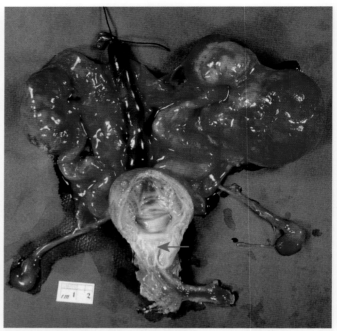

Fig. 7.38 Type 1 posterior urethral valve. A postmortem specimen of a baby who died of Potter syndrome secondary to posterior urethral obstruction. The intra-abdominal testes were prevented from entering the inguinal canals by the over-distended bladder. The urethra has been opened ventrally to reveal the large verumontanum with two posterior urethral valve leaflets extending from its inferior margin (arrow). The bladder is thick-walled and trabeculated and the ureters open into diverticula. The tortuous megaureters connect with dysplastic, hydronephrotic kidneys.

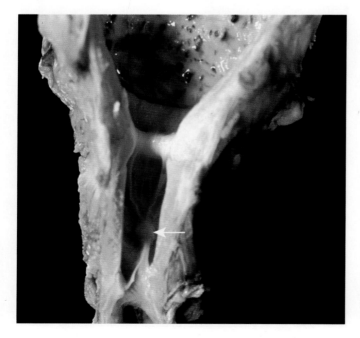

Fig. 7.39 Close-up view of the verumontanum (arrow) below which extend two posterior urethral valve leaflets. The bladder is thick-walled.

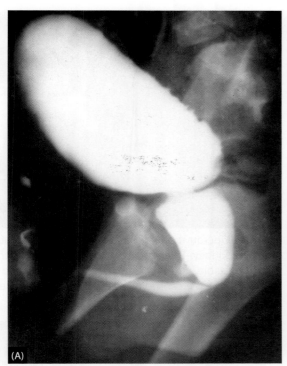
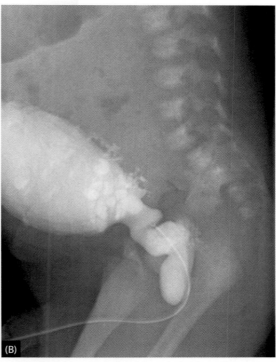

Figs. 7.40A, B (A) Posterior urethral valve (type 3). A micturating cystourethrogram (MCU) in a baby boy, demonstrating the persisting remnant of the urogenital membrane low in the posterior urethra. In normal development, the urogenital membrane covers the urogenital sinus and disintegrates around completion of the 7th week of development. Abnormal persistence is suggested to give rise to the obstructing valve leaflets, which here have caused massive proximal dilatation of the urethra and a trabeculated bladder. (B) Another posterior urethral valve demonstrated in an MCU. The posterior urethra is markedly dilated and tortuous above the level of the valve, and there is severe trabeculation of the bladder.

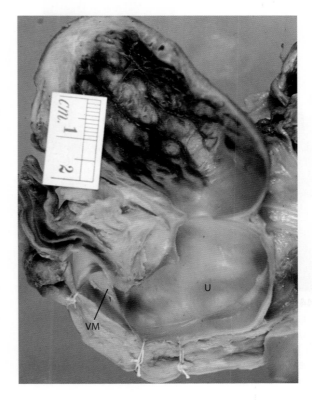

Fig. 7.41 Type 3 posterior urethral valve. A sagittal section of a postmortem specimen showing the obstructed thick-walled and haemorrhagic bladder. Below the bladder is a massively dilated posterior urethra (U). The verumontanum with its inferior crista (VM, arrow) is not as prominent as in type 1 valves. Near the urethral bulb is a windsock membrane with a central small opening (arrow) and a post-stenotic dilatation. This membranous obstruction is attributed to persistence of the urogenital membrane.

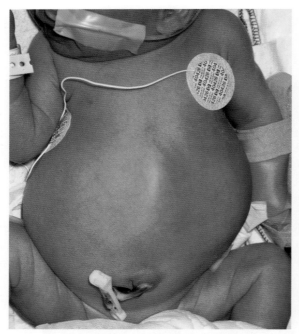

Fig. 7.42 Severe urethral or ureteric obstruction may lead to dysplasia during development of the kidney, and a multicystic kidney. This may be evident at birth by abdominal distension and palpable renal masses. This infant had a huge irregular mass in the left flank, which was the cause of the abdominal distension.

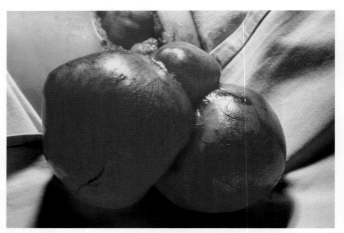

Fig. 7.43 Operative photograph showing a multicystic dysplastic kidney. The cysts are of variable size and there is no recognisable kidney outline. Severe dysplasia and cyst formation is often caused by atresia of the upper ureter.

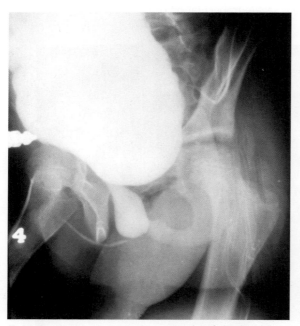

Fig. 7.44 A percutaneous contrast study of the bladder and urethra in an infant with type 1 posterior urethral valve. The needle can be seen entering a dilated and irregular bladder. The bladder neck is relatively well preserved but the posterior urethra is grossly dilated as far as the urethral valve. The anterior urethra is narrow.

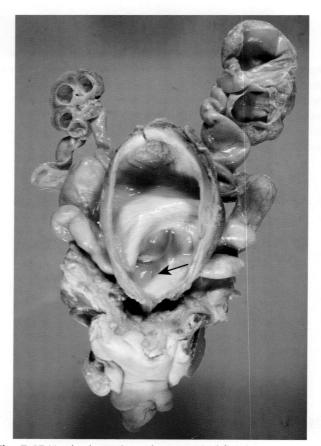

Fig. 7.45 Urethral atresia and rectovesical fistula. A postmortem specimen of a baby with an anorectal malformation in whom the urethral atresia forced the urine to drain through a rectovesical fistula (arrow). There are massive megaureters. The urethral obstruction caused gross cystic dysplasia of the kidneys and led to the child's death from Potter syndrome.

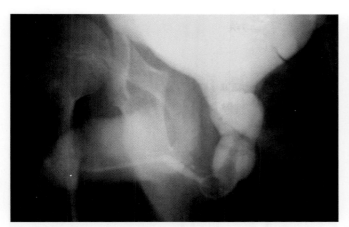

Fig. 7.46 Urethral polyp. A micturating cystourethrogram shows proximal dilatation of the posterior urethra and bladder with a narrow anterior urethra. A large polyp is visible occluding the bulbar urethra. The polyp is on a narrow stalk coming from the region of the verumontanum.

Fig. 7.47 Urethral polyp in an 8-year-old boy who presented with haematuria and intermittent difficulty passing urine. The polyp was found to be arising from the verumontanum.

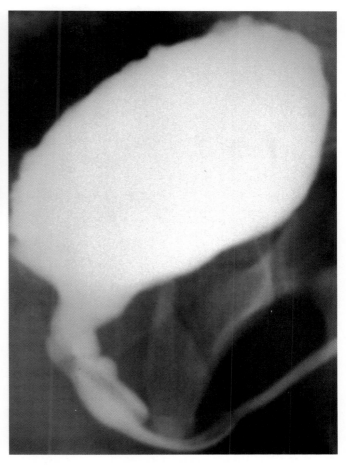

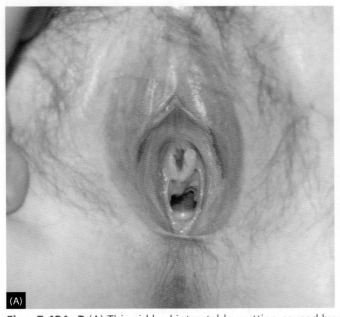

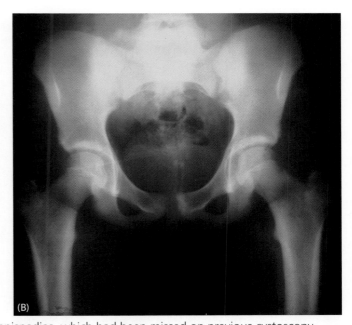

Figs. 7.48A, B (A) This girl had intractable wetting caused by epispadias, which had been missed on previous cystoscopy. Examination of the vestibule shows the abnormal U-shape of the urethral orifice caused by deficiency of the urethral sphincter anteriorly. (B) Plain radiograph of another girl with epispadias, which was also unrecognised at birth and presented with intractable wetting later in childhood. The wide gap between the pubic bones can be seen.

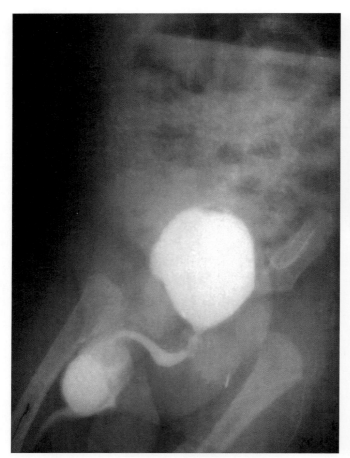

Fig. 7.49 Large anterior urethral diverticulum on urethrography.

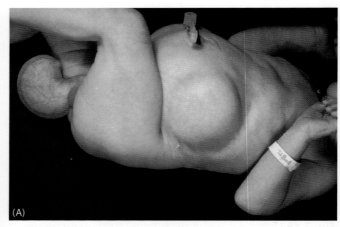

(A)

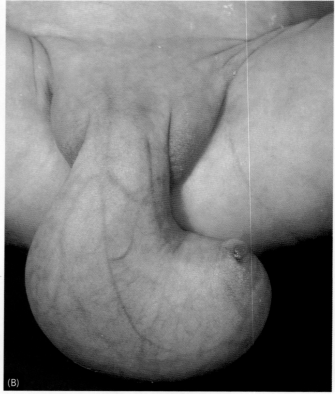

(B)

Figs. 7.50A, B Megalourethra in an infant with deficiency of the abdominal wall musculature (prune belly syndrome). A megalourethra is commonly associated with prune belly syndrome.

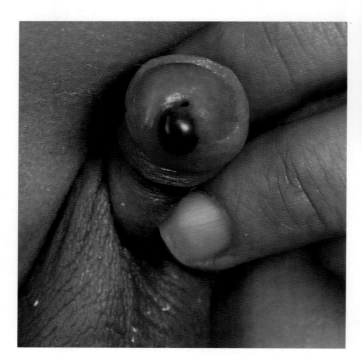

Fig. 7.51 Lateral cystic distal urethral duplication. This small boy presented with a 'blood blister' adjacent to his orthotopic urethral meatus, from haemorrhage into a cystic duplication.

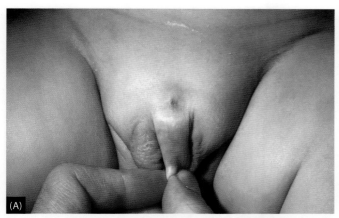 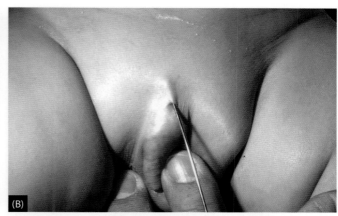

Figs. 7.52A, B Congenital prepubic urethral sinus. This may be a variant of a dorsal duplication of the urethra. The tract extended as far as the bladder wall but did not communicate with the lumen of the bladder.

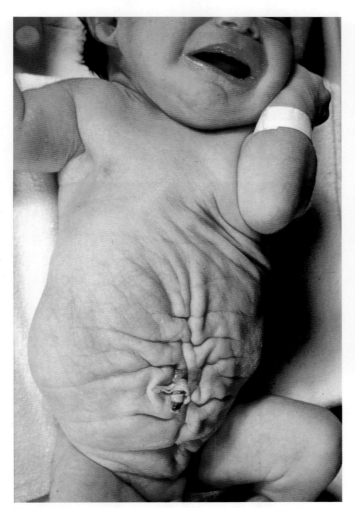

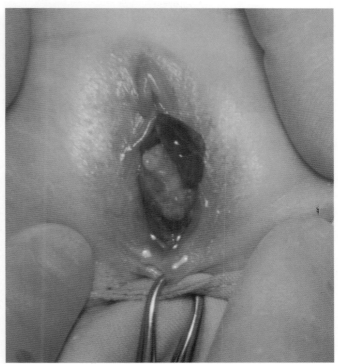

Fig. 7.54 Rhabdomyosarcoma, presenting as a growth appearing from the urethra. It needs to be distinguished from a urethral polyp, prolapse of the urethral mucosa and a prolapsing ureterocele.

Fig. 7.53 Prune belly syndrome. Prune belly is caused by *in-utero* transient obstruction (10–20 weeks' gestation) of the urethra between its penile and glanular parts. This caused massive dilatation proximal to the obstruction, including the wrinkled appearance of the abdomen, which is seen after birth.

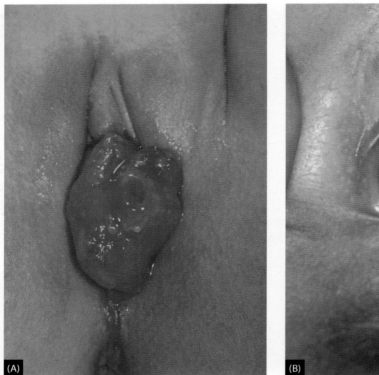
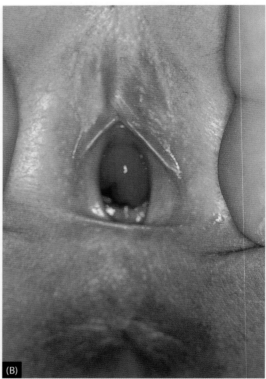

Figs. 7.55A, B (A) Urethral prolapse in a small girl. The urethral opening is in the middle of the prolapse. (B) Urethral prolapse of short duration.

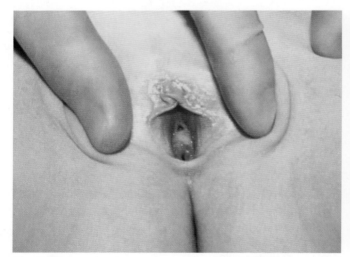

Fig. 7.56 A prolapsing ureterocele. It should be distinguished from urethral mucosal prolapse, urethral polyp and rhabdomyosarcoma protruding through the urethra.

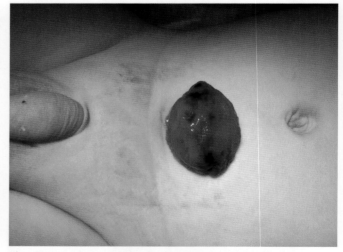

Fig. 7.57 Prolapsing vesicostomy in a boy who has a posterior urethral valve.

FEMALE GENITALIA AND GYNAECOLOGICAL CONDITIONS

Labial adhesions are an acquired condition of the labia minora, most likely from ulceration of the labia with subsequent adhesion formation during re-epithelialisation. They are usually discovered on routine examination, but may cause discomfort on micturition or a small amount of dampness after micturition if the fusion is almost complete. This condition may be misdiagnosed as being congenital absence of the vagina, a mistake that can cause parents much unnecessary anxiety. Labial adhesions are never observed at birth.

Developmental abnormalities are rare in girls. Imperforate hymen presents either at birth, when mucus secreted by the vagina accumulates beneath a bulging imperforate hymen to form a mucocolpos, or at puberty, with amenorrhoea and haematocolpos or haematometrocolpos, with or without cyclical attacks of abdominal pain. Removal of the membrane provides drainage and relief of symptoms.

In menarchal or pubertal girls, a variety of gynaecological problems may cause abdominal symptoms, including the exaggerated intraperitoneal bleeding of ovulation (Mittelschmerz bleeding), rupture of a small luteal cyst, tubal menstruation, torsion of the ovary, acute salpingitis and primary peritonitis. A pelvic ultrasound scan can detect even small ovarian cysts. Clinically, the distinction between rupture of a follicular or luteal cyst and acute pelvic appendicitis can be difficult. Simple ovarian cysts in the neonate often involute spontaneously.

PERINEAL MASSES

A number of masses may appear in the perineum, particularly in girls. They may appear from the urethra or the vaginal opening, and the external appearance may give little clue to the diagnosis. For example, a rhabdomyosarcoma protruding through the urethra may have a similar appearance to that of a urethral polyp, prolapse of the urethral mucosa or a prolapsing ureterocele. A lesion bulging from the vaginal introitus is more likely to be a rhabdomyosarcoma. This can be distinguished easily from the bulging hymen seen in the neonate with vaginal atresia.

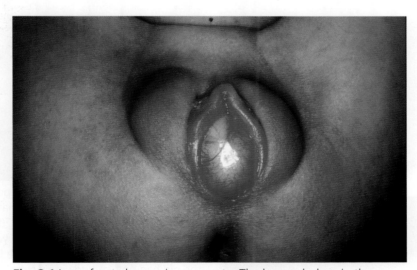

Fig. 8.1 Imperforate hymen in a neonate. The hymen bulges in the introitus because of distension of the vagina by mucus. Absence of maternal hormonal stimulation of mucus production after birth will allow spontaneous resorption of the mucus. However, it will re-present at the onset of puberty with haematometrocolpos. Treatment at birth is by simple incision of the hymen.

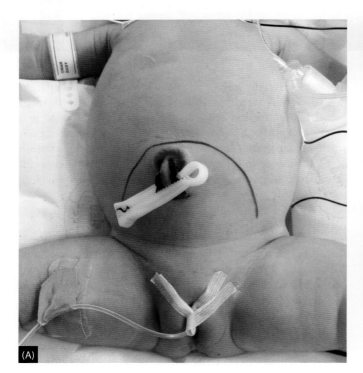

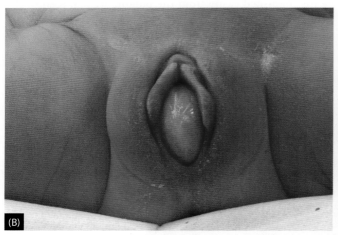

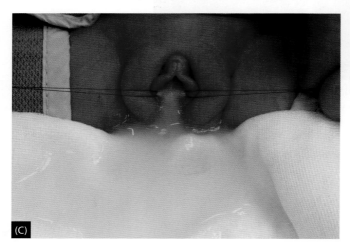

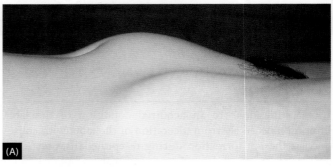

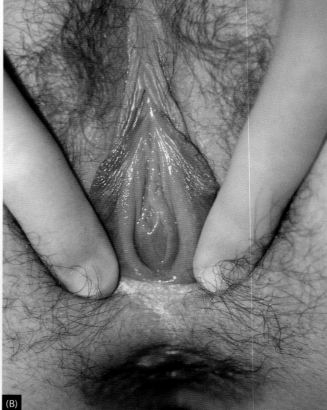

Figs. 8.3A, B (A) Haematometrocolpos in a 13-year-old girl who presented with lower abdominal pain and a mass that was easily palpable on examination. (B) On inspection of the perineum and introitus a blue tinge was visible beneath the bulging imperforate hymen. Despite being well into puberty, the girl had not yet knowingly started menstruating.

Figs. 8.2A–C (A) Mucometrocolpos presenting in an infant with a distended abdomen as a mass extending from the pelvis (the pen marking outlines its upper limit). (B) Examination of the perineum in the same baby reveals a bulging hymen and a vagina filled with mucus. (C) Incision of the imperforate hymen allowed drainage of a large volume of mucus.

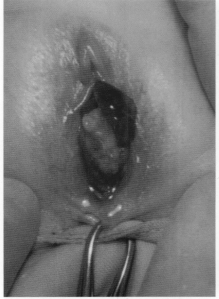

Fig. 8.4 Rhabdomyosarcoma, presenting as a growth appearing from the urethra. It needs to be distinguished from (1) a urethral polyp, (2) prolapse of the urethral mucosa and (3) a prolapsing ureterocele.

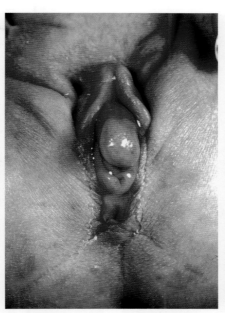

Fig. 8.5 Urethral polyp. The baby presented with a pedunculated polyp in the introitus, which was shown to be arising from the urethral meatus.

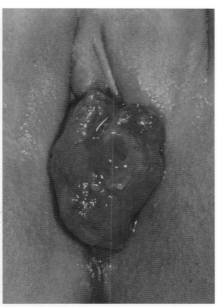

Fig. 8.6 Urethral prolapse in a small girl. The urethral opening is in the middle of the prolapse.

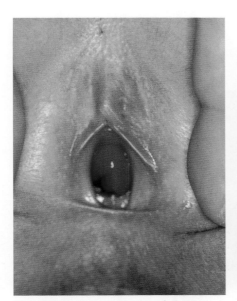

Fig. 8.7 Urethral prolapse of short duration, with less ulceration than in **Fig. 8.6.**

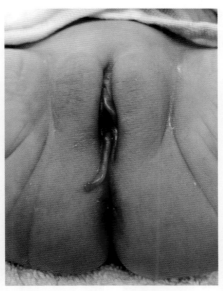

Fig. 8.8 Vaginal fibroepithelial polyp in a baby.

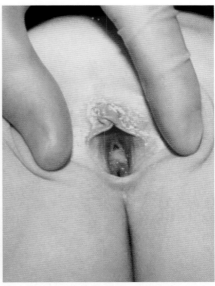

Fig. 8.9 A prolapsing ureterocele. It should be distinguished from urethral mucosal prolapse, urethral polyp and rhabdomyosarcoma protruding from the urethra.

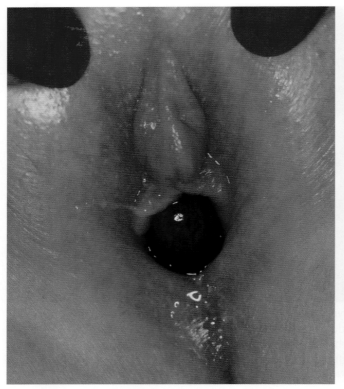

Fig. 8.10 Vaginal rhabdomyosarcoma. This 2-year-old girl presented with a mass protruding from the vagina, which was shown to be a tumour arising from the vault of the vagina.

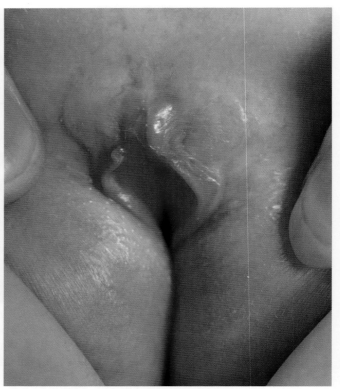

Fig. 8.11 Median cleft extending from the umbilicus to the clitoris; this is best considered a variant of epispadias.

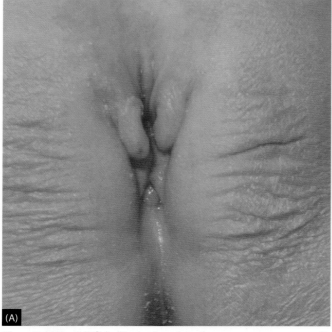

(A)

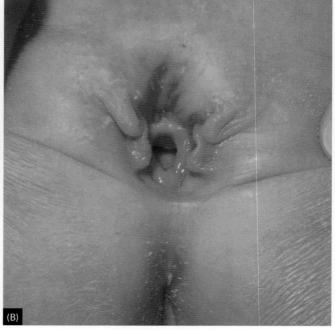

(B)

Figs. 8.12A, B Bifid clitoris showing the appearance normally (A) and with lateral retraction of the labia majora (B).

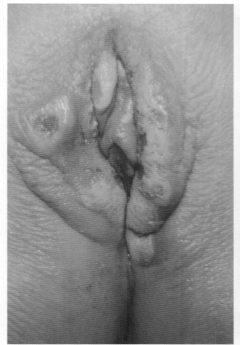

Fig. 8.13 Vulval ulcers may develop as a result of 'nappy rash' with local excoriation, or be the result of sexual abuse.

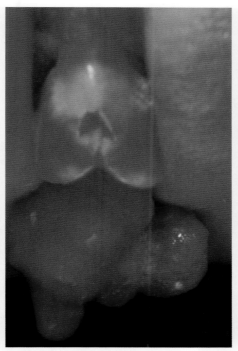

Fig. 8.14 A protuberant haemangioma of the vulva. This should be distinguished from a rhabdomyosarcoma.

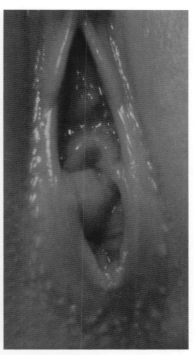

Fig. 8.15 A girl with an imperforate hymen between a normal urethral meatus and a rectovestibular fistula.

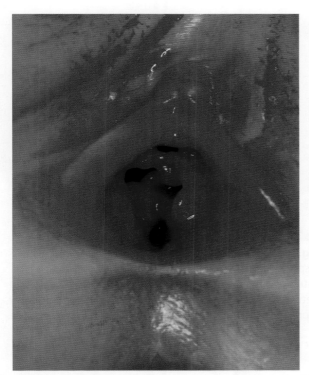

Fig. 8.16 Rectovestibular fistula in an introitus with a double vagina, producing four openings along with the urethra.

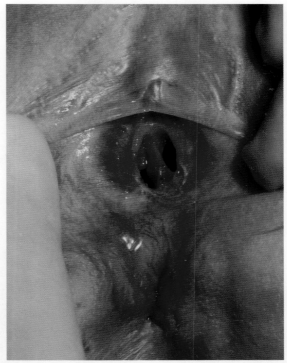

Fig. 8.17 Septate vagina. The sagittal vaginal septum extended upwards about 2 cm. The vagina and uterus were otherwise normal.

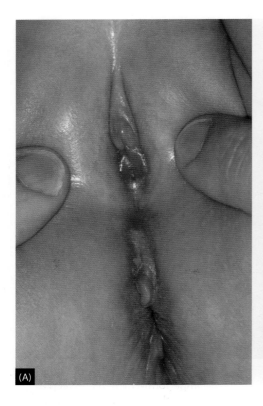

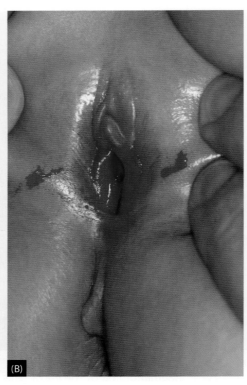

Figs. 8.18A, B (A) Labial adhesions are a common acquired condition of the labia minora, and are believed to occur when irritation and ulceration of the labia results in secondary adhesion between each labium minora during re-epithelialisation. (B) Same patient: the appearance following separation of the labia for labial adhesions. The raw area of the inner surface of each labium minora has caused minor bleeding. The introitus is now fully visible. Recurrence is common unless prevented by application of vaseline and regular sitz baths to prevent enteric flora colonising the skin.

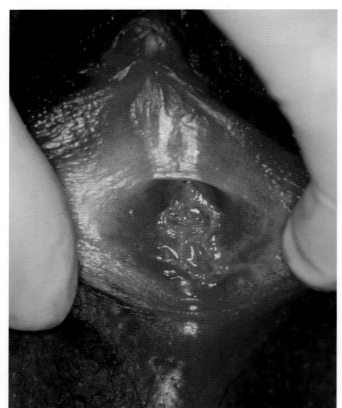

Fig. 8.19 Imperforate hymen may present at puberty with amenorrhoea and haematocolpos or haematometrocolpos.

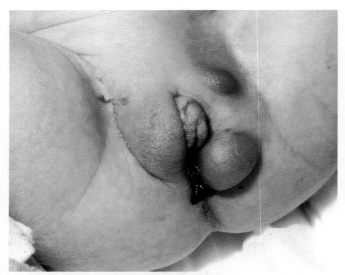

Fig. 8.20 An infant with a cloacal anomaly and partially displaced labium majora, which is likely to be caused by external pressure from the heel of the fetus. The pale skin between the two parts of the left labium majora probably represents scarring after healing of the fetal pressure sore.

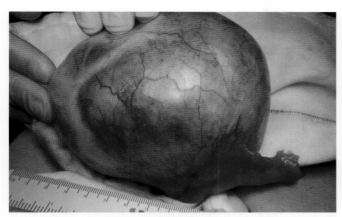

Fig. 8.21 Operative appearance of a large ovarian teratoma. These may be malignant.

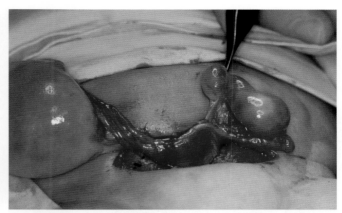

Fig. 8.22 Operative appearance of bilateral simple ovarian cysts exposed through a Pfannenstiel incision. Simple ovarian cysts are not infrequent in the neonate and may be diagnosed antenatally on ultrasonography. They tend to involute spontaneously, although large cysts (>5 cm) are at risk of torsion. They may be caused by maternal stimulation of the ovarian follicles *in utero*.

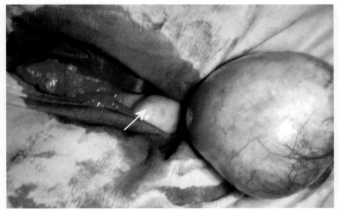

Fig. 8.23 A large follicular cyst of the ovary in a child presenting with precocious puberty. The normal contralateral ovary is arrowed.

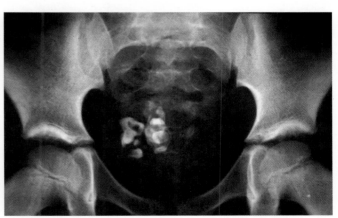

Fig. 8.24 A small ovarian teratoma with bone and teeth. These tumours commonly present in adolescence with abdominal pain secondary to torsion of the enlarged ovary.

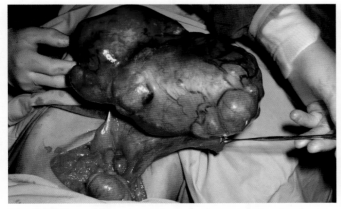

Fig. 8.25 Operative appearance of a large ovarian teratoma. These may be malignant as in this case.

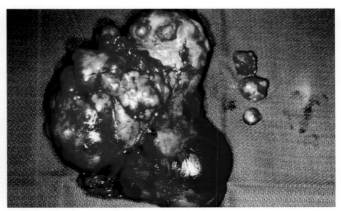

Fig. 8.26 A resected ovarian teratoma in which three 'teeth' have been removed.

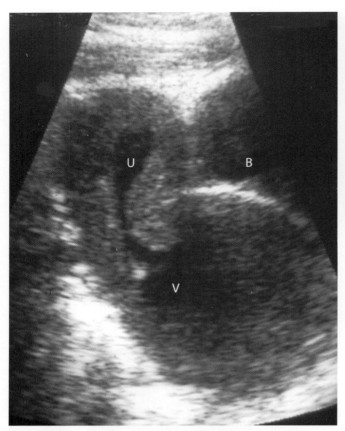

Fig. 8.27 Ultrasound scan of a pubertal girl with an imperforate hymen showing gross distension of the vagina with blood, with the bladder in front of it. U, uterus, V, vagina, B, bladder.

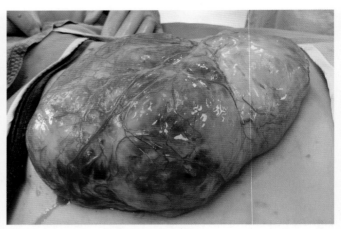

Fig. 8.28 Operative appearance of an ovarian Sertoli–Leydig cell tumour in an 11-year-old girl. These are rare sex-cord stromal tumours containing testicular tissues that produce androgens and may lead to virilising features. They may be benign or malignant.

The limbs and soft tissues | CHAPTER 9

HIPS

Congenital dysplasia with dislocation of the hip leads to severe deformity and abnormal gait unless it is recognised and treated shortly after birth. For this reason, it must be looked for actively at birth by clinical use of the Ortolani test: in a relaxed and warm baby the pelvis is held between the finger and thumb of one hand while the other hand holds the thigh with the thumb in the groin anteriorly and the fingers on the greater trochanter posteriorly. After flexion of the hip to 90 degrees it is abducted to 45 degrees, where forward pressure from the fingers will push a dislocated femoral head back into the acetabulum. Conversely, backward pressure will tend to dislocate the head posteriorly. Relocation of the femoral head may be associated with an audible and palpable 'clunk'. If clinical examination at birth produces an equivocal finding, the child should have an ultrasound scan of the hip joints and be referred to a specialist paediatric orthopaedic surgeon for a second opinion. Failure to diagnose congenital dysplasia +/− dislocation of the hip at birth is a serious error.

PERTHES DISEASE

Perthes disease is a form of osteochondritis in which there is partial or complete loss of the blood supply of the femoral head leading to aseptic necrosis but with preservation of the cartilaginous articular surface. This is followed by revascularisation. The femoral head becomes compressed and dense, and the child develops an intermittent painless limp and ill-defined aches in the legs. There is restriction of abduction in flexion, adduction in flexion and internal rotation. Long-standing disease produces wasting of the gluteal muscles, shortening of the limb and a positive Trendelenburg test. Radiography of the hip is diagnostic. The natural history is one of resolution over months and initial treatment may require bed rest with elevation of the legs in spring-loaded traction. Perthes disease should be distinguished from the 'irritable hip', multiple epiphyseal dysplasia (which is bilateral), tuberculosis of the hip and avascular necrosis of the femoral head in juvenile chronic arthritis.

SLIPPED UPPER FEMORAL EPIPHYSIS

In adolescent boys, particularly those who are obese, the upper femoral epiphysis may slip off the femoral neck downwards and posteriorly. This presents either insidiously or acutely with pain and a limp and the leg held in external rotation. Radiographs may be difficult to interpret unless good lateral views are taken to show the position of the epiphysis. In minor cases, bed rest may be sufficient treatment, although more severe forms require pinning of the epiphysis to prevent any further slippage.

Osgood–Schlatter disease affects the tibial tuberosity in early adolescence. Partial avulsion of the tuberosity leads to a painful and tender swelling. Less common forms of osteochondritis juvenilis include Köhler disease of the tarsal navicular and Panner disease of the humeral capitulum.

LEGS

Compression *in utero* can cause significant deformities in the legs, and may be secondary to anomalies in the fetus or an abnormal uterus.

Bow legs are seen frequently in early infancy but rarely require treatment, as the shaft of the tibia straightens with growth. Between 3 and 5 years, knock knees may become apparent as the medial femoral condyle grows a little faster than the lateral condyle. By 7 years of age, growth of the lateral condyle has caught up, re-establishing a horizontal knee joint and resolution of the knock knees.

In-toeing is a minor deformity, where the toes point medially. It can be caused by inset hips (femoral anteversion), internal tibial torsion or metatarsus adductus.

FEET

Flat feet is a common minor defect. In infancy, a thick fat pad in the sole may give the impression of a flat foot even though the arch is normal. Loose ligaments in infancy may suggest a flat foot but walking on tiptoes restores the normal arch.

Pes cavus, or a high arch to the foot, may be due to a minor inherited anomaly or may develop secondary to an unrecognised neurological disorder, such as tethering of the spinal cord. Neurological problems can be excluded by general examination and the Gower test, where the child sits on the floor and is asked to stand up. If there is leg weakness, the child can stand only by using the hands as well as the legs.

Talipes equinovarus may be secondary to postural compression of the foot during the third trimester or an underlying neurological defect (e.g. spina bifida), but is more often an intrinsic abnormality of the foot. The forefoot is adducted and the entire foot is inverted and supinated. If clinical examination reveals limitation of passive movement, immediate treatment is required since the joints are lax in the first few weeks after birth, allowing rapid correction by serial casting or splints.

Talipes calcaneovalgus may be associated with congenital dysplasia and dislocation of the hip. It is usually a simple postural abnormality that recovers shortly after birth and rarely a severe intrinsic deformity.

Abnormalities of the toes include syndactyly and polydactyly, hammer toes, hallux valgus and various forms of local gigantism.

HANDS AND FINGERS

Trigger thumb, which is often bilateral, is caused by a fusiform swelling of the flexor pollicis longus tendon opposite the metacarpophalangeal joint, which is being restricted in its range of movement by a narrow tendon sheath. The swelling is palpable as a hard nodule. Flexion of the thumb is full, but active extension may be prevented by the tendon swelling within the constricting sheath. Passive extension may produce an audible or palpable snap.

Other abnormalities of the fingers include incomplete separation of the digits (syndactyly), congenital duplication of the digits (polydactyly) and abnormalities of growth of the digits producing abnormally bent fingers. Syndactyly may be part of an inherited syndrome, such as Apert syndrome. Aplasia or hypoplasia of the radius may occur, often in association with oesophageal atresia or an anorectal malformation, as part of the VACTERL (Vertebral defects, Anorectal malformations, Cardiac defects, Tracheo-oEsophageal fistula, Renal anomalies, and Limb abnormalities) association.

SCOLIOSIS

Scoliosis, or lateral curvature of the spine, may be compensatory, postural or structural in origin. The distinction can be made on clinical examination. Compensatory scoliosis may occur secondary to a variety of conditions, including torticollis, unequal leg length or, occasionally, following thoracotomy involving rib resection, where chest asymmetry has developed. Structural scoliosis is often associated with a degree of kyphosis and has a number of causes including hemivertebrae, fractured vertebrae or neurological imbalance, or it is idiopathic (commonest). Kyphoscoliosis may occur in certain dysplasias of bone.

OSTEOMYELITIS

Organisms may reach the metaphysis of a long bone from the blood or a local injury, producing local pain and tenderness and loss of spontaneous movement. If the infection is unrecognised and not treated, progression of the disease may produce elevation of the periosteum to form an abscess and even ischaemic necrosis of the adjacent bone to form a sequestrum. Late signs of osteomyelitis include severe generalised signs of toxicity and an immobile limb with obvious tenderness and swelling. There may be fluctuance over a subperiosteal abscess. Delayed diagnosis is common in neonates because of poor localising signs. In adolescents it may be misdiagnosed initially as a sprain. The child will have signs of sepsis and local tenderness on percussion or compression of the involved bone, with an effusion in the neighbouring joint. There may be enlarged lymph nodes and splenomegaly. Cultures of the blood and subperiosteal abscess should be taken. *Staphylococcus aureus* is the usual organism, although *Haemophilus influenzae* and *Streptococcus* spp. also may be responsible.

SEPTIC ARTHRITIS

The signs and symptoms of septic arthritis are similar to those of osteomyelitis. The pain and tenderness are localised over the distended capsule of the joint and there is restriction of all movement. In infants the inflammatory signs may spread to the overlying skin. The treatment of septic arthritis is surgical lavage of the joint cavity and high-dose intravenous antibiotics.

SEMIMEMBRANOSUS BURSA

A semimembranosus bursa lies between the gastrocnemius and the semimembranosus muscle. Enlargement produces a cystic swelling on the medial side of the popliteal fossa. Sometimes, a cyst in this region may be an extension into the popliteal fossa from the knee joint. These lumps are painless, but produce an obvious cosmetic deformity in the extended leg. The cyst resolves spontaneously over some months or years.

GANGLION

A cystic swelling of the tendon sheath is a common abnormality on the wrist or hand, or the foot. Occasionally there may be extrusion of the synovium from within the joint cavity. The lesion may resolve spontaneously.

MISCELLANEOUS DEFORMITIES

There are many rare causes of deformity of the limbs, including limb deficiency. Phocomelia, or telescopic foreshortening or a limb, is a rare congenital abnormality that became well known because it was the characteristic defect produced by thalidomide toxicity in the 1960s. Sprengel shoulder is a rare condition caused by failure of the scapula to descend from its original cervical position in the embryo. Craniocleidodysostosis, and cervical rib are seen occasionally. Scurvy once was common but now is rare. Another rare genetic cause of deformity is osteogenesis imperfecta. Birth injuries or other accidents can produce secondary deformity. In the leg, aplasia of the fibula

may occur as part of the VACTERL association analogous to radial aplasia. Intrauterine compression causes severe growth failure in the leg. Lumps on the toes may be an exostosis or a digital fibroma.

NEOPLASMS

Abnormal bone growth may occur with congenital benign exostosis or simple cyst formation. Aneurysmal bone cyst is an example of more aggressive cystic disease of the bone, and usually presents as a painful, swollen long bone with or without a pathological fracture. Benign tumours are uncommon in childhood: one that presents with severe pain in the bone is osteoid osteoma.

Malignant neoplasms of the bone include osteosarcoma, which usually affects the long bones, or Ewing tumour, which more commonly affects the bones of the trunk. Osteosarcoma presents with pain and swelling, most commonly in the distal femur, proximal tibia or proximal humerus. However, it can occur in any bone and it may be difficult to distinguish from Ewing tumour if it occurs in the pelvis. Plain radiographs show typical features of destruction of the bony cortex with soft tissue swelling and/or ectopic calcification as well as infiltration of the medullary cavity. Dissemination of osteosarcoma is quite common, and lung metastases may appear many years after the primary diagnosis (see Chapter 4).

Ewing tumour is a slightly less aggressive sarcoma affecting the shorter bones of the trunk. A large soft tissue extension of the tumour may be present prior to diagnosis, and initially it may not be obvious that the primary lesion is within a bone. The histological characteristics of Ewing tumour are not dissimilar to those of other small cell tumours such as neuroblastoma, which makes histological confirmation of the diagnosis more difficult. Recently recognised chromosomal translocations have improved diagnostic accuracy. Ewing tumour responds well to chemotherapy, and the aim of treatment is to excise the bone containing the tumour once the soft tissue lesion has resolved. If the lesion arises in a rib this is relatively straightforward; however, in other bones, such as the vertebrae or the pelvis, this may be more difficult.

Rhabdomyosarcoma of the muscles of the limbs or trunk is an important abnormality to distinguish from benign cysts and inflammatory lesions. Any child with a soft tissue swelling that is not immediately recognisable as a congenital cyst or inflammatory lesion should undergo biopsy to exclude rhabdomyosarcoma.

SUPERFICIAL INFECTION

Infection of the skin and subcutaneous tissues is common in children. Certain infections have surgical significance (e.g. hand infections) and failure to treat them promptly and adequately may result in their rapid progression and long-term deformity. Other superficial infections may include mycobacterial ulceration, erysipelas or the mundane ingrown toenail. Skin necrosis may occur because of emboli. Axillary lymphadenopathy is common following minor skin trauma to the arm or hand, and occasionally occurs after thrombosis or BCG vaccination.

VASCULAR ANOMALIES

Vascular anomalies comprise a spectrum of vascular tumours and vascular malformations that range from simple angiomatous birthmarks to life-threatening lesions. Their classification has changed over the years but the International Society for the Study of Vascular Anomalies divides them into two broad groups: vascular tumours (proliferative lesions including common haemangiomas) and vascular malformations (relatively static lesions arising from defective vascular morphogenesis).

Vascular tumours

Most vascular tumours are benign. The most common is the infantile haemangioma (previously known as a 'strawberry naevus'), which appears within the first few weeks of life as a solitary skin lesion (typically a pale pink or bright red spot). Over the next 3–6 months it rapidly increases in size, following which there is a stable period for a year or so before it begins to involute gradually. Most will disappear by the age of 5 years, leaving a small area of redundant pale skin. Infantile haemangiomas may be focal or multifocal and are most commonly found around the head and neck. Rarely, they are segmental and associated with other anomalies (e.g. PHACE syndrome – **P**osterior fossa brain malformations, **H**aemangioma, **A**rterial lesions in the head or neck, **C**ardiac abnormalities/coarctation of the aorta, and **E**ye abnormalities). Cutaneous infantile haemangiomas do not require treatment (e.g. propranolol) unless they interfere with vision: where involvement of the eyelids causes occlusion of the visual axis for even a few weeks it can produce an amblyopic eye. They may also require treatment if they create major problems in management because of bleeding, infection or ulceration (especially with lesions exposed to urine).

Congenital haemangiomas are less common than infantile haemangiomas. They are fully grown at birth and often regress rapidly in infancy (rapidly involuting congenital haemangioma = RICH) but can remain stable in size (noninvoluting congenital haemangioma = NICH) or show only partial regression. Other vascular tumours include the rare Kaposiform haemangioendothelioma, which may involve tissues deep to the skin and behave as a locally aggressive tumour. It can be associated with potentially life-threatening thrombocytopaenia and consumptive coagulopathy (Kasabach–Merritt phenomenon).

A pyogenic granuloma is a reactive proliferation of capillaries that presents as a solitary shiny red skin lump with a raspberry-like irregular surface. They are most common on the head or neck but may be found on the lips, hands and feet, and elsewhere. Pyogenic granulomas are friable and can bleed profusely. In children, development of a pyogenic granuloma may be the result of minor local trauma or infection.

Vascular malformations

Vascular malformations are present at birth and are composed mainly of capillaries, veins, lymphatics, arteries or a combination of vessel types. Simple vascular malformations typically consist of one vessel type:

1   Capillary malformations affect the skin and mucosa (the 'port wine' stain) and are generally persistent throughout life, although those on the forehead and nape of the neck (the so-called 'salmon patch' or 'stork bite') may fade. They may be associated with underlying tissue anomalies such as bone and soft tissue overgrowth or central nervous system and ocular anomalies (Sturge–Weber syndrome).
2   Venous malformations are soft and compressible. They may be focal, multifocal or diffuse (e.g. involving a lower limb or affecting the skin, soft tissue and gut [blue rubber bleb naevus syndrome]).
3   Arteriovenous malformations may be sporadic or occur as part of hereditary haemorrhagic telangiectasia.
4   Lymphatic malformations consist of dilated lymphatic channels and are classified as macrocystic, microcystic and mixed varieties. They are most common in the cervicofacial (previously called cystic hygroma) and axillary regions where they present with soft subcutaneous swellings. Rarely, lymphatic malformations are more widespread involving viscera and bone or causing chylous effusions. Primary lymphoedema is due to lymphatic dysgenesis and is considered to be a subtype of lymphatic malformation.

More complex vascular malformations affect multiple vessel types and may be associated with numerous other anomalies. A good example is Klippel–Trenaunay syndrome in which the lower limb and sometimes the pelvis and abdomen are affected by capillary, venous and lymphatic malformations with soft tissue and limb overgrowth.

VASCULAR OBSTRUCTION

Arterial obstruction may be traumatic, iatrogenic (e.g. a complication of arterial cannulation for diagnostic or monitoring purposes [usually in the neonate]), embolic (including septic emboli) or secondary to vascular compression from a tumour or abscess. Permanent occlusion may cause an acute compartment syndrome, tissue necrosis and subsequent functional impairment.

MELANOCYTIC NAEVI

Melanocytic naevi (moles) may be congenital or acquired and arise as a result of a benign proliferation of melanocyte type cells within the lower epidermis and/or dermis.

Acquired melanocytic naevi are common in children because of a genetic predisposition and/or sun exposure. They are more common in individuals with a light complexion. Lesions vary considerably in appearance but they tend to be round or oval, less than 6 mm in diameter, have a sharp, regular border and be evenly pigmented. They are found typically on the trunk or limbs but may be seen occasionally on the palms or soles or under the nails (causing melanonychia). Acquired melanocytic naevi are classified histologically into three types:

1   Junctional naevi where the nests of melanocytes are at the epidermal/dermal junction.
2   Compound naevi where the melanocytes are also in the dermis.
3   Intradermal naevi where the melanocyte nests are in the dermis. Intradermal naevi produce less melanin and usually manifest as skin-coloured or tan papules.

Pigmented naevi that change significantly in appearance (e.g. enlarge rapidly), develop irregular borders or variable pigmentation require excision biopsy to exclude malignant melanoma (which is rare in children).

A 'halo' naevus is a melanocytic nevus surrounded by a rim of depigmentation. This appearance often heralds spontaneous regression of the naevus by a process thought to involve a T-cell-mediated immune response. A Spitz naevus is a benign pink, tan or red-brown papule that develops on the face or limbs and often causes anxiety because of its initial rapid growth.

Congenital melanocytic naevi are present from birth, may be solitary or multiple, are variable in size and appear as brown or black lesions sometimes containing dark hairs. Rarely, they cover a large area of skin, when they are known as a giant naevus. Because of their distribution, the latter are often referred to as a 'bathing trunk' naevus, although they may be seen on the limbs or scalp; they tend to grow with the child and may become raised and verrucous. These lesions are at high risk of developing a melanoma, which tends to be aggressive and often metastasises.

An ephelis ('freckle') is a a small, light brown or tan mark on the skin, most often seen in individuals with light complexions. Café-au-lait spots are coffee-coloured skin patches. Many children have one or two, but if more than six have developed by the time the child is five years, then neurofibromatosis should be excluded. The Mongolian spot is a classic blue naevus. It is a flat blue/grey birthmark with diffuse margins most often found on the lower back, buttocks or limbs. Mongolian spots may last for months or years, but they usually disappear by the time a child reaches school age. They are harmless and do not need treatment.

Blueberry muffin syndrome refers to a neonate or infant with multiple blue/purple skin nodules. These either arise from clusters of blood-forming cells in the skin (extramedullary erythropoiesis) or from bleeding into the skin (purpura) or cutaneous tumour deposits. The differential diagnosis therefore includes tumours (e.g. leukaemia, neuroblastoma, Langerhan cell histiocytosis), blood disorders, such as haemolytic disease of the newborn, and congenital infections.

EPIDERMAL NAEVI

Epidermal naevi are benign, hamartomatous skin lesions that may be seen in early childhood. They are composed of epidermal cells and structures, including keratinocytes, sebaceous glands and hair follicles. Keratinocytic epidermal naevi, also called linear epidermal nevi, are the most common form. Rarely, skin cancers may arise in these lesions in adult life. Epidermal naevus syndrome refers to the association of an epidermal naevus with other malformations.

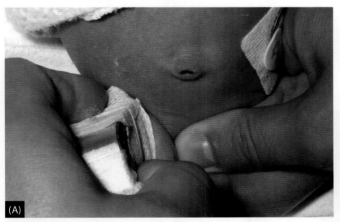
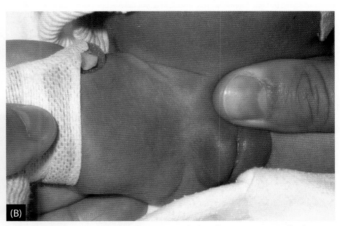

Figs. 9.1A, B Ortolani test. The leg is held with the thumb anteriorly on the shaft of the femur and the fingers posteriorly over the greater trochanter. The hip is flexed to 90 degrees (A) and then abducted to 45 degrees (B). The fingers over the posterior trochanter attempt to push the dislocated femoral head into the acetabulum. Posterior pressure by the thumb when the leg is adducted can dislocate the hip in some infants.

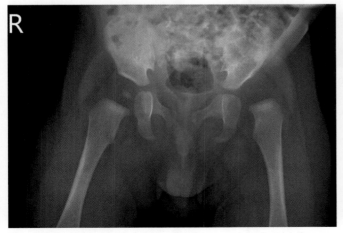
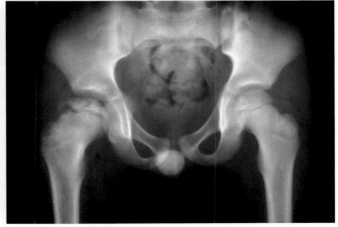

Fig. 9.2 A dislocated left hip, which was missed at birth, is shown on a radiograph of a 5-month-old infant. The acetabulum is shallow and the ossification centre in the head of the femur delayed relative to the normal right hip.

Fig. 9.3 Perthes disease is caused by avascular necrosis and secondary compression of the femoral head. This young boy with involvement of the right femur presented with an intermittent painless limp.

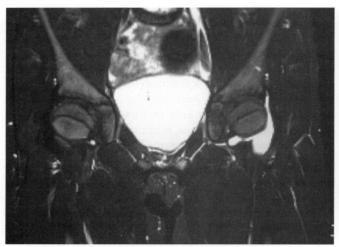

Fig. 9.4 Irritable hip with transient synovitis on MRI in a 12-year-old who presented unable to weight-bear on the left leg.

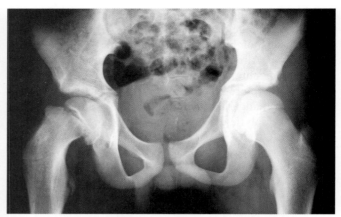

Fig. 9.5 Slipped upper femoral epiphysis can present as an acute slip with sudden pain and immobility of the hip joint, or as a chronic slip with gradual onset of symptoms. In this child with a chronic presentation, bed rest with no weight-bearing was required initially, but operative pinning of the head of the femur to prevent further slipping is sometimes required.

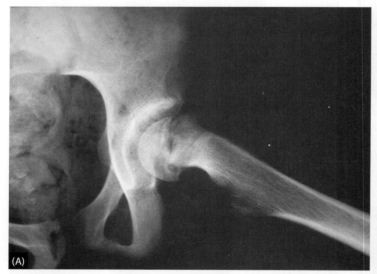

(A)

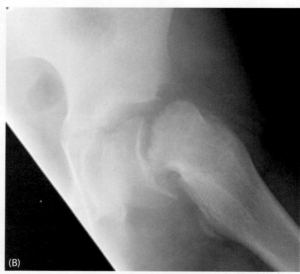

(B)

Figs. 9.6A, B Slipped upper femoral epiphysis. (A) Special radiographic views may be required to demonstrate the degree of slip of the femoral head. (B) Radiograph of the hip with the leg abducted reveals that the head of the left femur has slipped posteroinferiorly. This disorder is more common in obese adolescents.

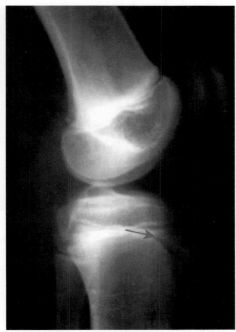

Fig. 9.7 Osgood–Schlatter disease in a 13-year-old boy. Although considered an osteochondritis, Osgood–Schlatter disease is really a fracture displacement of the tip of the tibial tuberosity (arrow).

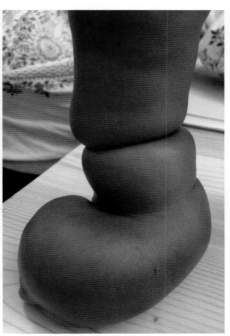

Fig. 9.8 Amniotic band causing a tourniquet constriction of the limb with chronic lymphoedema.

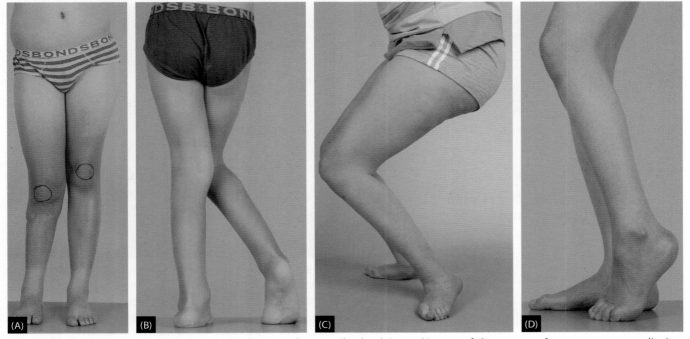

Figs. 9.9A–D (A) Congenital short leg in this boy produces a tilted pelvis, and is one of the causes of compensatory scoliosis. Note that the marks on the patellae are at different heights. (B) A boy with cerebral palsy demonstrating toe-walking on the right leg. (C) In this child with severe cerebral palsy there are flexion deformities at both hips and knees, as well as toe-walking on the left side. (D) A lateral view of a child with left-sided toe-walking caused by significant imbalance between the flexor and extensor muscles in the left calf.

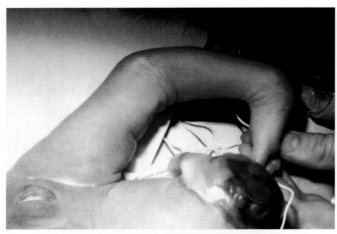

Fig. 9.10 Genu recurvatum. The hyperextension of the knee joint is visible, demonstrating that the *in-utero* position of the leg was hyperextended along the trunk of the fetus. The foot was probably near the face or shoulder. Note the associated exomphalos.

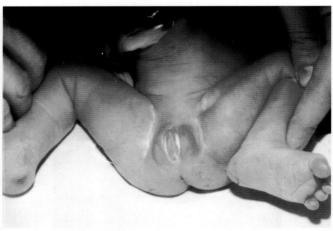

Fig. 9.11 Genu recurvatum. The right leg of this baby has been hyperextended *in utero* so that there is relative limitation of flexion of the right leg compared with the left when passive flexion at both knees is attempted.

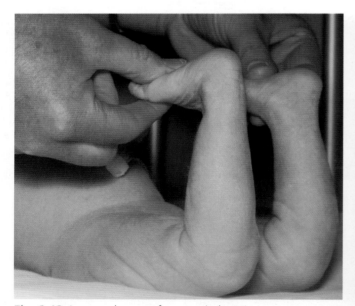

Fig. 9.12 A gross degree of congenital genu recurvatum.

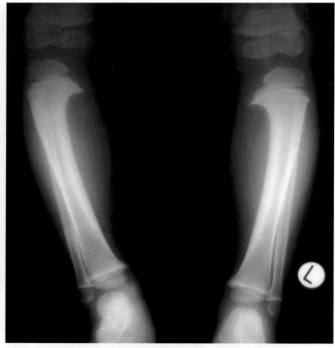

Fig. 9.13 Bow legs is a transient phase during normal growth of the tibia in infancy. It usually straightens spontaneously in the first 2 years of life. This radiograph shows an unusually severe degree of bow legs that required osteoclasis of the tibias to get the legs straight.

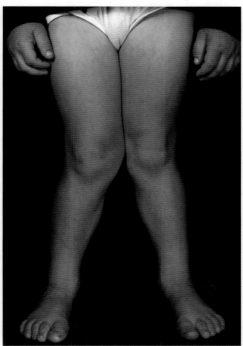

Fig. 9.14 Knock knees is a normal variant of growth in 3–4-year-old children when the medial femoral condyle grows more quickly than the lateral condyle. The valgus deformity of the leg means that the medial malleoli are not touching when the knees are together. In normal postural knock knees, the distance between the medial malleoli should be less than 10 cm. This anomaly tends to resolve spontaneously by 6–7 years with catch-up growth of the lateral condyle producing a horizontal knee joint. In this child with severe knock knees, surgical intervention was required.

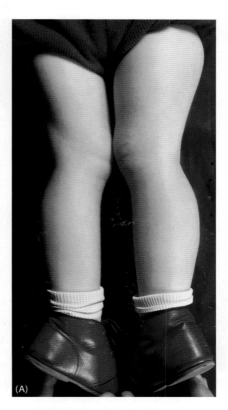

(A)

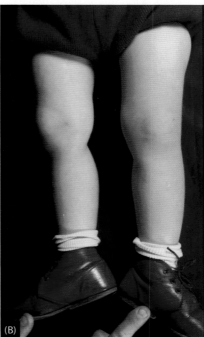

(B)

Figs. 9.16A, B Inset hips in a child who presented with in-toeing. Femoral anteversion is characterised by increased anteversion of the femoral neck relative to the femur and compensatory internal rotation of the femur (A), such that the knees are 'facing' each other; (B) shows the degree of external rotation achieved.

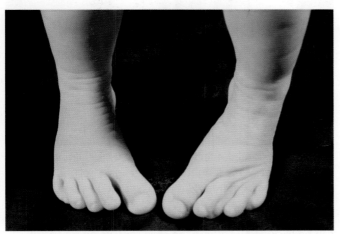

Fig. 9.15 In-toeing can be caused by (1) 'inset hips' (femoral anteversion), (2) internal tibial torsion or (3) foot deformity. This child has metatarsus varus, where the forefoot is adducted and in the varus position, and is relatively fixed. In most cases of in-toeing, no surgical intervention is required.

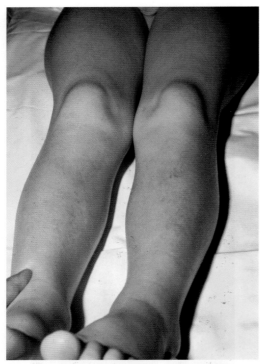

Fig. 9.17 Internal tibial torsion. The patellae tend to point slightly outwards, while the toes point directly forwards. This indicates that there is a longitudinal rotational deformity of the tibia.

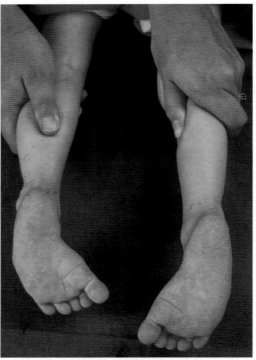

Fig. 9.18 Metatarsus adductus. The medial deviation of the forefoot is particularly conspicuous in the left foot. This is generally a benign abnormality, although a few children have a fixed bony deformity and require orthopaedic surgery to straighten the forefoot.

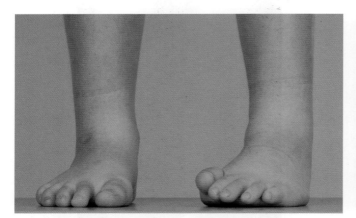

Fig. 9.19 Metatarsus varus, the other term given to metatarsus adductus, is where there is both fixed adduction and varus abnormality. Many orthopaedic surgeons use the terms interchangeably.

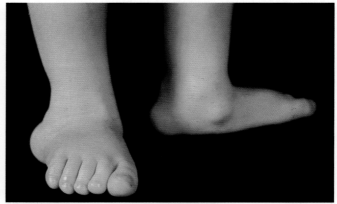

Fig. 9.20 Bilateral flat feet (pes planus). This child has complete loss of the longitudinal arch and a secondary valgus deformity. In infants, the arch is filled with a fat pad and the longitudinal ligaments may be lax so that the arch is not conspicuous. In older children normal variants can be excluded by asking the child to walk on tip-toe. If there is merely laxity of the ligaments, contraction of the tendons during tip-toe walking demonstrates that the bony structures are normal with a normal longitudinal arch. Flat feet rarely require surgical treatment. If they cause aching with prolonged exercise, special arch supports or a heel cup in the shoes may be indicated.

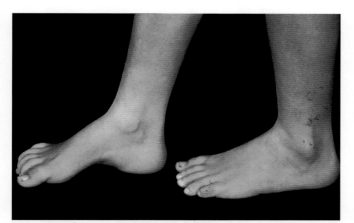

Fig. 9.21 Pes cavus. This child has a small right foot and a high arch. Asymmetrical pes cavus, particularly associated with growth failure of the foot, is highly suggestive of a progressive neurological lesion caused by tethering of the spinal cord. This is a common consequence later in childhood in children with occult spinal dysraphism. Inspection of the spine of this child may reveal a hairy patch, pigmented naevus, haemangioma or a lipoma. There may be associated urinary symptoms, such as abnormal voiding. Neurosurgical release of the tethered spinal cord should prevent progression of the abnormality.

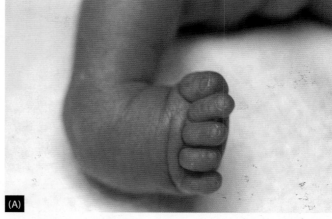

(A)

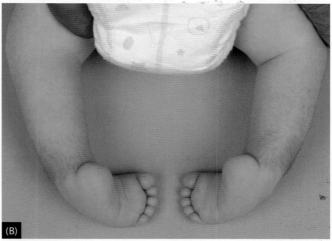

(B)

Figs. 9.22A, B (A) Talipes equinovarus is one of the commonest congenital anomalies of the feet, affecting approximately 1:1,000 live children. This abnormality is more common in boys. Also known as club foot, it is a combination of a number of deformities: equinus, varus, adductus and cavus. Talipes equinovarus may be caused by compression of the fetal feet without any fixed deformity. Treatment is indicated where a fixed deformity is present, preventing a full range of passive movement. If serial casting in the neonatal period fails to correct the abnormality, surgical release of the soft tissues may be necessary. (B) An infant with bilateral talipes equinovarus.

Fig. 9.23 Talipes equinovarus can be caused by *in-utero* compression. Shown is an infant with the legs folded into the position occupied *in utero*, demonstrating the equinus position of the left foot. The bruised perineum is consistent with a breech delivery. Intrauterine compression is not usually associated with an intrinsic abnormality of the foot. At birth, the foot has a full range of passive movement and rapidly recovers in the first few weeks postnatally.

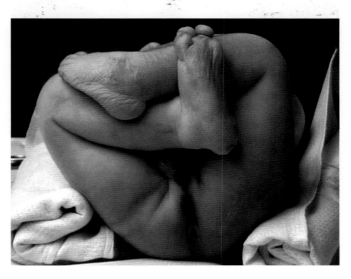

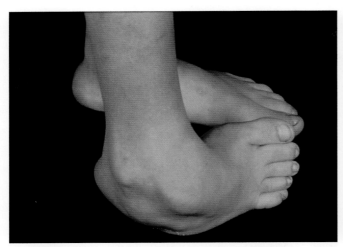

Fig. 9.24 Severe talipes equinovarus in an older child affecting the right foot. Surgical release of the soft tissues will be required. Clinical examination should exclude disorders of the nervous system, such as spina bifida, as causes of this abnormality. Sometimes, severe equinovarus is associated with other neuromuscular or bony defects, such as arthrogryposis.

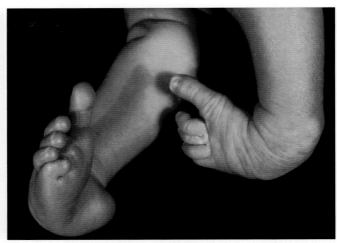

Fig. 9.25 Arthrogryposis multiplex congenita is a systemic disorder causing multiple deformities and restriction of joint movement. It is considered to develop as a result of decreased movement *in utero*, which may be caused by neurological or muscle problems, connective tissue disorders, oligohydramnios or a genetic disorder. Treatment requires a multidisciplinary team of orthopaedic surgeons, physiotherapists and orthotists.

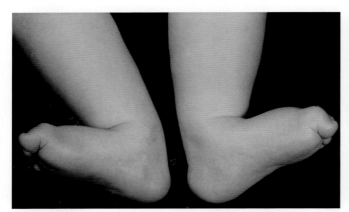

Fig. 9.26 Talipes calcaneovalgus in an infant with spina bifida. The legs have reduced muscle bulk that has been replaced by fat. There are bilateral hammer-toe deformities and the dorsum of each foot shows characteristic lymphoedema caused by an absence of the muscle pump from paralysis. Calcaneovalgus may be associated with congenital dislocation of the hip.

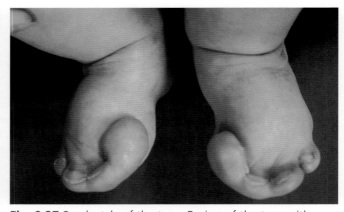

Fig. 9.27 Syndactyly of the toes. Fusion of the toes with some local overgrowth of the soft tissue.

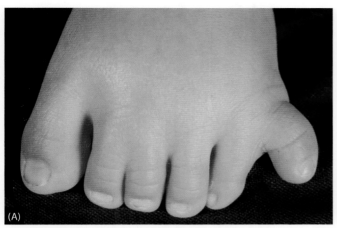

(A)

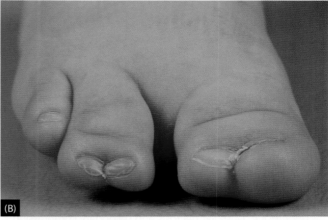

(B)

Figs. 9.28A, B (A) Syndactyly combined with polydactyly of the toes. (B) A complex form of syndactyly, with fusion of the first and second toes and the third and fourth toes.

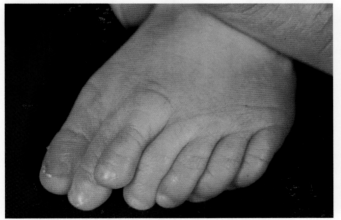

Fig. 9.29 Polydactyly of the toes, with secondary compression of the toes in the shoe causing overriding of the third toe.

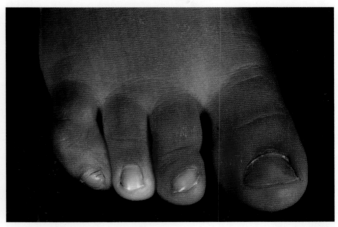

Fig. 9.30 Congenital absence of one toe. This child with four toes had no other abnormalities.

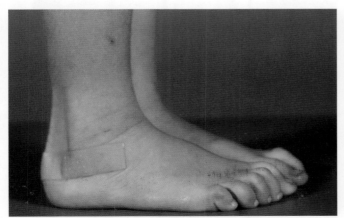

Fig. 9.31 Curly toes. Sometimes these may be caused by inadequate footwear or an underlying neurological lesion.

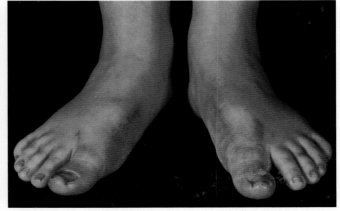

Fig. 9.32 Bilateral infected ingrowing toenails with overgrowth of granulation tissue. There is a minor degree of hallux valgus of the right foot.

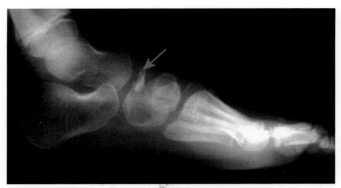

Fig. 9.33 Köhler disease in a 6-year-old boy who presented with a painful right foot and a limp. The tarsal navicular (arrow) has undergone avascular necrosis and secondary compression.

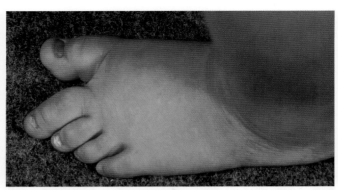

Fig. 9.34 Local gigantism of the second toe.

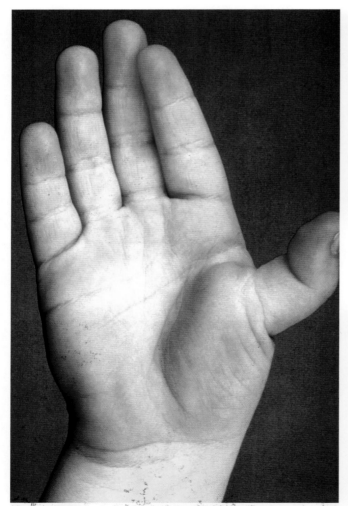

Fig. 9.35 Trigger thumb. The thickened tendon of flexor pollicis longus is limited in its movement within the tendon sheath, preventing full extension of the thumb.

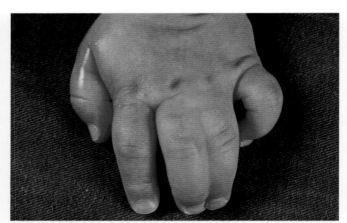

Fig. 9.36 Syndactyly of the middle and ring fingers. In this simple variety, there is fusion of the skin only. It is due to failure of the connecting ectoderm between the digital rays to undergo programmed cell death.

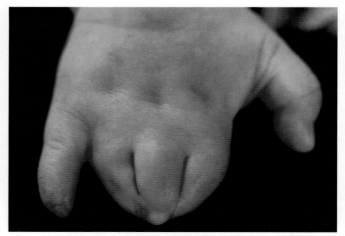

Fig. 9.37 Syndactyly with bony fusion. The index, middle and ring fingers are joined in an abnormal manner with bony and skin fusion.

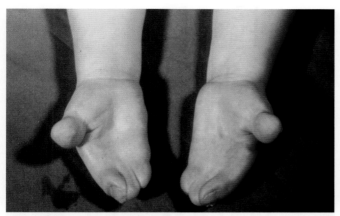

Fig. 9.38 Syndactyly with bony fusion and hypoplasia. There are only four identifiable digital rays in these hands.

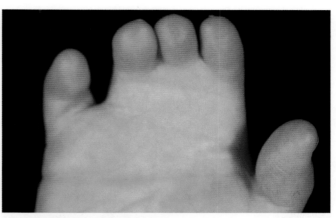

Fig. 9.39 Syndactyly with hypoplasia. There is hypoplasia of the middle three digital rays with partial syndactyly.

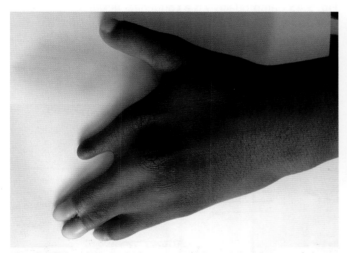

Fig. 9.40 Syndactyly with associated partial absence of the index finger.

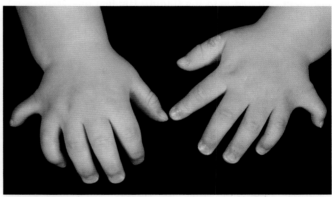

Fig. 9.41 Polydactyly. Extra digital rays occur most commonly on the ulnar side of the hand. This child has symmetrical polydactyly with an extra little finger. There is a bony connection between the accessory finger and the rest of the hand.

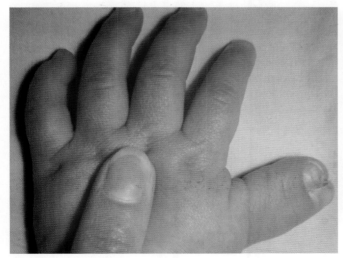

Fig. 9.42 Partial duplication of the thumb on the left hand.

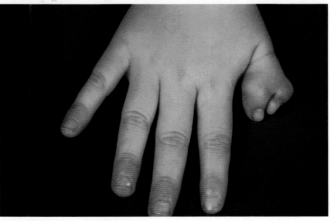

Fig. 9.43 Duplication of the right thumb. In contrast to **Fig. 9.42**, one of the thumbs is naturally larger than the other, allowing the smaller duplication to be excised, and leaving a normal functional and cosmetic appearance.

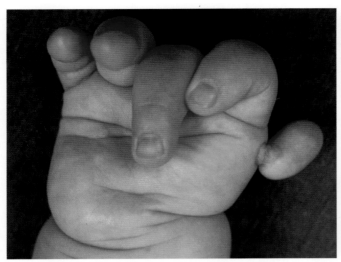

Fig. 9.44 Hypoplasia of the thumb. The first digital ray, which would normally make the thenar eminence of the thumb, has become significantly hypoplastic, leaving a small pedunculated remnant. Pollicisation of the index finger is required to make a functional hand.

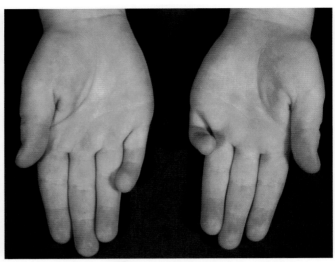

Fig. 9.45 Camptodactyly is a congenital flexion deformity that usually affects the little finger. This prevents the hand from being held completely flat. Camptodactyly is usually sporadic but may be inherited.

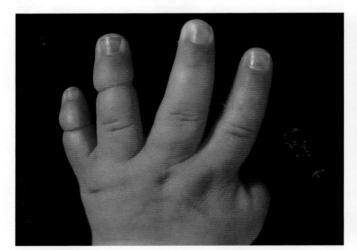

Fig. 9.46 Congenital constriction ring strictures of the fingers. There is controversy as to whether these are caused by amniotic bands or are an intrinsic abnormality in the development of the digital rays. The condition is readily corrected by excision of the ring and re-suturing with multiple Z-plasties.

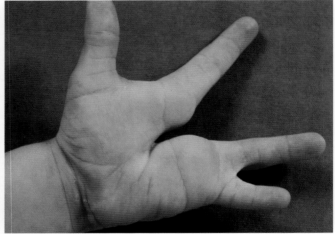

Fig. 9.47 Ectrodactyly with aplasia of the middle ray of the hand. The function of the hand is not impeded as much as might be expected. This is also known as split hand (or foot) malformation, cleft hand or 'lobster claw hand'.

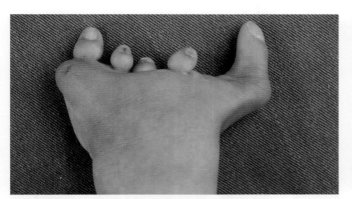

Fig. 9.48 A complex hand deformity with abnormal development of all digital rays.

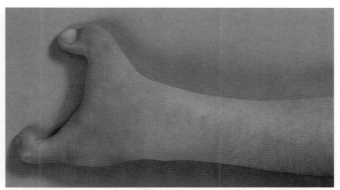

Fig. 9.49 Complex hand deformity with aplasia of the second, third and fourth digital rays, with associated deformity of the first and fifth digital rays.

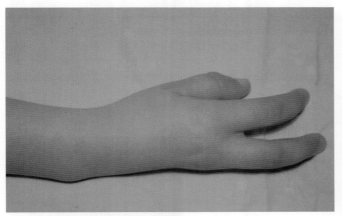

Fig. 9.50 Aplasia of the ulnar rays of the hand, leaving a thumb, index and middle finger only. This hand has a normal pincer grip but deficient power, since power is usually greatly augmented by the fourth and fifth fingers.

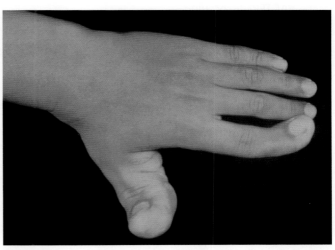

Fig. 9.51 Hamartomatous enlargement with secondary deformity of the index finger and thumb.

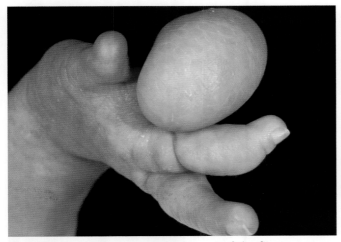

Fig. 9.52 Hamartomatous enlargement of the fingers may be caused by overgrowth of fatty and neural tissues.

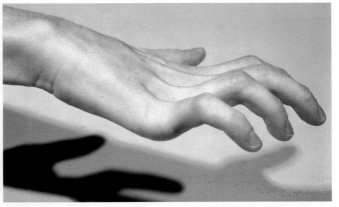

Fig. 9.53 Claw hand. This is the characteristic claw hand deformity seen in a Volkmann contracture following a supracondylar fracture of the humerus with secondary ischaemic necrosis of the forearm flexors.

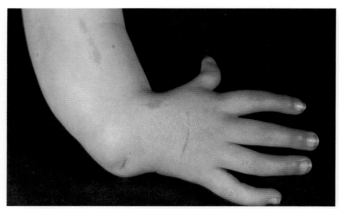

Fig. 9.54 Radial club hand. Partial radial aplasia causing radial deviation of the hand and abnormality of the thumb. This anomaly may be seen in patients with Fanconi anaemia or the VACTERL association.

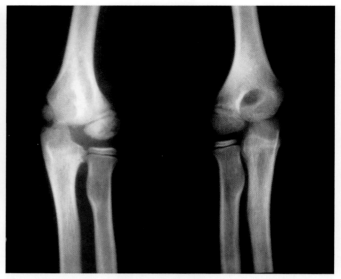

Fig. 9.56 Panner disease in an 8-year-old boy who presented with painful swelling of the elbow for several weeks. There was a limitation of extension and swelling over the head of the radius. There is osteochondritis of the right capitulum and adjacent widening of the joint space. The capitulum recovered with conservative therapy over several years.

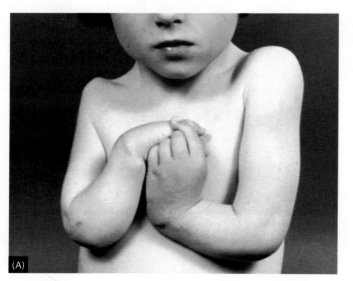

(A)

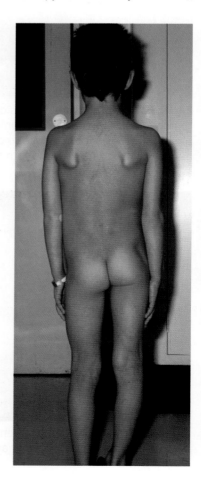

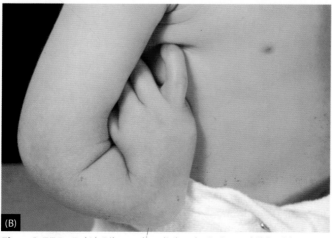

(B)

Figs. 9.55A, B (A) Bilateral radial aplasia in a child with VACTERL association. (B) Severe radial aplasia in a child with VACTERL association.

Fig. 9.57 Compensatory scoliosis. This boy has a congenital short leg, producing tilting of the pelvis and secondary compensatory scoliosis.

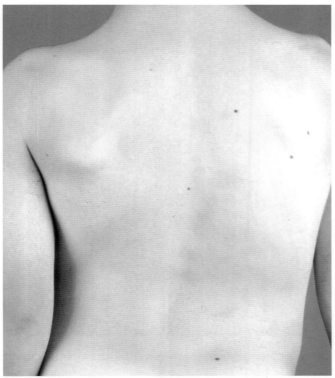

Fig. 9.58 Scoliosis is evident from inspection of the back; postural scoliosis cannot be excluded until further examination is carried out.

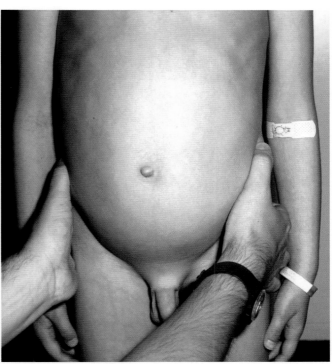

Fig. 9.59 During physical examination, the first thing to check is that the hips are horizontal. This is conveniently done by observing that the levels of the anterior superior iliac spines are horizontal when the child is standing.

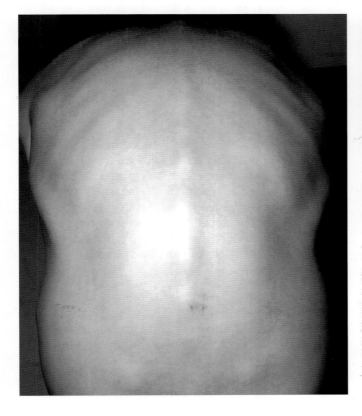

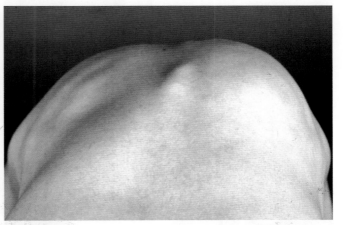

Fig. 9.61 In an intrinsic abnormality, as seen in **Fig. 9.59**, the spinal deformity persists. There may be associated asymmetry of the chest wall.

Fig. 9.60 The child then bends forwards to touch the toes. If the scoliosis is postural, the deformity disappears completely on flexion.

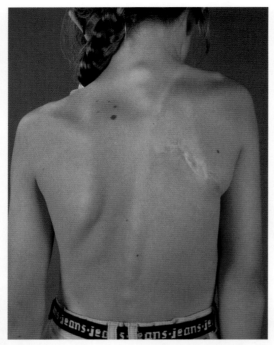

Fig. 9.62 Scoliosis secondary to multiple thoracotomies. This girl required several thoracotomies to correct oesophageal atresia, including through a rib bed approach. This has caused a secondary scoliosis.

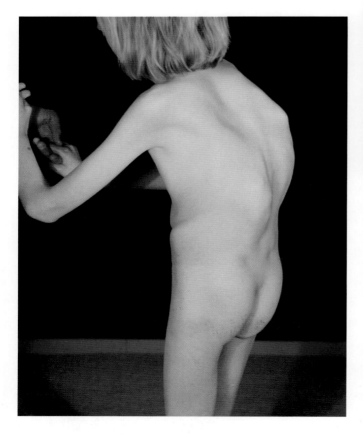

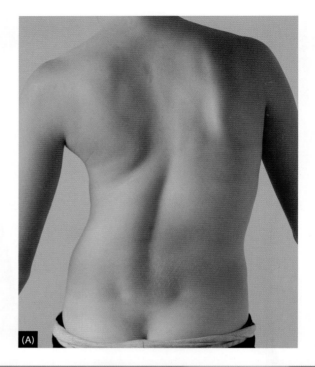

(A)

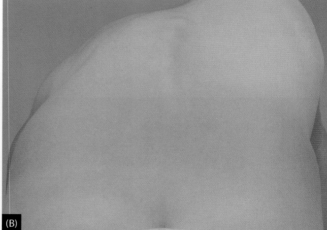

(B)

Figs. 9.63A, B Intrinsic scoliosis in an adolescent girl. (A) Unequal growth of the vertebral epiphyses during adolescence has led to kyphoscoliosis. Treatment consists initially of exercises to strengthen the back muscles, followed by the use of various braces. If these measures fail, operative intervention with fixation of the spine with metal rods may be required. (B) The intrinsic deformity is obvious on bending forward.

Fig. 9.64 Severe kyphoscoliosis, with a major rotational defect, so that the right side of the chest is more prominent. This degree of scoliosis is commonly associated with underlying neuromuscular disorders, which may accentuate any growth defects in the vertebrae.

Fig. 9.65 Kyphoscoliosis in spina bifida. In this child with a thoracolumbar myelomeningocele, there is inadequate growth of both the skeleton and soft tissues at and below the level of the lesion. Inequality of the postural muscles of the spine leads to gross and progressive kyphoscoliosis. Many children with spina bifida require open fusion of the spine before they reach adolescence.

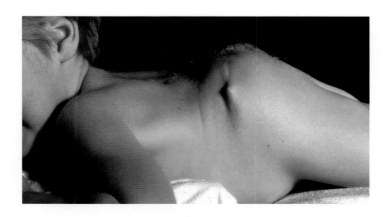

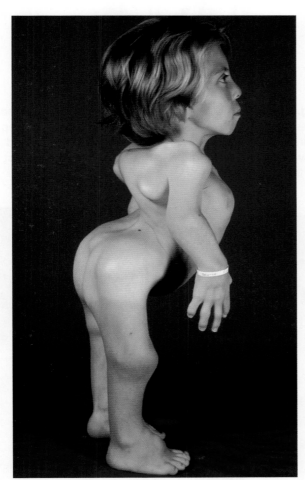

Fig. 9.66 Morquio disease, (a mucopolysaccharide storage disease) is a rare form of osteochondrodysplasia, causing severe deformities of the skeleton, including kyphoscoliosis.

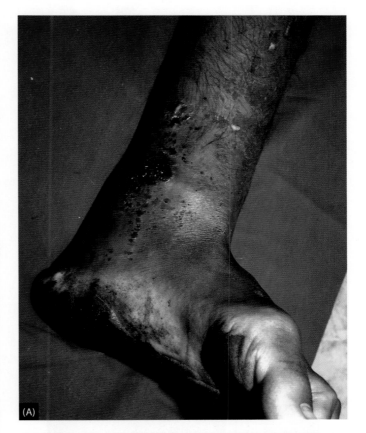

Figs. 9.67A, B Osteomyelitis. (A) This 12-year-old girl had a 3-month history of left ankle swelling, which had been producing a purulent discharge for 2 months. There is a chronic discharging sinus secondary to osteomyelitis. (B) The radiological features of osteomyelitis in the same child.

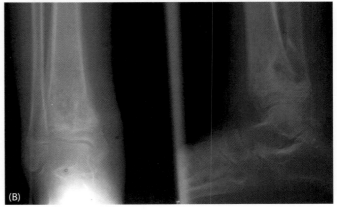

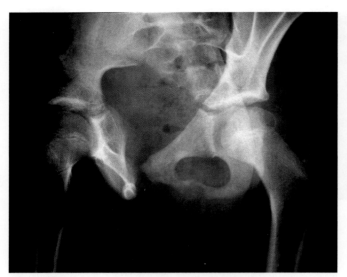

Fig. 9.68 Osteomyelitis of the inferior pubic ramus. This oblique radiograph of the pelvis shows a local destructive lesion caused by infection in the pubic ramus.

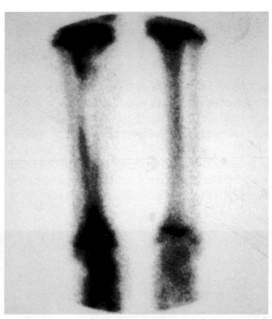

Fig. 9.69 Osteomyelitis of the tibia in a 9-year-old boy who presented with a swollen leg, initially thought to be a deep vein thrombosis. This nuclear scan shows decreased blood flow in a sequestrum in the shaft of the tibia, with the rest of the tibia hyperaemic.

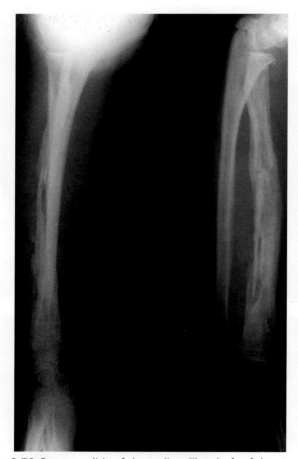

Fig. 9.70 Osteomyelitis of the radius. The shaft of the radius has become chronically infected, with formation of a sequestrum and secondary new bone formation. There is significant distortion of the bone.

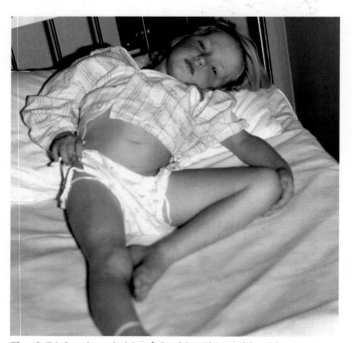

Fig. 9.71 Septic arthritis of the hip. This child, with obvious systemic symptoms, has a painful swollen left hip joint held in flexion and abduction, the so-called 'frog position'. Clinically, there are signs of septicaemia associated with local pain and tenderness. Diagnosis is confirmed by blood cultures and aspiration of the joint under an anaesthetic, at which time the pus can be evacuated by arthrotomy.

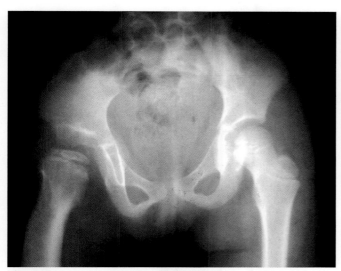

Fig. 9.72 Radiographic appearances in a child who has septic arthritis of the right hip with secondary necrosis of the upper femoral epiphysis.

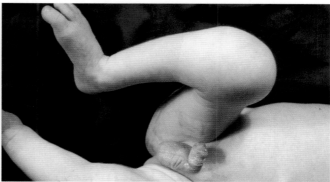

Fig. 9.73 Septic arthritis of the knee, presenting as a swelling of the right knee. The inflammatory process is not obvious externally, but the signs are more conspicuous because of their chronicity. The inflammatory reaction has not yet spread through to the skin. Aspiration of the joint allows a diagnosis to be made and the pus can be evacuated by joint lavage. High-dose systemic antibiotics are needed for several weeks to eradicate the infection.

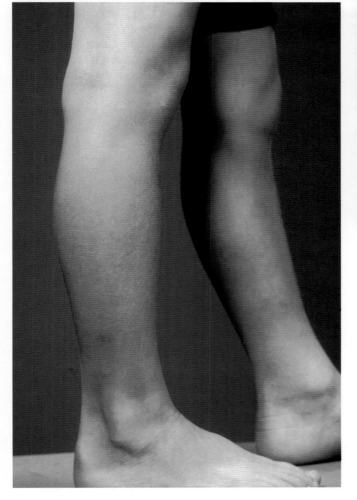

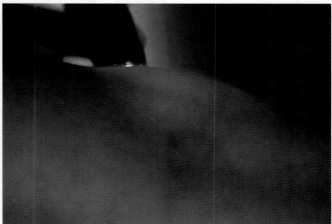

Fig. 9.75 Transillumination of the popliteal cyst (same child as in **Fig. 9.74**) confirms that it contains clear fluid.

Fig. 9.74 Popliteal cyst. There is a cyst present in the popliteal fossa behind the right knee. This is usually on the medial side of the popliteal fossa, protruding from beneath the semimembranosus muscle. A Baker cyst or a semimembranosus bursa are alternative names for what is probably the same disease. The cyst is lined by synovial membrane and contains joint fluid. When the knee is extended the lesion is more conspicuous and feels tense. On flexion of the knee, the cyst becomes more difficult to see but easier to feel. The cyst usually resolves spontaneously within a year or two, and because recurrence is uncommon, surgery is usually best avoided.

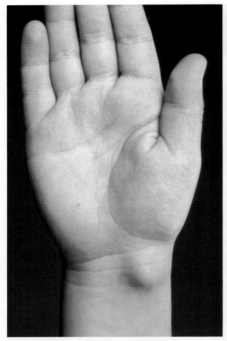

Fig. 9.76 Ganglion of the wrist.

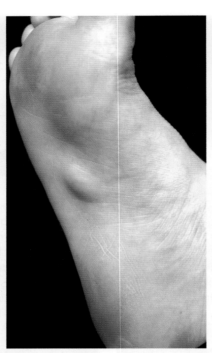

Fig. 9.77 Ganglion of the foot.

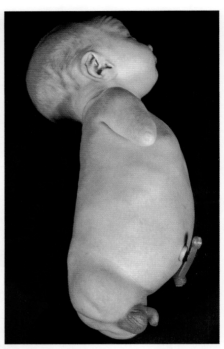

Fig. 9.78 Limb deficiency. This infant has been born with general deficiency of all limbs. In some cases, it is presumed to be caused by congenital amputation from amniotic bands.

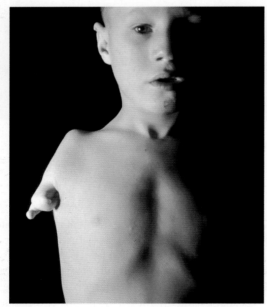

Fig. 9.79 Phocomelia. This boy demonstrates the classic telescopic foreshortening caused by thalidomide toxicity during gestation. Phocomelia has been a rare but sporadic abnormality, both before and after the thalidomide problem in the early 1960s. Children suffering thalidomide toxicity usually have bilateral phocomelia of either upper or lower limbs. Sporadic phocomelia is more commonly unilateral.

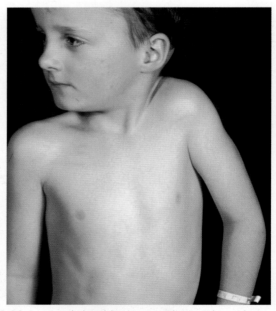

Fig. 9.80 Sprengel shoulder is a condition where there is congenital elevation of the scapula, in this case on the left side. The scapula has remained near its original high cervical position, where it forms in the embryo. When the abnormality is bilateral, the neck is very short and often webbed.

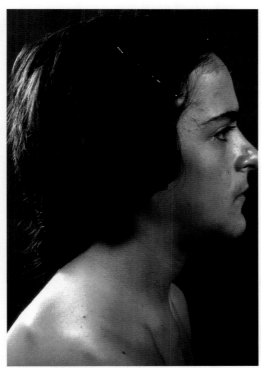

Fig. 9.81 Craniocleidodysostosis. Deficiency of ossification of the vault of the skull leads to the top of the head feeling flat, soft and flabby.

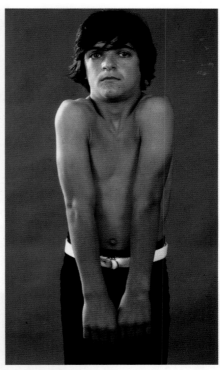

Fig. 9.82 Craniocleidodysostosis. There is absence of ossification of the clavicle as the abnormality affects membranous bones. Deficiency can be confirmed by the demonstration of extreme mobility of the shoulder girdle.

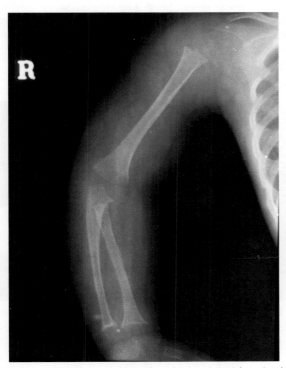

Fig. 9.83 Scurvy. The epiphyseal widening is evident in this infant with scurvy.

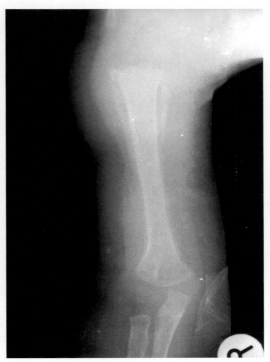

Fig. 9.84 Progression of the vitamin C deficiency in scurvy may lead to subperiosteal haemorrhage with secondary ossification, seen here in the proximal humerus.

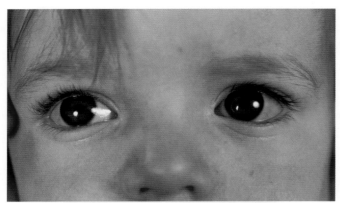

Fig. 9.85 Osteogenesis imperfecta. This rare metabolic disorder of the bone matrix produces a fragile skeleton, which may be fractured *in utero*. A classical physical sign of one of the variants of this group of diseases is blue sclera.

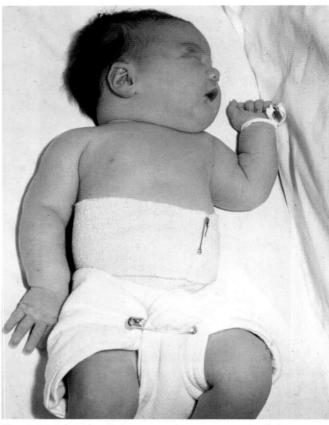

Fig. 9.86 Erb palsy. Damage to the upper trunk of the brachial plexus is usually caused by traction on the shoulder while attempting to deliver the head during breech delivery. Note the 'waiter's tip' position of the right hand and the bruise caused by application of forceps over the right eyebrow.

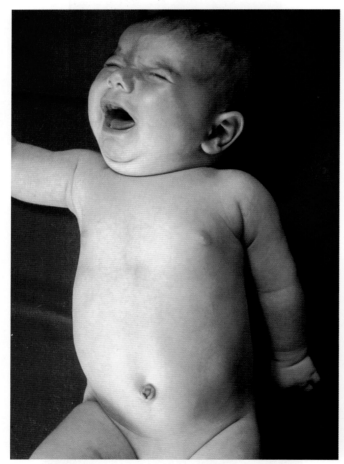

Fig. 9.87 Erb palsy. Most neonates with Erb palsy have suffered a neuropraxia from traction on the upper trunk of the brachial plexus during a traumatic delivery. This resolves spontaneously within a few weeks or months. Occasionally, there is a more severe injury of the brachial plexus, causing persistence of the Erb palsy, as in this baby.

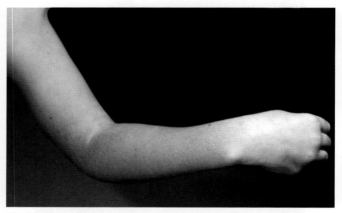

Fig. 9.88 Radial nerve palsy. The withered forearm and wrist drop shown here are secondary to radial nerve palsy caused by a previous humeral fracture.

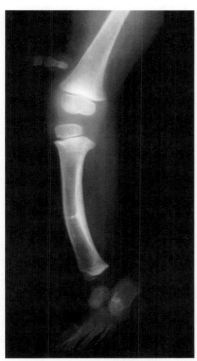

Fig. 9.89 Absent fibula. Radiograph showing lower leg deformity caused by absence of the fibula. This is analogous to radial aplasia and may be part of the VACTERL association.

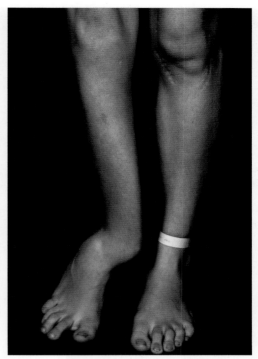

Fig. 9.90 Absent fibula. The ankle is destabilised by this congenital anomaly, which may produce secondary deformity.

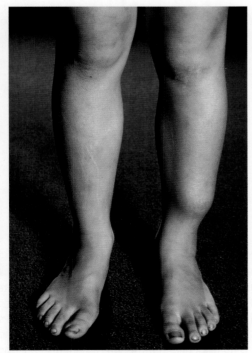

Fig. 9.91 Tibial exostosis. This boy has a major deformity of the subcutaneous border of the left tibia, which on x-ray was shown to be a benign exostosis.

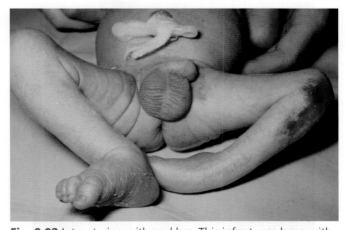

Fig. 9.92 Intrauterine withered leg. This infant was born with a small withered left leg, with apparent pressure necrosis over the knee. This was most likely caused by intrauterine compression interfering with the blood supply of the limb.

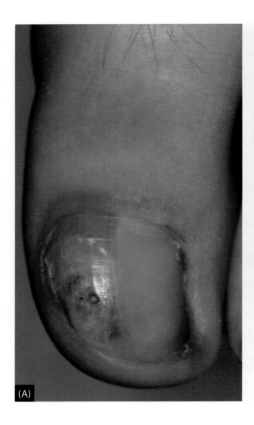

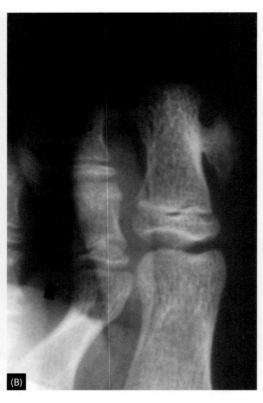

Figs. 9.93A, B Subungual exostosis. (A) Benign exostosis under the medial edge of the left great toenail has caused distortion and maldevelopment of the nail. (B) Radiograph of the same child showing the bony exostosis on the distal phalanx.

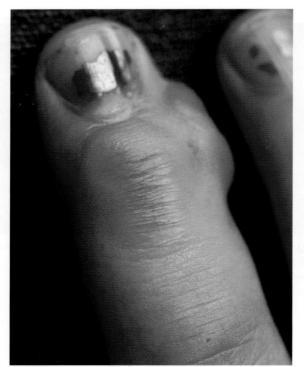

Fig. 9.94 Digital fibroma. A firm fibrous, subcutaneous nodule is present on the side of the digit. This may be part of a multiple fibrous dysplasia syndrome or it can be an isolated deformity. Occasionally, it is a neurofibroma related to a digital nerve.

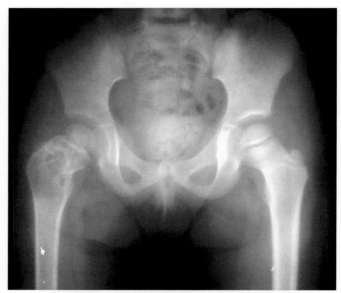

Fig. 9.95 Simple bone cyst. This 5-year-old girl presented with a 1-week history of a limp. Radiography of the femur showed a cyst, which was aspirated and injected with steroid, but the limp persisted, necessitating biopsies. On pathology, there was no evidence that this was an aneurysmal bone cyst, and a final diagnosis of a simple cyst was made.

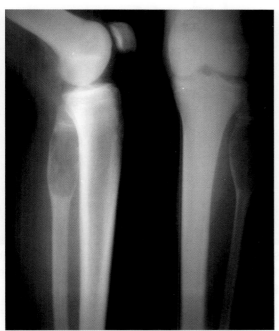

Fig. 9.96 Aneurysmal bone cyst in a 15-year-old boy who presented after being knocked on the lateral side of the left calf. He complained of tenderness for a month, and was able to walk but not run. Physical examination showed a painful swelling over the left upper fibula. Aneurysmal bone cysts are benign tumour-like osteolytic lesions composed of blood-filled channels.

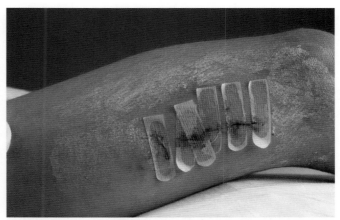

Fig. 9.97 Osteosarcoma. This 10-year-old girl has an obvious mass in the lower end of her right femur. There is a biopsy scar laterally.

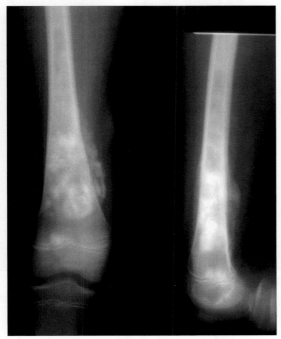

Fig. 9.98 Osteosarcoma in an 11-year-old boy who developed a painful swelling in the lower thigh. Radiography showed an osteosarcoma with ectopic calcification in the soft tissues, elevation of the periosteum and destruction of the medullary cavity of the distal femur.

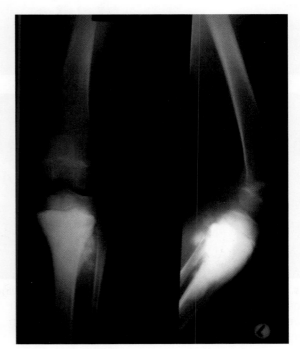

Fig. 9.99 Osteosarcoma in a 13-year-old boy who presented with a 2-month history of pain in the distal left thigh and a 2-week history of swelling in the proximal tibia. On examination there was a swelling in the proximal left tibia, with shiny skin and limitation of knee extension.

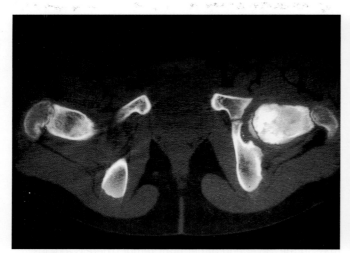

Fig. 9.100 CT scan of a 12-year-old boy with left hip pain waking him at night; the scan demonstrates an osteosarcoma of the left femoral neck.

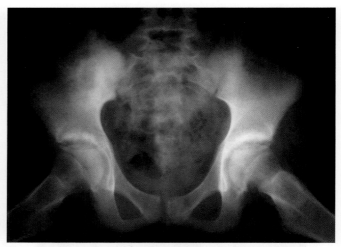

Fig. 9.101 Osteosarcoma. This adolescent presented with a lesion in the right ilium, which was initially thought to be a Ewing tumour on the plain film.

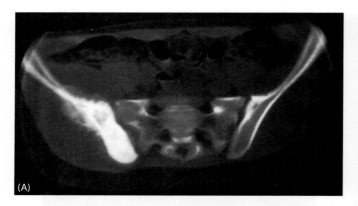

(A)

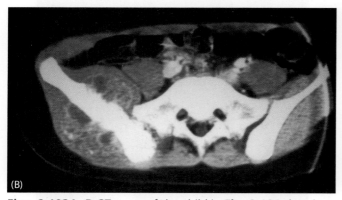

(B)

Figs. 9.102A, B CT scans of the child in **Fig. 9.101** showing an osteosarcoma of the ilium with calcification in the soft tissue. Histology showed this to be an osteosarcoma with chondroid differentiation.

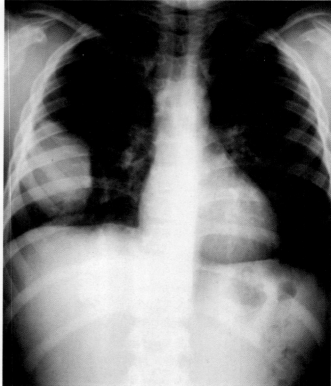

Fig. 9.103 Pulmonary metastasis from an osteogenic sarcoma. A chest radiograph showing a large cannon-ball metastasis.

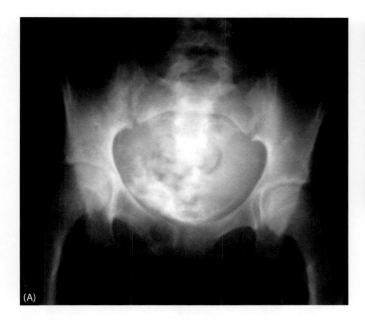

(A)

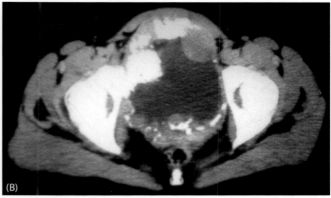

(B)

Figs. 9.104A, B Ewing tumour. (A) This 16-year-old girl presented with a large suprapubic mass. The plain radiograph shows a lytic lesion in the right superior pubic ramus and adjacent soft tissue calcification. (B) A CT scan of the same patient shows the extent of the lesion bulging into the pelvis and surrounding the bladder.

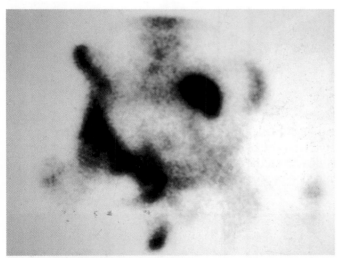

Fig. 9.105 A nuclear bone scan showing uptake in the right pubis and ilium from a Ewing tumour.

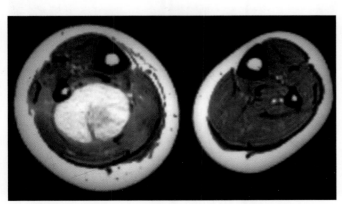

Fig. 9.106 Rhabdomyosarcoma of the calf of the patient in **Fig. 9.107** on MRI.

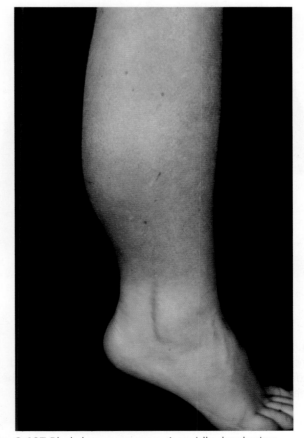

Fig. 9.107 Rhabdomyosarcoma. A rapidly developing swelling in the lower calf muscle is associated with some erythema but no limitation of movement. Note the child is able to stand on tip-toe, which excludes an acute inflammatory cause.

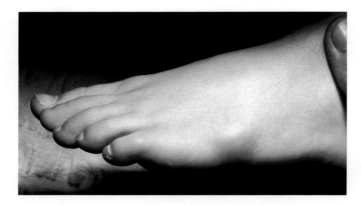

Fig. 9.108 Rhabdomyosarcoma. A painless, slightly erythematous lump on the side of the foot which, on biopsy, was found to be a rhabdomyosarcoma.

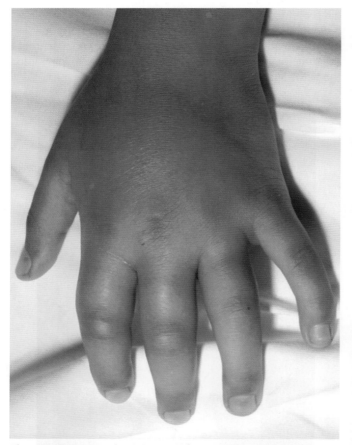

Fig. 9.109 Deep palmar space infection. The back of the hand is red and swollen and the fingers cannot be moved readily. This was a haemolytic streptococcal infection of the deep palmar space.

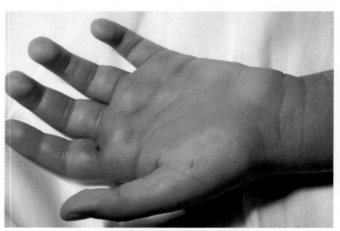

Fig. 9.110 The same child as in **Fig. 9.109**, showing erythema and oedema of the palmar surface of the hand. Erythema on the palmar surface is indicative of severe infection because the skin of the palm is so thick.

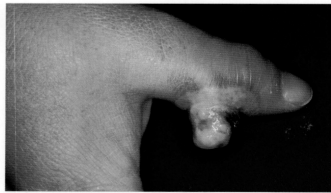

Fig. 9.111 Granuloma of the thumb. A nasty, infected granuloma on the side of the thumb suggests an unrecognised foreign body that is preventing the normal process of healing. The lesion needs debridement and exploration under anaesthesia to exclude a concealed foreign body.

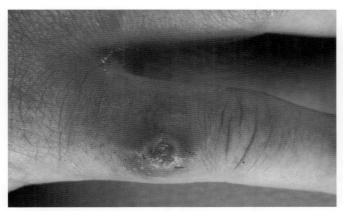

Fig. 9.112 Orf is a zoonotic viral disease that normally affects sheep. It is transmitted to humans who handle sheep, such as farmers, shearers or farmers' children.

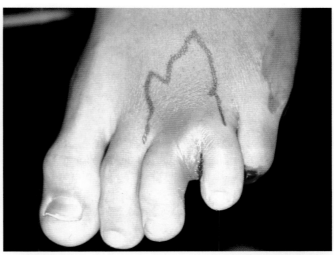

Fig. 9.113 Web-space infection of the foot. There is cellulitis and oedema with separation of the third and fourth toes. To prevent permanent damage to the tendons of the toes, this deep-seated abscess needs immediate drainage.

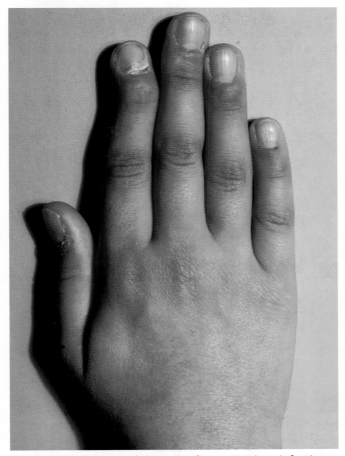

Fig. 9.114 Deformity of the index finger. Previous infection around the terminal phalanx can produce a deformity, either by damaging the distal attachments of the long flexor tendons or by osteomyelitis of the distal phalanx.

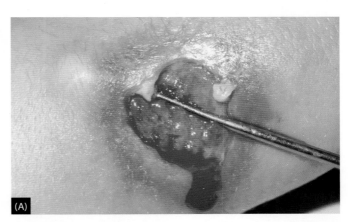

(A)

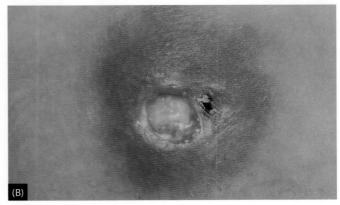

(B)

Figs. 9.115A, B Bairnsdale ulcer. (A) This subcutaneous infection (also known as a Buruli ulcer) is caused by *Mycobacterium ulcerans*. It presents with an indolent, subcutaneous ulcer with undermining edges, most often on the limbs. Note the probe extending under the edge of the ulcer for several centimetres. (B) A close-up view of a Bairnsdale ulcer on the thigh.

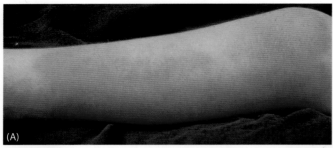 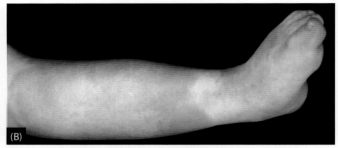

Figs. 9.116A, B Erysipelas. (A) A rapidly spreading infection with a characteristic red flare is seen with certain strains of *Streptococcus* spp. (B) In recent years a rare infection, but is now increasing in frequency.

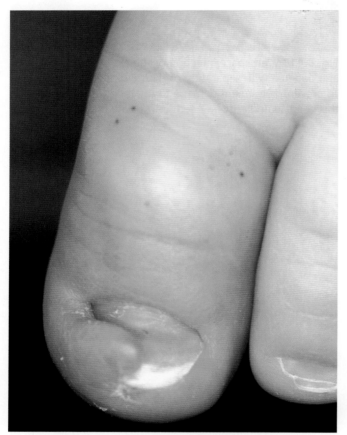

Fig. 9.117 Ingrown toenail with secondary infection. The corner of the nail has become embedded in the side of the nail fold. Recurrent and chronic infection has caused granulation tissue and lymphoedema of the nail fold, which is now overgrown and concealing the edge of the nail.

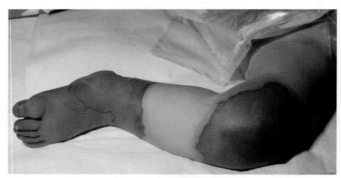

Fig. 9.118 Skin necrosis caused by septic emboli secondary to a central line used for total parenteral nutrition.

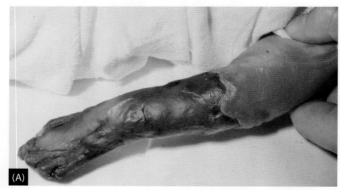

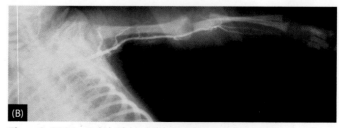

Figs. 9.119A, B (A) This child was born with gangrene of the left forearm, presumably caused by prenatal vascular obstruction. A thromboembolic event was suspected and the infant is likely to have a congenital prothrombotic disorder. (B) Angiogram of the same infant showing distal occlusion of the left forearm vessels.

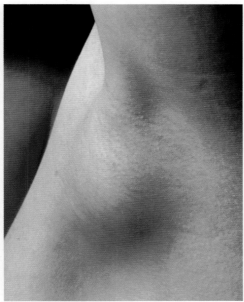

Fig. 9.120 Enlarged, slightly tender lymph nodes in the axilla of a child after recent BCG vaccination.

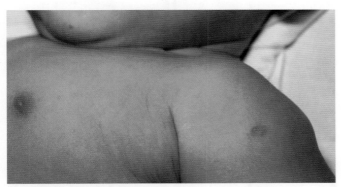

Fig. 9.121 BCG lymphadenitis. Note the scar of the BCG vaccination and the enlarged axillary lymph node in the anterior fold. There is also some erythema in the region.

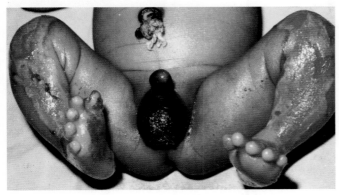

Fig. 9.122 Staphylococcal 'scalded-skin' syndrome predominantly affects neonates. The scalded-skin appearance may be extensive, and occasionally may cover most of the body. Exotoxins released by *Staphylococcus aureus* attack the desmosomes that enable skin cells to bind together.

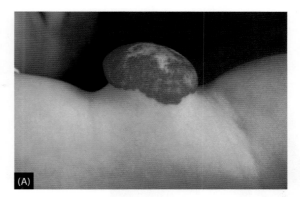

(A)

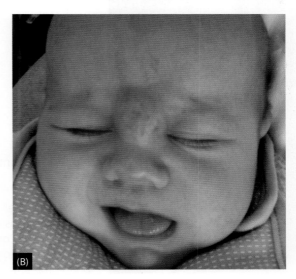

(B)

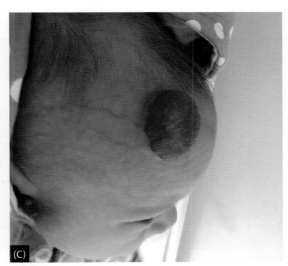

(C)

Figs. 9.123A–C (A) Infantile haemangioma on the left arm in a 6-month-old infant. There is some central scarring indicating that involution is already taking place. (B) Rapidly growing infantile haemangioma, where propranolol needs to be given. (C) Infantile haemangioma on the scalp. The decision to use propranolol would be debatable here unless the lesion becomes ulcerated or bleeds.

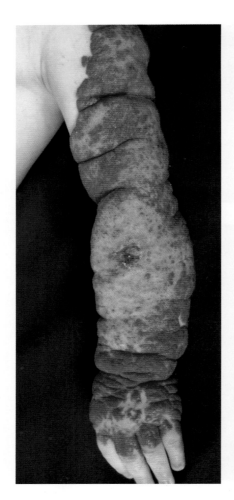

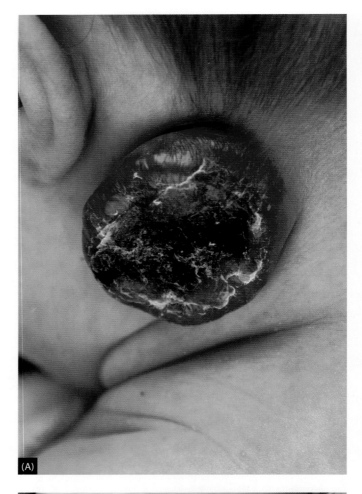

Fig. 9.124 Infantile haemangioma affecting the entire left upper limb, with areas of involution and one area of ulceration on the forearm.

(A)

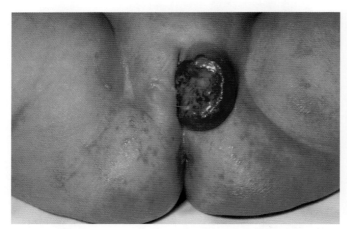

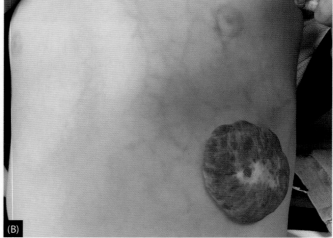

(B)

Fig. 9.125 Infantile haemangioma of the labium major, with secondary ulceration caused by nappy rash (ammonia dermatitis).

Figs. 9.126A, B (A) Involuting infantile haemangioma. There is a large, circumscribed lesion in the posterior triangle of the neck. Involution may be associated with ulceration. Regression of the central area first is common. (B) There is a leash of superficial vessels supplying this incompletely involuted infantile haemangioma on the chest wall of this 5-year-old girl.

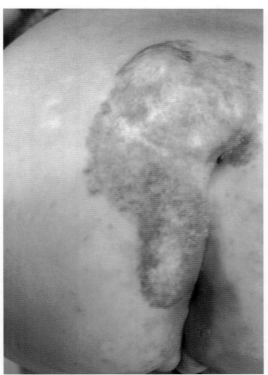

Fig. 9.127 Resolving infantile haemangioma of the perineum. Note that there is a congenital sacral sinus. Infantile haemangiomas arising in the perineum may be associated with abnormalities of the renal tract, pelvis or spine, and this child warrants a renal and spinal ultrasound scan.

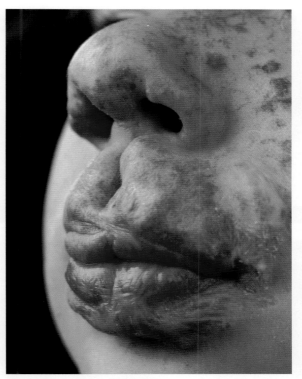

Fig. 9.128 Resolving infantile haemangioma of the face, leaving wrinkled skin that may need secondary plastic surgery later in childhood. These days facial haemangiomas would be treated with propranolol to prevent this complication.

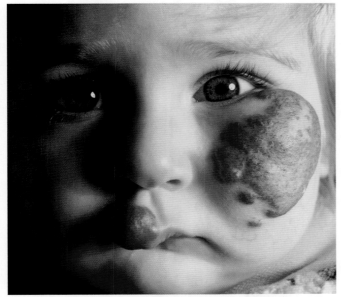

Fig. 9.129 Infantile haemangiomas of the face before the era of propranolol treatment. The left cheek lesion is close to the eye but not occluding the visual axis.

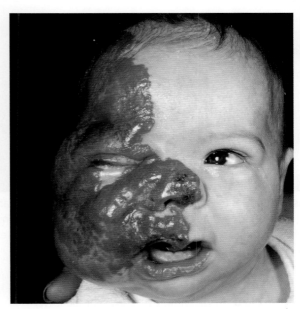

Fig. 9.130 A large, plaque-like infantile haemangioma of the face raises the possibility of PHACE syndrome (Posterior fossa brain malformations, Haemangiomas [particularly large, segmental facial lesions], Arterial anomalies, Coarctation of the aorta or cardiac anomalies, and Eye anomalies).

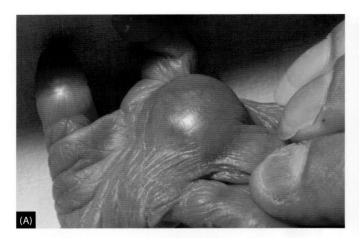

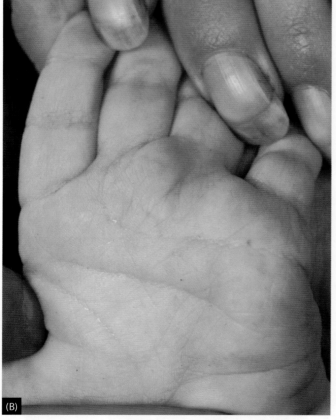

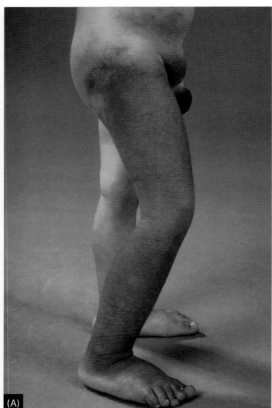

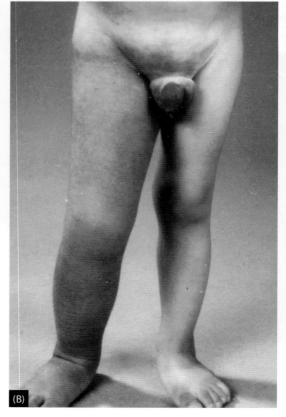

Figs. 9.131A, B (A) Vascular anomaly of the palm of the hand with no abnormal capillaries but a slight blue discolouration. (B) The palm of the same child, 13 months after birth. There has been almost complete resolution of the lesion.

Figs. 9.132A, B (A) Idiopathic overgrowth of the lower limb associated with a vascular malformation, which may be caused by mutations in the *PIK3CA* gene. (B) Same child showing increased diameter of the entire lower limb, as well as overgrowth of the genitalia.

Fig. 9.133 A large congenital haemangioma was present from birth in this infant, shown here at 5 weeks. This is the rare RICH lesion (Rapidly Involuting Congenital Haemangioma) which, unlike the common infantile haemangioma, is already present at birth. In this child the lesion involuted early, leaving just redundant skin by 1–2 years of age.

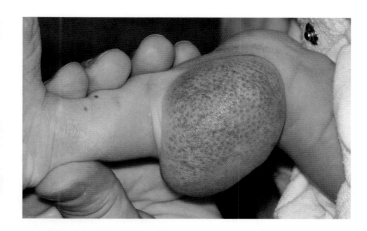

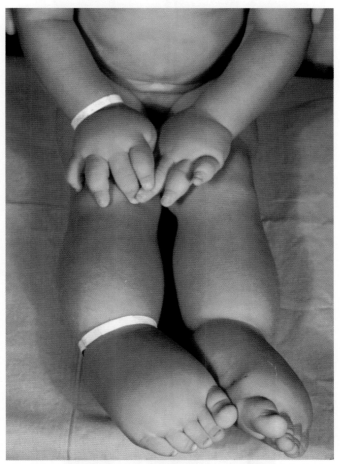

Fig. 9.134 Chronic lymphoedema of the legs, which is likely to be a congenital anomaly of the lymphatic system in the lower trunk and legs.

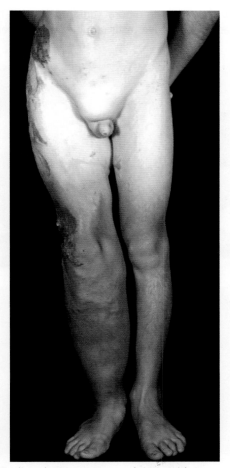

Fig. 9.135 Klippel–Trenaunay syndrome with a vascular malformation of the lower trunk and lower limb with overgrowth. Most case are related to mutations in the *PIK3CA* gene.

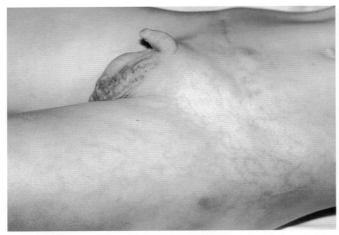

Fig. 9.136 Idiopathic iliofemoral vein thrombosis. This child also had an undescended testis requiring orchidopexy.

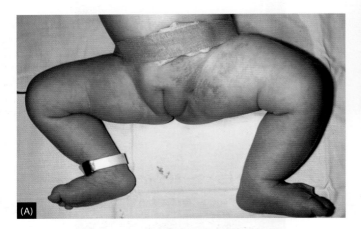

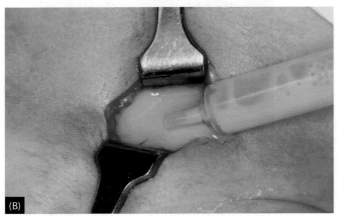

Figs. 9.137A, B (A) Acute venous obstruction and lymphoedema of the left leg caused by a deep-seated iliac abscess. (B) Same child: a mass in the left iliac region was thought to be a tumour. However, at exploration a large volume of pus was drained and the venous occlusion in the leg resolved rapidly.

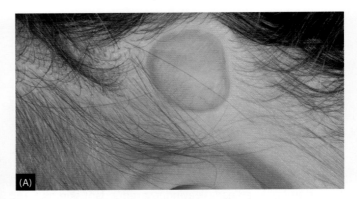

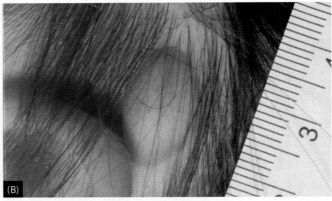

Figs. 9.138A, B Vascular malformation on the scalp, which was present at birth and has not changed with age.

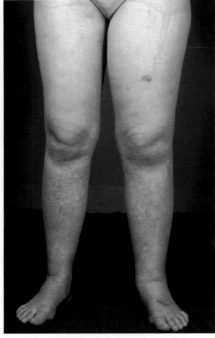

Fig. 9.139 Long-standing venous obstruction of the external iliac vein has left this patient with a chronically swollen left lower limb, secondary to presumed lymphoedema.

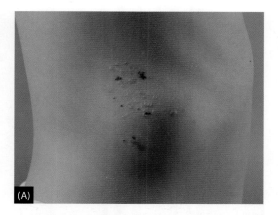

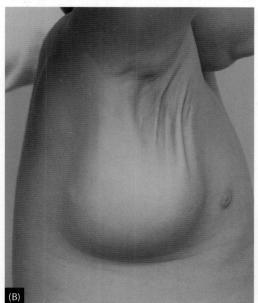

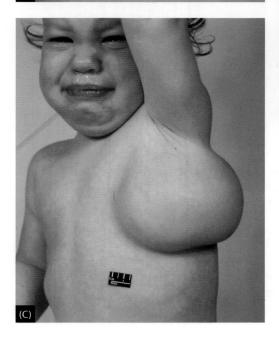

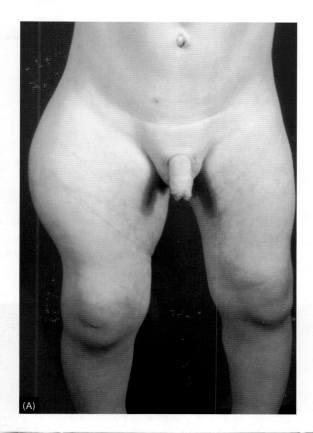

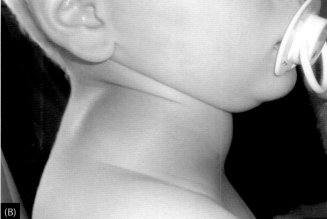

Figs. 9.141A, B (A) Lymphatic malformation of the upper thigh. (B) Lymphatic malformation in the side of the neck with secondary infection.

Figs. 9.140A–C (A) Lymphatic malformation of the chest wall with overlying cystic blebs in the skin, which are the result of dilated, abnormal lymphatics within the skin itself. (B) A more deeply placed lymphatic malformation on the chest wall with no overlying abnormal lymphatics in the skin. (C) Lymphatic malformation of the left chest wall and axilla.

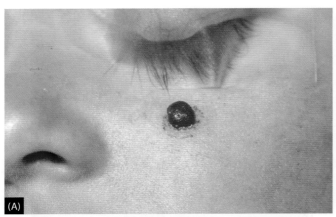

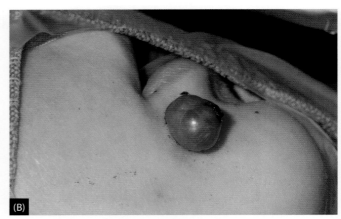

Figs. 9.142A, B (A) This pyogenic granuloma probably resulted from local trauma and secondary infection, producing an overgrowth of granulation tissue. There is often a small arteriole supplying the lesion, which produces recurrent bleeding. (B) A pyogenic granuloma near the corner of the mouth.

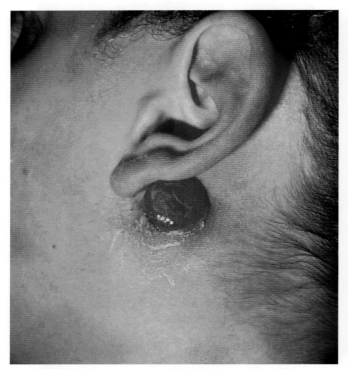

Fig. 9.143 Pyogenic granuloma. A larger lesion behind the left external ear. A chronic inflammatory lesion in this site would be suggestive of a first branchial sinus anomaly.

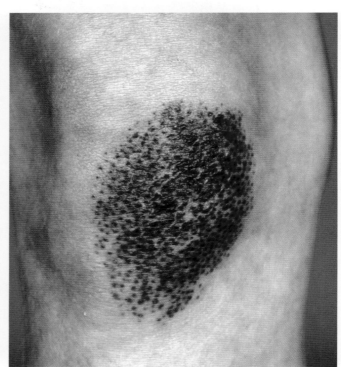

Fig. 9.144 Pigmented naevus of the left knee.

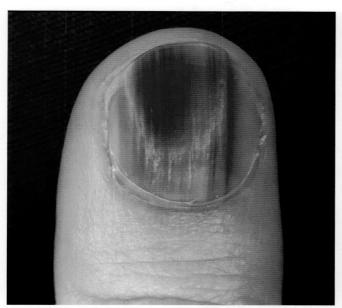

Fig. 9.145 Junctional naevus in the nail matrix producing melanonychia.

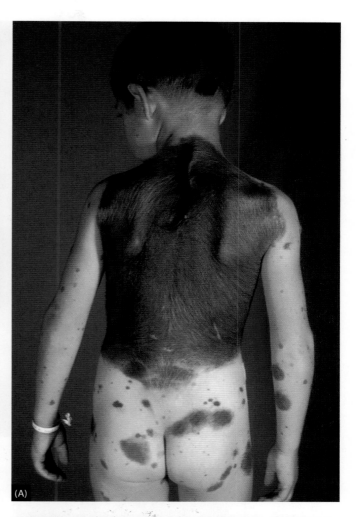

(A)

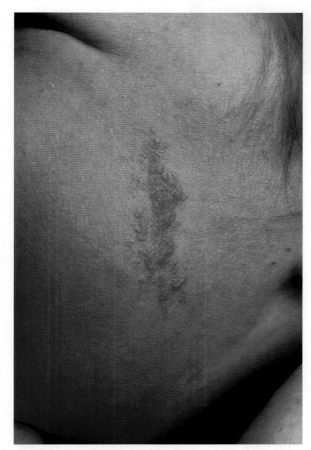

Fig. 9.146 A linear epidermal naevus.

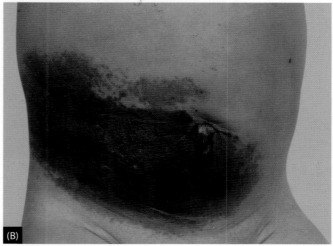

(B)

Figs. 9.147A, B (A) A giant hairy naevus. (B) A giant congenital melanocytic naevus, showing the tendency for them to be distributed in a pattern similar to the dermatomes.

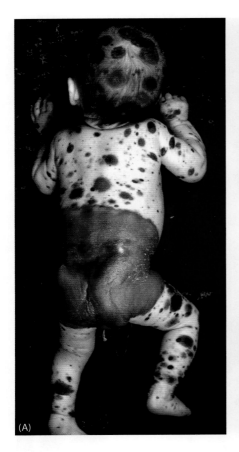

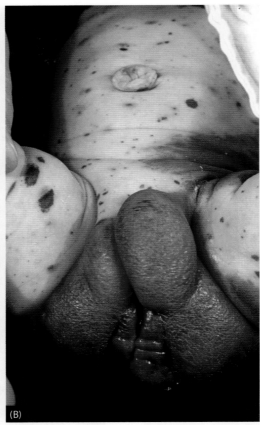

Figs. 9.148A, B (A) A 'bathing trunk' naevus. Note the multiple other naevi over the rest of the body (satellite lesions). (B) The same child, showing secondary local gigantism of the genitalia.

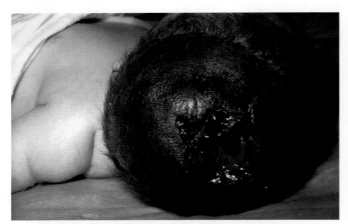

Fig. 9.149 A giant congenital melanocytic naevus of the scalp, with secondary ulceration.

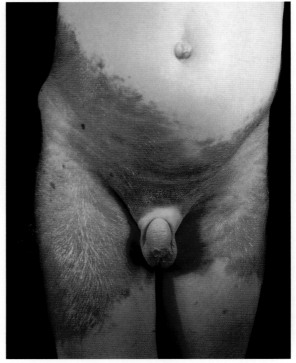

Fig. 9.150 A bathing trunk naevus with secondary malignant degeneration (melanoma) near the right anterior superior iliac spine.

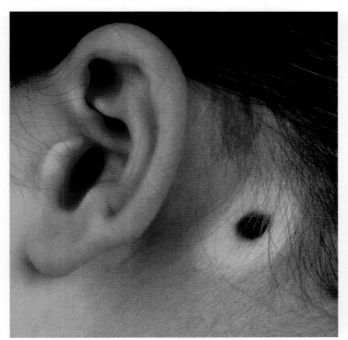

Fig. 9.151 A halo naevus showing the dark central pigmentation surrounded by the area of vitiligo.

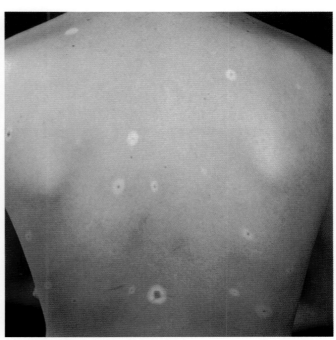

Fig. 9.152 Multiple halo naevi.

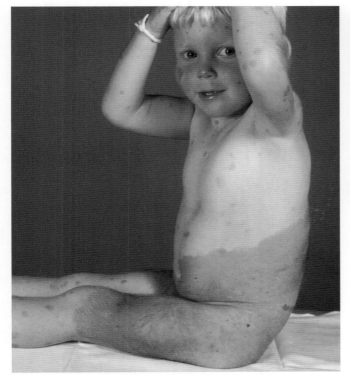

Fig. 9.153 A boy with neurofibromatosis type 1 (NF1, or von Recklinghausen disease), showing multiple areas of 'cafe-au-lait' pigmentation.

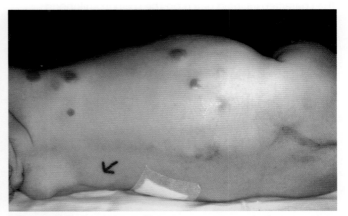

Fig. 9.154 'Blueberry muffin baby'. A congenital neuroblastoma has metastasised to the skin, producing multiple pigmented nodules.

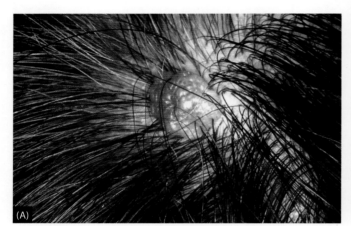

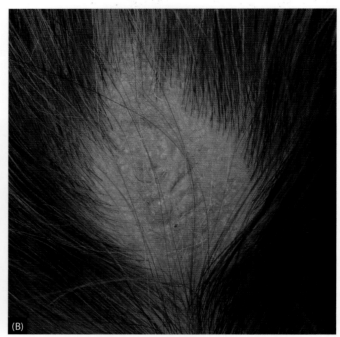

Figs. 9.155A, B (A) Fibroma, appearing as a brown, wart-like lesion on the scalp. (B) A naevus sebaceous of Jadassohn is a variety of congenital epidermal naevus predominantly composed of sebaceous glands. It appears as a hairless plaque that is yellow and typically on the scalp or face. They may be removed to prevent the risk of neoplastic change and also to remove the characteristic bald patch on the scalp in childhood.

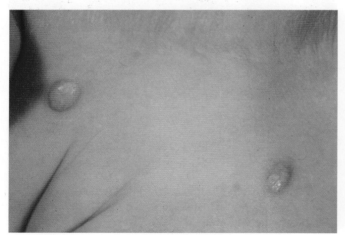

Fig. 9.156 Juvenile xanthogranuloma. These are benign asymptomatic red, yellow or brown nodules composed of fat-containing histiocytes. They occur in infancy and early childhood and usually disappear within a few years.

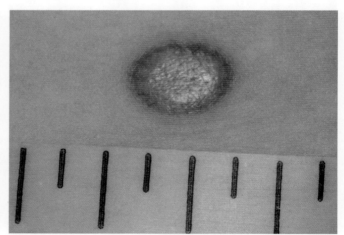

Fig. 9.157 Benign fibrous histiocytoma, which is similar on histology to a xanthogranuloma. It contains large number of histiocytes. The lesion turns yellow on blanching.

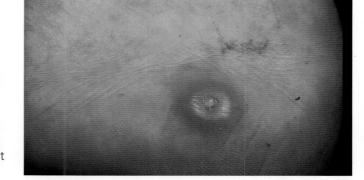

Fig. 9.158 Molluscum contagiosum. This is caused by a poxvirus, which in this child has affected the left heel. The umbilicated papules tend to be more numerous and persistent in children with atopic eczema or immunodeficiency.

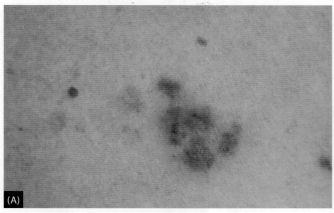

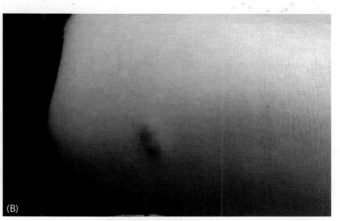

Figs. 9.159A, B (A) Glomangioma. The blue–black nodules in the skin are painful to touch because of histamine release. (B) Glomangioma or glomus tumour on the arm. The common sites for this rare tumour are under the nail, on the fingertip or on the foot. This girl had multiple glomus tumours as part of a hereditary condition that affected at least five members of her family.

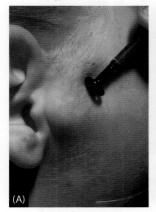
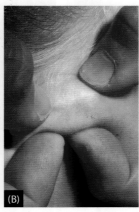
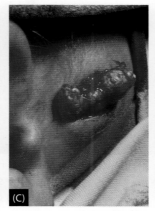
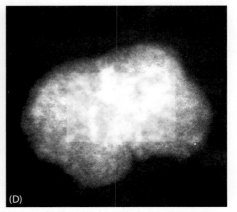

Figs. 9.160A–D (A) Pilomatrixoma. This is a benign subcutaneous nodule affecting the hair follicles. The lesion is tethered to the skin and is usually nodular, hard and irregular. (B) Same patient showing the skin tethering and the irregular shape of the lesion. It can vary in size from a few millimetres to a few centimetres in diameter. (C) A pilomatrixoma during excision, showing calcification. (D) A radiograph of an excised pilomatrixoma showing the calcification. There is death of the hair follicles in the centre of the lesion, eliciting an inflammatory reaction with secondary calcification. Pilomatrixomas occur most often in the head and neck but may be found subcutaneously at other sites.

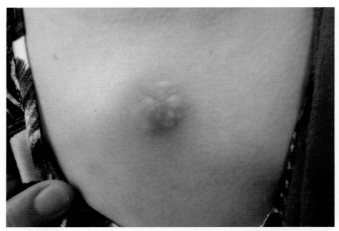

Fig. 9.161 Pilomatrixoma in the neck, showing the characteristic slightly yellow nodular lesion, which feels as if it is attached to the back of the skin, rather than feeling like it is under the skin.

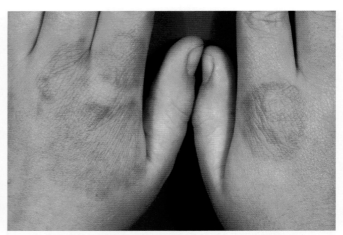

Fig. 9.162 Granuloma annulare. The typical appearance is of reddish bumps arranged in a ring on the back of the forearm, hands or feet. The condition usually resolves without treatment.

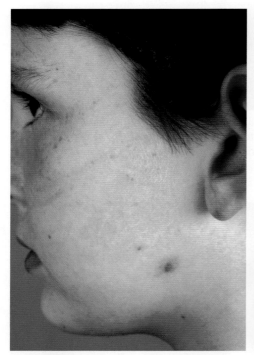

Fig. 9.163 Spider naevus. The lesion is characterised by a central red arteriole (the spider's body) surrounded by radial thin-walled capillaries (the spider's legs). Single lesions are common and do not denote underlying liver disease. In children spider naevus may be secondary to minor trauma, but this is speculative.

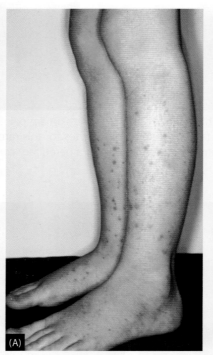

(A)

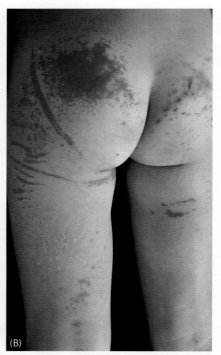

(B)

Figs. 9.164A, B Henoch–Schönlein purpura. (A) This vasculitis has caused multiple lesions on the shins. (B) Characteristically, Henoch–Schönlein purpura causes a vasculitic rash over the buttocks, as shown in this child.

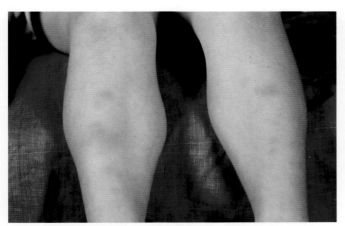

Fig. 9.165 Erythema nodosum. These tender nodules over the shins may be idiopathic or can be associated with several chronic gastrointestinal or respiratory diseases, including TB.

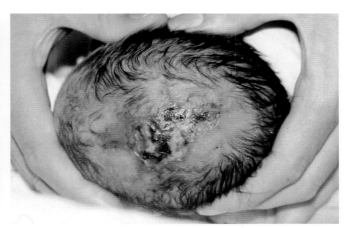

Fig. 9.166 Aplasia cutis congenita. Note the congenital skin defect on the scalp in this neonate.

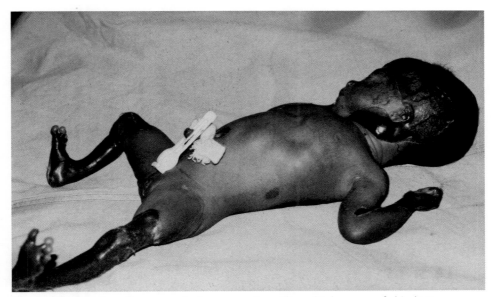

Fig. 9.167 Aplasia cutis congenita in a neonate with multiple areas of skin loss. The differential diagnosis includes epidermolysis bullosa.

ABDOMINAL AND THORACIC INJURIES

Torso trauma in children is second only to head trauma in frequency and associated mortality. The vast majority of abdominal and thoracic injuries are due to blunt trauma such as falls, transport-related incidents (motor vehicle accident, pedestrian versus vehicle) and sporting activities. Penetrating injuries, including stab wounds or bullet wounds, are relatively uncommon in most developed countries, apart from the USA. Non-accidental injury should always be considered if the history is inconsistent with the observed trauma or when the presentation is delayed.

A child's ribs are elastic and compliant, such that compressive forces are readily transmitted through to the underlying thoracic and abdominal organs. As a consequence, rib fractures are uncommon, but torso organ injuries are much more common. Thoracic injuries due to compression include pulmonary contusion, haemothorax, pneumothorax or pneumomediastinum. A pneumothorax under tension necessitates immediate decompression of the pleural cavity. An early chest radiograph will delineate the nature and extent of thoracic injury in most instances, but some may also benefit from chest CT imaging. Aortic rupture from rapid deceleration is rare in childhood because of the low frequency of high-velocity collisions and the greater elasticity of the vessels. Diaphragmatic rupture from acute compression is also rare in children, and while clinical features can be subtle, the plain radiological or CT chest findings are often diagnostic. Sustained torso compression causes traumatic asphyxia.

Lateral impacts over the costal margin can cause splenic, hepatic or renal injury, resulting in haemoperitoneum or an extraperitoneal haematoma and often an ileus. Referred pain to the left shoulder tip from irritation of the phrenic nerves on the peritoneal surface of the diaphragm is suggestive of splenic trauma. There may be signs of hypovolaemic shock, such as tachycardia, prolonged capillary return and cool peripheries. Children effectively compensate for hypovolaemia with tachycardia, and a low systolic blood pressure is a late and concerning feature. In children, demonstration of haemoperitoneum *per se* is not an indication for surgery. Nowadays, initial imaging in major abdominal trauma is with a contrast enhanced CT scan. Diagnostic peritoneal lavage is virtually never undertaken. Renal injuries are usually associated with an extraperitoneal haematoma (because of their retroperitoneal location) and haematuria (see below). Non-operative management is the mainstay of most blunt hepatic, splenic and renal injuries, and is successful in >95% of cases. Uncommon cases of ongoing major bleeding may necessitate intervention such as angioembolisation or laparotomy. Preservation of the spleen obviates the risk of post-splenectomy pneumococcal sepsis.

Anterior compression of the epigastrium puts the pancreas and duodenum at risk of injury. Pancreatic trauma may lead to the development of a pseudocyst in the weeks that follow. Perforation or haematoma of the duodenum may be associated with avulsion of the right renal artery where it crosses the lumbar spine. Compression of the lower abdomen anteriorly occurs with lap-belt injuries. During rapid deceleration, the small bowel is compressed by the lap-belt against the spine, causing perforation or mesenteric vascular injury, which may lead to secondary perforation following necrosis. The child with a lap-belt injury is also at risk of a hyperflexion injury of the spine, producing ligamentous instability, or even multiple fractures of the lumbar vertebrae (Chance fracture). Clinical examination may reveal a bruise over the lumbar region and lumbar spine radiographs will demonstrate any instability. Proven or suspected injury to the bowel with perforation is an indication for laparoscopy and/or laparotomy.

Compression of the pelvis with a fracture suggests a severe injury, such as a high-velocity motor vehicle crash or a fall from a height. Both the bladder and membranous urethra may be injured.

UROLOGICAL INJURIES

Injury to the urinary tract can occur anywhere from the kidney to the distal urethra. Blunt abdominal trauma is more likely to cause renal injury, whereas straddle injuries in males may produce urethral damage. In all suspected intraabdominal injuries, the presence or absence of blood in the urine must be determined. Absence of haematuria virtually excludes injury to the urinary tract, except where the ureter has been transected. Clinically, there may be signs of extravasation of urine and blood in the flank or loin, and contrast urography will confirm the diagnosis.

Falls and kicks to the loin are the usual cause of renal trauma. The clinical features include tenderness and muscular rigidity over the loin and, in time, a mass may become palpable through the anterior abdominal wall. Macroscopic haematuria is usual. A CT scan with intravenous contrast will delineate the injury. The severity of the injury ranges from renal contusion to complete avulsion of the vascular pedicle of the kidney. Lacerations to the pelvicalyceal system, or through the renal parenchyma into the calyces, may lead to urinary extravasation into the perinephric space. A renal laceration may involve disruption of the vascular supply to one pole of the kidney, with necrosis. Renal injuries may cause significant retroperitoneal blood loss and must always be considered in blunt abdominal trauma. Haematuria following a relatively minor accident suggests that there may be a pre-existing abnormality in the kidney (e.g. hydronephrosis or Wilms tumour). Renal ultrasound scan or other urinary tract investigation must be performed in these children.

Bladder injuries, which are rare in children, may be either extraperitoneal or intraperitoneal, as the bladder is anatomically related to both spaces. Extraperitoneal bladder rupture and injury to the posterior urethra may occur with pelvic fractures. When the urethra is injured, a male child is unable to pass urine and a small amount of frank blood may appear at the external urethral meatus. Urinary extravasation in the perineum extending into the scrotum may be seen, and in time the bladder will become palpable in the suprapubic region. This sign may be obscured by haematoma and tenderness in the lower ventral abdominal wall from the concomitant pelvic injury. Straddle injury is another major cause of urethral injury, especially in males, such as occurs when a child slips on a wet floor while climbing out of a bath. In boys this ruptures the bulbar urethra. There will be a bruise in the perineum, but urine extravasation is limited by Scarpa's fascia (known as Colles' fascia in the perineum). A retrograde urethrogram must be obtained in any child who is suspected of having a urethral injury.

SOFT TISSUE INJURIES

Lacerations are sustained during falls or play, when handling dangerous objects, or are incurred during major trauma. Assessment of a child with a laceration may be difficult. Firstly, the child may be too small to cooperate, and secondly, bruising or stretching of nerves may cause a neuropraxia with temporary loss of function of that nerve, mimicking transection. Likewise, tendons may be incompletely severed but appear to have intact function on clinical examination. Examination for sensory deficit can be particularly unrewarding. For these reasons, it is mandatory that all wounds in children are explored adequately, especially those that are likely to involve nerves, vessels or tendons. There may be a related fracture. All non-viable tissue and foreign material should be removed at the time of exploration. Lacerations may become secondarily infected.

Infants, particularly those wearing woollen booties or mittens, may get a strand or wool of hair encircling a digit, causing hair-thread tourniquet syndrome. This can also rarely affect other parts of the body, including the penis, clitoris and uvula.

FRACTURES

Fractures are common because children play vigorously and often fail to take adequate precautionary or evasive measures. Fractures are misdiagnosed frequently as sprains because they are so close to the joint. However, since the ligaments are relatively stronger than the bones in childhood, sprains are rare. Two features that make fractures in childhood different from those in adults are the flexibility of the bone and the presence of a growth plate. Simple, deforming injuries usually produce greenstick fractures, rather than comminution. Healing is rapid,

and delayed union and non-union are rare. The fracture can be reduced by manipulation under regional or general anaesthesia, and remodelling during growth will ensure a satisfactory long-term result. When the growth plate has been injured the fracture may need precise anatomical reduction, by open surgery and internal fixation. Growth arrest may occur around the knee, even when the growth plate has not been fractured.

Upper limb fractures

Fractures of the clavicle are extremely common in children, and usually follow a fall. Reduction is rarely required, and the fracture heals satisfactorily with the arm in a sling. Local bruising on the arm indicates a soft tissue injury, while obvious deformity and local tenderness suggest a fracture.

A supracondylar fracture of the humerus may occur after a fall on to the outstretched hand. The elbow joint is pushed posteriorly and the distal humerus is tilted backwards. There is severe pain and swelling with immobility of the elbow joint. The brachial artery may be damaged by the bone end leading to spasm or direct vascular injury. Clinically, the radial pulse may be absent. If ischaemia persists, there will be pain, pallor, paralysis and puffiness of the forearm, which ultimately leads to muscle infarction and secondary fibrosis (Volkmann contracture). Key signs of vascular injury include loss of the radial pulse and increased pain in the forearm when the fingers are extended passively. In this situation the fracture needs to be reduced rapidly and, if reduction does not relieve the vascular spasm, the artery may need exploration.

A capitellar fracture of the humerus occurs when the lateral condyle of the humerus is fractured following a fall on to the outstretched hand. It may be misdiagnosed as a sprain unless the small flake of distal metaphysis is recognised, indicating a fracture through the cartilaginous growth plate.

Of the forearm fractures the most common is a greenstick fracture of the lower end of the radius and ulna. Mid-shaft breaks of the radius and ulna occur with more severe trauma. Mid-shaft fracture of the ulna may be associated with dislocation of the radial head if there is a direct blow to the back of the forearm. Dislocation or subluxation of the radial head my also occur in infants from pulling the arm too hard ('pulled elbow').

Lower limb fractures

Mid-shaft fractures of the femur are seen after pedestrian or cycle accidents. In small children, bleeding from the femur may not be severe. Hence, if there is evidence of hypovolaemia, it may reflect significant injury elsewhere, such as a ruptured spleen.

Toddlers running about may suffer a twisting injury to the tibia, producing a spiral fracture. Diagnosis may be delayed if the child is still able to walk and is not old enough to describe any physical symptoms. It is therefore one cause of a limp in a small child.

Trauma | CHAPTER 10

NON-ACCIDENTAL INJURY (CHILD ABUSE)

Sadly, child abuse is endemic in all sectors of society. It comes in many guises, and it is essential that the clinician is able to recognise the features that are suggestive of non-accidental injury (NAI).

Sexual abuse is a specific form of maltreatment in children and may go unrecognised unless the clinician maintains a high index of suspicion. Occasionally, there may be a direct report of abuse from the child. More often, the presentation is relatively obscure and includes: venereal disease; genital or rectal trauma; precocious sexual interest; pregnancy; inappropriate sexual activity; indiscrete masturbation; or genital inflammation and discharge. Sexual abuse needs to be distinguished from other causes of vaginal discharge, urinary tract infection, perineal and perianal abnormalities, and simple accidents involving the perineal region (e.g. straddle injury). Medicolegal considerations make a detailed examination under controlled conditions essential.

BURNS

Approximately two-thirds of burns in childhood are due to hot liquids (scalds) and occur in the home. Knowledge of the causative agents is helpful in anticipating the likely severity of the burn. In general, the depth of a thermal burn depends on the temperature generated by the causative agent, the length of time the skin was exposed and the physical characteristics of the heat source. For example, petroleum products generate very much more heat than hot water for a given length of time of exposure. In electrical burns, all tissues between the entry and exit points of the current may be damaged. Skin is a poor conductor, so is less affected than the underlying muscle, nerves and blood vessels, masking the true seriousness of the injury.

The severity of the burn depends on the depth of the tissue damaged and the percentage surface area of the body affected:

1 The metabolic upset is greater with deeper burns.
2 Healing occurs more slowly in deep dermal burns.
3 Deep burns require skin grafting.
4 Deep circumferential burns involving limbs or the chest wall may require urgent decompression with escharotomy.

Estimation of the depth of epidermal burns (evident as erythema only but very painful) and full-thickness burns (white, leathery and insensate) is easy, whereas the depth of thermal burns (superficial, mid or deep dermal) may be initially difficult to establish (*Table 10.1*). Depth can be difficult to estimate in the first few hours after the burn, but a more accurate assessment is possible on day 3 post injury. In the mid or deep dermal burn, coagulative necrosis and thrombosis of underlying vessels is seen as dark red puncta, although there may be islands of surviving skin between them. Superficial burns are typically painful and tender, but discomfort reduces as the burn deepens due to damage to the dermal nerve endings, such that full-thickness burns are pain-free and insensate. Alongside the

TABLE 10.1 Clinical features according to the depth of burn.

Classification	Depth characteristic	Clinical features
Superficial	Epidermal	Erythema only, very painful
	Superficial dermal	Blisters +/− intact, brisk capillary return, moist, painful
	Mid dermal	Less moist, sluggish capillary return, less painful
Deep	Deep dermal	Dry, fixed staining (no capillary return), reduced sensation
	Full thickness	White, charred, leathery, insensate

depth of burn, estimating the percentage of total body surface area (TBSA) burned is crucial, as it affects both management and outcome. The area of epidermal burns is discounted from TBSA estimations. Young children have a proportionally larger head and smaller limbs than the older child or adult, and accurate TBSA calculation is possible with tools such as a 'Lund and Browder' chart. Despite this, there is a tendency to overestimate the area burned. Late sequelae of burns include hypertrophic scars, contractures, psychological consequences and, depending on their location, microstomia or loss of digits.

Inhalation injury

Burn injuries sustained in a closed environment may be associated with the inhalation of hot gases and products of combustion. The presence of an inhalation injury should be suspected where:

1 There are burns to the nose or hairs in the nostrils or oedema of the mucous membrane of the mouth and pharynx.
2 There is a hoarse voice (suggestive of vocal cord oedema).
3 There is an audible wheeze, confirmed on auscultation.
4 There are signs of hypoxia – restlessness, confusion, disorientation or a change of behaviour; these features may be difficult to distinguish clinically from pain, fear and anxiety.

CAUSTIC INGESTION

Swallowing corrosive fluids or solids is nearly always accidental in the toddler between 1 and 3 years of age. Cleaning agents (e.g. dishwashing powder or detergents) are swallowed often, and the oesophagus is the organ injured. Alkalis are more commonly ingested than acids. Circumferential oesophageal burns may lead to severe strictures, which usually need repeated dilatations and may ultimately require resection.

Clues to the diagnosis of oesophageal injury can be obtained from the history (observation of the child having swallowed a corrosive, excessive drooling and dysphagia) and from evidence of burns on the lips, buccal mucosa, soft palate or tongue. If these structures are burned, it is likely that the oesophagus will be involved as well. The definitive diagnosis is made by oesophagoscopy performed at about 24 hours after the injury. This will determine the severity of the burn and the likelihood of subsequent stricture formation.

FOREIGN BODIES

Accidental swallowing of a foreign body is most frequent in the first years of life. The vast majority of ingested foreign bodies are asymptomatic, and once they reach the stomach they will pass spontaneously without danger to the child. Ingested foreign bodies that become stuck are most often encountered in the post-cricoid region of the distal pharynx at the level of the cricopharyngeus muscle. Less often, ingested foreign bodies arrest in the lower oesophagus. Radiographs identify the position of a radiopaque foreign body, but plastic toys, which may be jagged and angular, are radiolucent and this may lead to delay in diagnosis. If a foreign body becomes impacted in the oesophagus and remain unrecognised, oesophageal ulceration may progress to perforation and potentially fatal sequelae such as mediastinitis, an acquired tracheo-oesophageal fistula or an aorto-oesophageal fistula. Dysphagia, dyspnoea, pain and swelling in the neck, and fever or pleuritic pain may be the first signs that a complication has developed.

Long straight foreign bodies (e.g. bobby-pins) may get stuck at the duodenojejunal flexure and require surgical extraction. 'Button' or 'disc' batteries used in many household devices may release strong alkali, resulting in a chemical burn that may cause local necrosis and perforation if its passage through the gut is delayed. A button battery lodged in the oesophagus is particularly dangerous as severe injury can occur within several hours. Heavy metal poisoning (mercury, cadmium, nickel, zinc or magnesium) has been reported.

Inhaled foreign bodies typically present with sudden onset of coughing, spluttering and gagging, with a residual wheeze. The clinical picture varies with the size of the object, the site of lodgement and the time elapsed since the object was inhaled. Inspiratory stridor and retraction of the supraclavicular and intercostal areas suggest that the object is in the larynx or subglottic area. Tracheal or bronchial foreign bodies produce a wheeze with radiological evidence of a ball-valve type of obstruction on expiratory and inspiratory radiographs. Distal impacted objects tend to present late with chronic chest infection from lobar or segmental consolidation.

Foreign bodies may also become lodged in the external auditory canal, the nose and the piriform fossa. The knee and foot are common sites for foreign bodies (e.g. pins or glass fragments on to which the child has walked or crawled). Radiopaque objects can be identified readily on radiographs and removed with the assistance of an image intensifier. Unrecognised foreign bodies may lead to infection.

OCULAR INJURIES

In children with head injuries and facial abrasions, especially to the middle third of the face, an eye injury should be suspected. An open eye injury needs to be excluded, even if it requires a general anaesthetic to do so. Failure to recognize an open eye injury is likely to result in blindness. Subconjunctival haemorrhages occur from a number of causes. These include remote thoracic and head injuries and direct local trauma to the eye, as well as orbital or frontal fractures. The cause of the haemorrhage can usually be determined by searching for a posterior limit to the haemorrhage, which is not present when it is caused by a posterior orbital fracture.

Mechanical injuries of the eye are classified according to the Birmingham Eye Trauma Terminology and are divided into closed and open globe injuries. Open globe injuries may result from rupture as the result of blunt trauma or injuries from sharp objects. Open injuries to the globe are frequently associated with damage to intraocular structures, particularly the lens and retina. A foreign body may be retained within the eye in some instances. The primary surgical management is to remove any retained intraocular foreign body, close the defect in the eye wall and prevent intraocular infection. The prognosis is related to the amount of intraocular damage.

Hyphemas are caused by blunt force that distorts the globe and tears iris blood vessels. In general, they are managed conservatively, the blood clearing from the anterior chamber with rest alone. Secondary haemorrhage occurs in some cases and is often associated with raised intraocular pressure, requiring intervention.

Chemical injury to the eye is common in childhood and frequently involves accidental exposure to cleaning agents or explosive devices such as fireworks. Management consists of initial first aid to remove the chemical with irrigation, and then subsequent management is directed at preventing infection, encouraging normal healing and, if needed, rectifying any permanent damage.

Full-thickness lacerations of the eyelid require meticulous primary repair of the skin and tarsal plates. Associated trauma to the globe or lacrimal drainage apparatus must be excluded. Lacerations involving the medial aspect of either eyelid should prompt thorough examination to exclude injury to the canalicular system. Isolated division of the superior canaliculus may not warrant repair as an intact lower system will allow adequate tear drainage. Primary repair is required if the lower canalicular system is divided.

Blow-out fractures of the orbit in childhood are uncommon. Imaging usually delineates the nature of the orbital injury. Entrapment of inferior rectus or medial rectus in the fracture or significant enophthalmos associated with a large bony defect in the orbital floor indicates a need for intervention. Diplopia in the absence of bony entrapment of a muscle will usually resolve with conservative management. If it persists, then surgical intervention is required.

Penetrating injury to the orbit can occur with a variety of different objects. Imaging is required to delineate the extent of the injury. Care must be taken to determine the extent of any associated eye and intracranial injuries. Management requires removal of a foreign body, antibiotic prophylaxis and repair of the associated injury.

The ocular features of non-accidental injury are varied. Retinal haemorrhage is the most common, and is believed to be due to shaking the child. Such retinal haemorrhages are often associated with intracranial haemorrhage. Traumatic retinoschisis and perimacular retinal folds have very high specificity for non-accidental injury in the absence of a severe closed head injury such as observed with crushing injuries or falls from a significant height. Haemorrhage within the optic nerve sheath is seen rarely, and occurs with severe and generally fatal shaking injury. Hyphema and lens damage may result from direct blows to the eye. Management is usually expectant. Mandatory reporting of suspected non-accidental injury is required in most countries.

HEAD INJURIES

Head injuries are the main cause of morbidity and mortality from trauma in children. They are responsible for 80% of the deaths, and most children with multiple system injuries have a head injury.

Injury to the brain occurs in two phases: first, at the time of the accident (primary brain damage) and secondly, as a consequence of both local and distant injuries causing additional brain injury (secondary brain damage). Therapeutic measures may influence the severity of the secondary brain injury. The child's brain is more susceptible to injury than the adult's because the cranial bones are thinner and afford less protection, the brain is less myelinated, making it more easily damaged, and the brain may develop marked hyperaemia and swelling. Major

associated chest and intra-abdominal injuries may produce hypoxia, hypercarbia and hypovolaemia, factors that adversely affect cerebral perfusion. Oxygenation of the brain may be compromised by airway obstruction, poor ventilation, hypotension, brain swelling and intracranial haemorrhage.

The initial neurological assessment determines the urgency of neurosurgical care and provides baseline information for the assessment of subsequent progress. The level of consciousness is best assessed using the Glasgow Coma Scale, which records eye-opening, best verbal response and best motor response (*Table 10.2*). This scale enables the clinician to assess conscious level objectively and to monitor its progress with time. A cumulative score of ten or less (out of 14) signifies a serious head injury. In the absence of shock, a decrease of three or more in the score strongly suggests development of a major intracranial complication. Children under 4 years of age do not have fully developed verbal skills, and a modified scale is required.

Pupillary size and reactivity should be recorded, with the diameter of the pupil measured in millimetres. Causes of fixed dilated pupils include traumatic iridoplegia, direct nerve damage, cerebral ischaemia or increased intracranial pressure. Detailed examination of the optic fundi can be delayed, but retinal haemorrhages suggest a major head injury and in a child less than 1 year of age, are strongly suggestive of non-accidental injury. Acute papilloedema developing within 2 hours of a head injury signifies grossly elevated intracranial pressure, which is usually fatal. Limbs are examined for their resting position, spontaneous movement and tone. Complete flaccidity ('loss of muscle tone') is seen with severe injury of the brainstem or high spinal cord transection. There is no spontaneous movement of the limbs. Patterns of rigidity include decerebrate rigidity and decorticate rigidity. In high brainstem lesions, rigidity usually is bilateral, whereas in injuries to one cerebral hemisphere, it is unilateral, with the head turned to the contralateral side. A down-going plantar response is considered normal except in infants. Where the response is equivocal, the examination should be repeated periodically. Bradycardia in the presence of increasing blood pressure is a late sign of increasing intracranial pressure. Hypotension associated with a head injury is usually caused by internal haemorrhage elsewhere, except (1) where there is obvious external haemorrhage from the scalp; (2) where a scalp haematoma is present in an infant; or (3) where intracranial haemorrhage occurs in the neonate and infant.

Cerebrospinal fluid (CSF) otorrhoea and rhinorrhoea reflect a dural tear and are associated with an increased risk of meningitis. CSF otorrhoea usually stops spontaneously, but CSF rhinorrhoea may require definitive surgical repair of the dura.

A foreign body penetrating the skull and lodged in the brain should initially be left *in situ* as it may be acting as a tamponade controlling cerebral bleeding. The object can be removed by the neurosurgeon in theatre.

An extradural haematoma results from a tear in a dural vessel and is usually seen in association with a skull fracture. The patient develops a headache and becomes drowsy. There may be boggy swelling in the temporal region and

Response	Degree	Score
Eye opening	Never	1
	To pain	2
	To speech	3
	Spontaneously	4
Best verbal response	None	1
	Garbled	2
	Inappropriate	3
	Confused	4
	Oriented	5
Best motor response	None	1
	Extension	2
	Abnormal flexion	3
	Withdrawal from painful stimuli	4
	Localises painful stimuli	5

TABLE 10.2 Glasgow Coma Scale.

the ipsilateral pupil becomes dilated and fixed. The level of consciousness decreases. A CT scan confirms the diagnosis and accurately locates the haematoma. Subdural haematomas result from injuries to the brain surface, including the bridging veins between the cerebral cortex and dura. They are seen in young children after high speed injuries, or after violent shaking in child abuse. The concomitant severe primary brain injury may make deterioration less obvious. The outlook is not as good as with an extradural haematoma. An intracerebral haematoma presents with slow neurological deterioration over several days following a severe head injury.

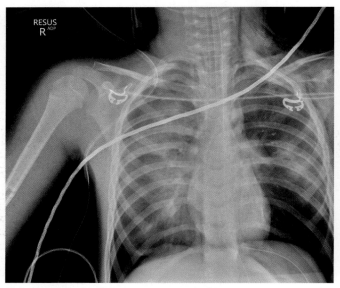

Fig. 10.1 Bilateral traumatic pneumothoraces following a motor vehicle accident. Note the right-sided rib fractures of ribs 1–4 and the right humeral shaft fracture. The first rib fracture is an important finding as such fractures are rare in the compliant, paediatric chest wall and should prompt a thorough assessment for both thoracic and extrathoracic injuries associated with extreme force to the chest of the child.

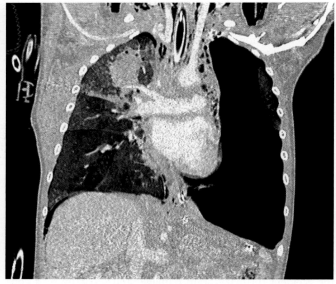

Fig. 10.2 Tension pneumothorax in a young child following a run-over accident with catastrophic lung injuries. It is unusual to image a tension pneumothorax, even more so on CT imaging. However, this child deteriorated during CT scanning, with tension of the left-sided pneumothorax evidenced by flattening of the left hemi-diaphragm, superior displacement of the heart off the diaphragm and displacement of the trachea to the right. Serious left lung injuries are also present.

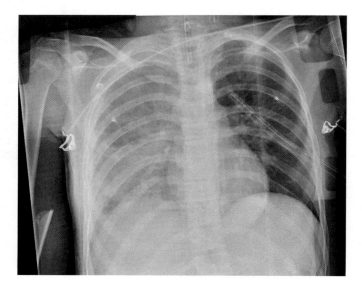

Fig. 10.3 Large right-sided haemothorax following severe blunt truncal trauma. A clinically obvious left-sided pneumothorax has already been addressed with an intercostal drain insertion prior to any imaging. Bilateral pneumocath insertion was performed prior to arrival at the hospital, but has been ineffective. Note the associated right humeral fracture and fractured ribs.

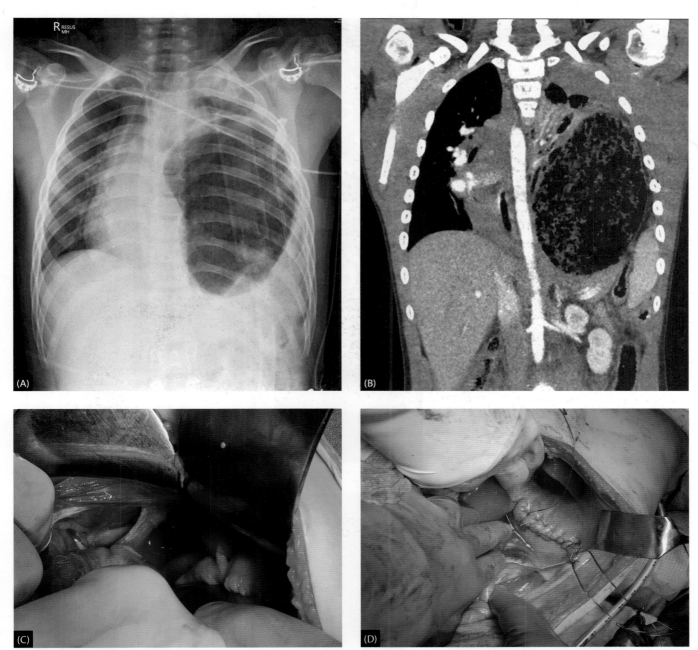

Figs. 10.4A–D (A) Traumatic diaphragmatic hernia on chest radiograph, with gas in displaced stomach. This appearance can be mistaken for a pneumothorax, with risk of iatrogenic gastric injury should intercostal drain insertion be attempted. This is a rare but important injury in children, typically following severe blunt trauma but may also occur with penetrating trauma. (B) Traumatic diaphragmatic hernia now shown on CT. This child has escaped associated solid organ injury. (C, D) Trauma laparotomy showing the appearance of the reduced diaphragmatic hernial defect prior to (C) and after (D) repair.

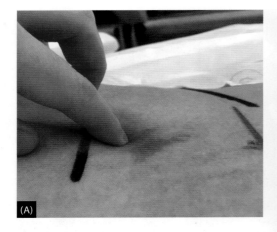

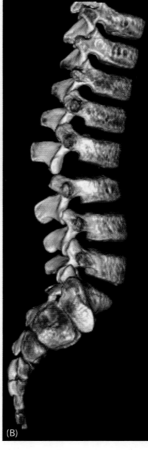

Figs. 10.5A, B (A) Chance fracture caused by hyperflexion injury, with a bruise over the lumbar spine and a depression where the longitudinal ligaments have been disrupted. This injury is often caused by a motor accident where the child is only wearing a lap seat-belt. (B) CT reconstruction showing the gap in the dorsal spines caused by rupture of the longitudinal ligaments in a hyperflexion injury.

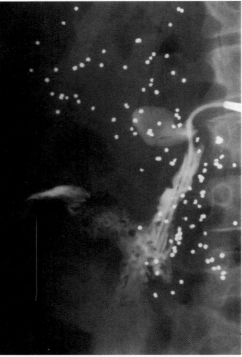

Fig. 10.6 This child previously sustained a shotgun blast to the abdomen and multiple pellets remain *in situ*. This study is a sinogram, performed to outline the tract of a chronic discharging osteomyelitis of the lumbar vertebra.

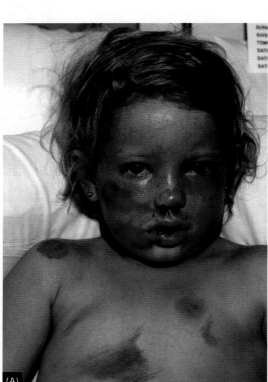

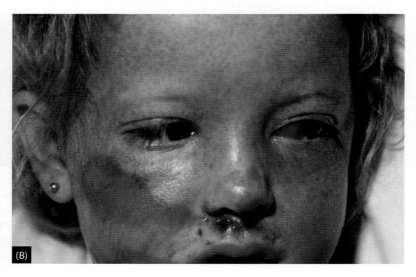

Figs. 10.7A, B (A) Traumatic asphyxia in a small child who was backed over by a car in the driveway. There are multiple petechial haemorrhages of the head, neck and shoulders secondary to compression of the chest, causing transient obstruction of the superior vena cava. There are also a number of superficial skin abrasions. Traumatic asphyxia may be accompanied by cerebral oedema. (B) Close-up view showing the facial petechial and subconjunctival haemorrhages.

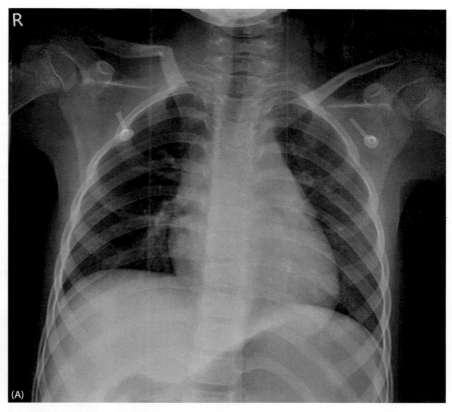

Figs. 10.8A–C Acute gastric dilatation is very common in children following multi-trauma, and in the absence of a gastric decompression tube presents a significant risk of vomiting and aspiration. The trauma chest radiograph (A) provides the first opportunity for recognition, but the stomach appearance is often overlooked. The CT appearance (B, C) is unequivocal and demands immediate action to prevent morbidity. Gastric decompression, which can be achieved by aspiration through a wide bore nasogastric tube, is an essential consideration in all children following multi-trauma.

(A)

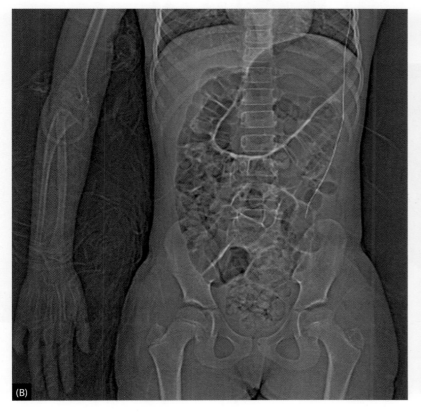

(B)

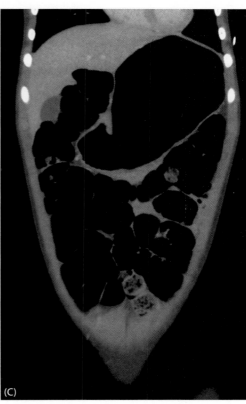

(C)

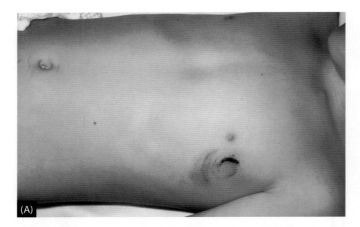

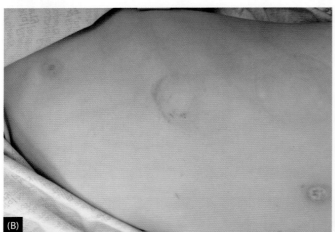

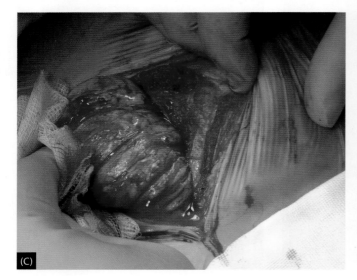

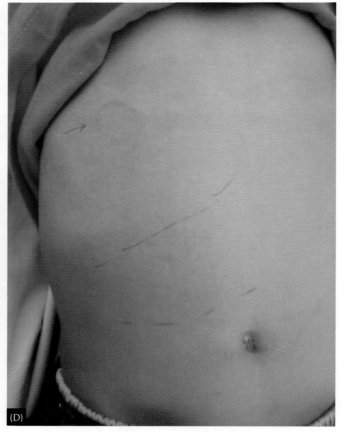

Figs. 10.9A–D Handlebar injuries. (A) A handlebar injury to the left lower chest wall in this child caused a ruptured spleen. The child presented with signs of hypovolaemia and marked tenderness in the left upper quadrant, which extended across the whole abdomen with time. He also complained of intermittent left shoulder-tip pain. There was no rib fracture, reflecting the elasticity of the child's chest wall. (B) Handlebar injury to the epigastrium, which resulted in transection of the pancreas. (C) Bike handlebar injury caused this transected pancreas. (D) Blunt trauma to the liver after a handlebar injury, with the site of the handlebar mark indicated. The dotted lines on the abdomen show the progressive enlargement of the liver as the intrahepatic bleeding continues.

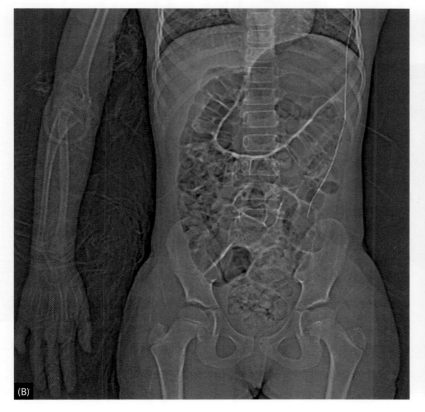

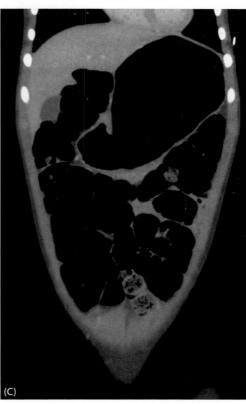

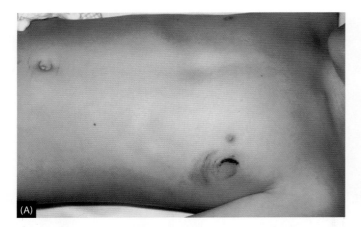

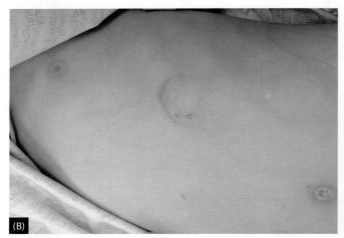

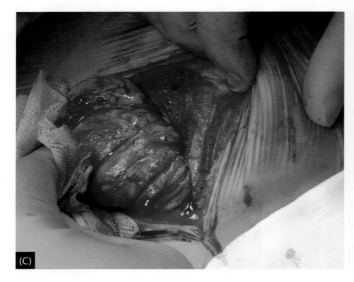

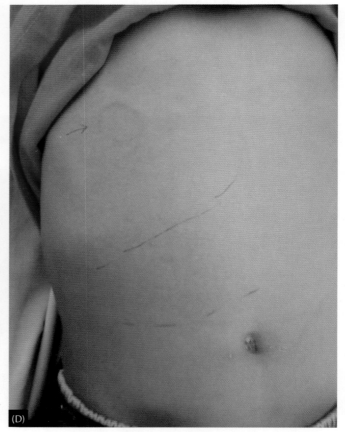

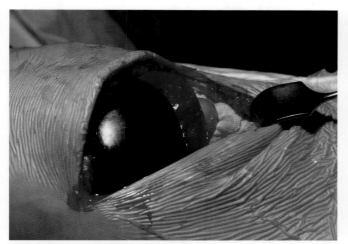

Fig. 10.10 A large hepatic haematoma replacing most of the right lobe of the liver. These injuries resolve spontaneously without surgery, although haemobilia is an occasional complication.

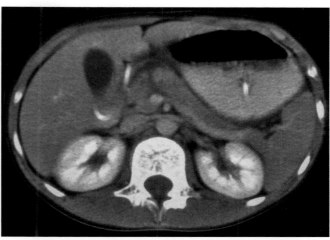

Fig. 10.11 Abdominal CT showing a fracture through the neck of the pancreas.

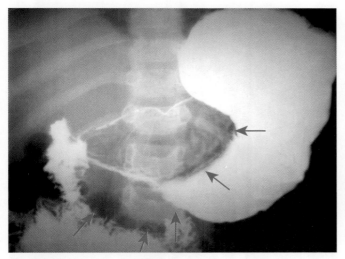

Fig. 10.12 A moderate-sized pancreatic pseudocyst causing compression of the body and antrum of the stomach, pushing the stomach anteriorly and to the left. The arrows mark the limit of the pancreatic pseudocyst. This is an historical image, and this pathology would now be demonstrated by CT and/or ultrasound imaging.

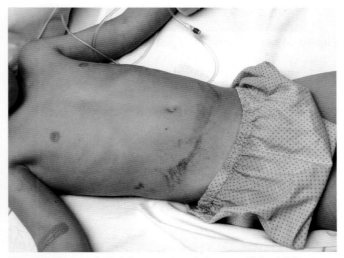

Fig. 10.13 Seat-belt injury to the abdomen. This child was involved in a rapid deceleration motor vehicle accident while wearing a lap-belt only, and sustained a lumbar vertebral (Chance) fracture and perforation of the ileum due to the hyperflexion. (See also **Fig. 10.5**.)

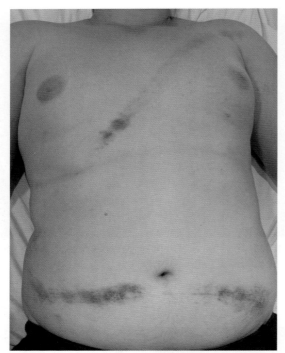

Fig. 10.14 Marked abdominal and chest wall bruising in the classical distribution of a lap-sash seat belt, which may herald significant intra-abdominal and thoracic injuries.

Figs. 10.15A, B (A) Application of a pelvic binder may be life-saving, but must be performed correctly with the pelvic binder positioned at the level of the femoral greater trochanters, as shown here. (B) This child with pelvic trauma has had a pelvic binder applied, but it is not correctly positioned and so is ineffective. The contrast in the bladder is from renal excretion of intravenous contrast given for a CT scan earlier during the child's care.

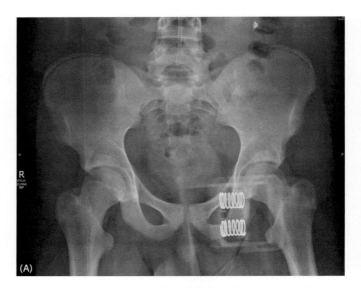

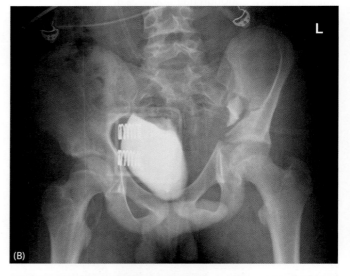

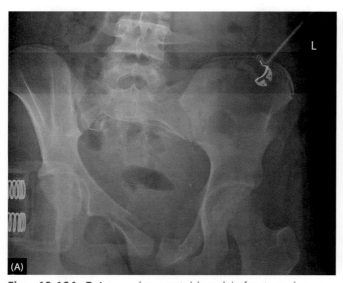

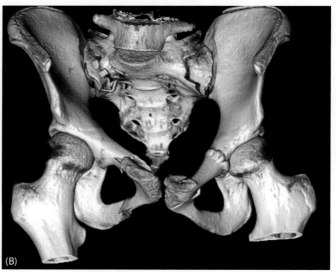

Figs. 10.16A, B A complex, unstable pelvic fracture shown on a plain radiograph (A) and CT reconstruction (B).

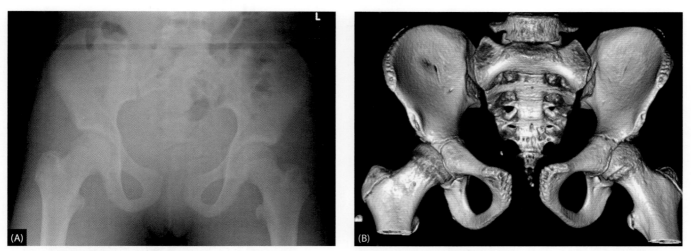

Figs. 10.17A, B 'Open book' pelvic fracture, with disruption of the sacroiliac joints and symphysis pubis shown on a plain radiograph (A) and CT reconstruction (B).

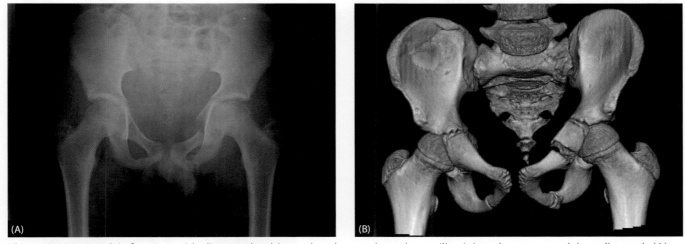

Figs. 10.18A, B Pelvic fracture with disrupted pubic rami and contralateral sacroiliac joint, shown on a plain radiograph (A) and CT reconstruction (B).

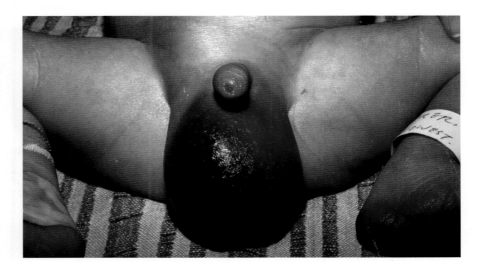

Fig. 10.19 Massive inguinoscrotal haematoma associated with a pelvic fracture in an infant.

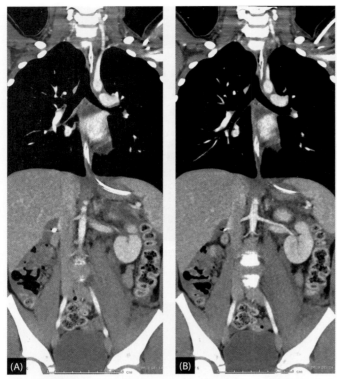

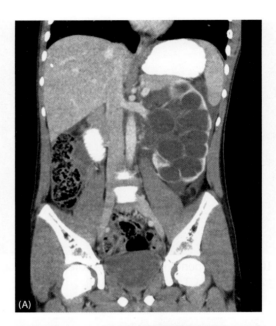

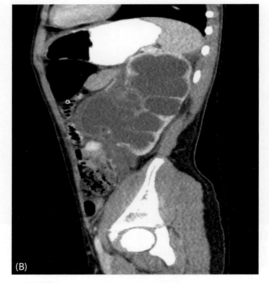

Figs. 10.20A, B (A) CT with contrast of a child with a disruption of the upper pole of the left kidney that extends down to the hilum. (B) Another view of the same patient demonstrating the rent into the renal pelvis, but the renal artery is intact.

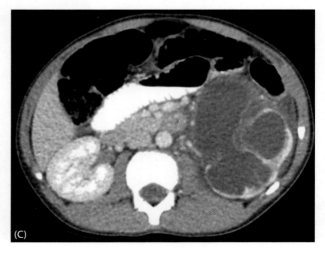

Figs. 10.21A–C Renal injury after minor trauma is one of the presentations of hydronephrosis. This CT scan revealed an extremely enlarged left kidney with extravasation in a child with a severe pelviureteric junction obstruction.

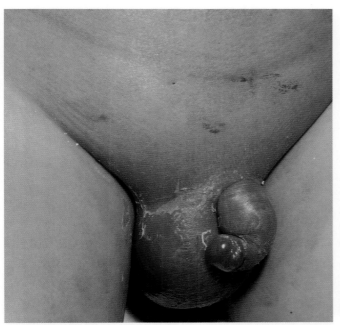

Fig. 10.22 Extraperitoneal bladder rupture in association with pelvic fractures showing extravasation of urine. There is woody induration of the lower abdominal wall with extension of the extravasation to the perineum, scrotum and penis.

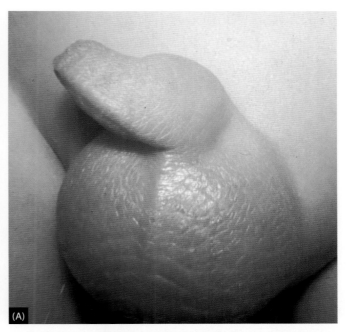

(A)

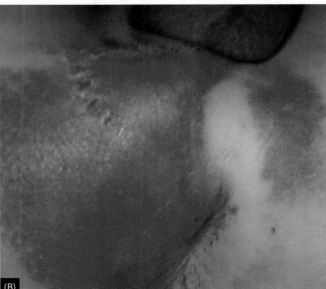

(B)

Figs. 10.23A, B (A) A straddle injury causing urethral disruption, with extravasation of urine in the perineum and scrotum. The child was unable to pass urine and had a palpable bladder in the suprapubic region. A carefully performed urethrogram delineated the injury. (B) Straddle injury in a different boy who was attempting to jump a fence. There is an extensive perineal haematoma. Urethral injury was suspected but not confirmed on a urethrogram.

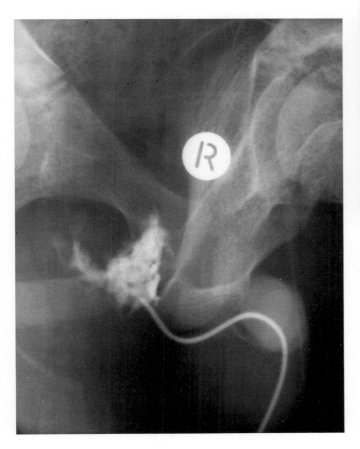

Fig. 10.24 Bulbar urethral injury demonstrated by extravasation of contrast-containing urine on urethrography.

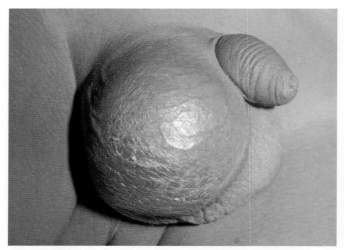

Fig. 10.25 Scrotal haematocele in a child who developed acute enlargement of the scrotum following trauma. The swelling did not transilluminate.

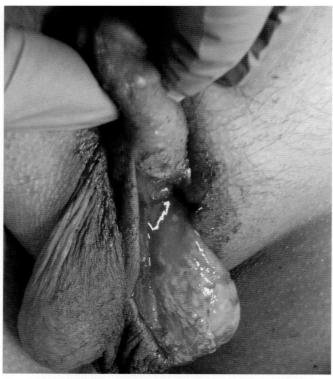

Fig. 10.26 Local trauma to the scrotum exposing the tunica vaginalis and its contained testis, which 'rides' up with the injury and is undamaged.

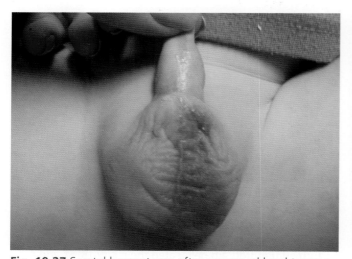

Fig. 10.27 Scrotal haematoma after presumed local trauma.

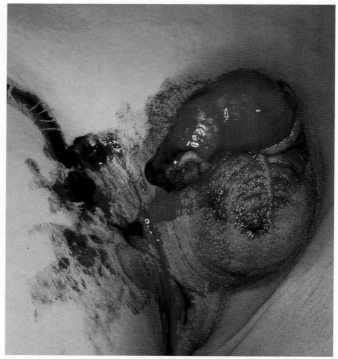

Fig. 10.28 Dog bite to the penis, which has caused a degloving injury to the shaft.

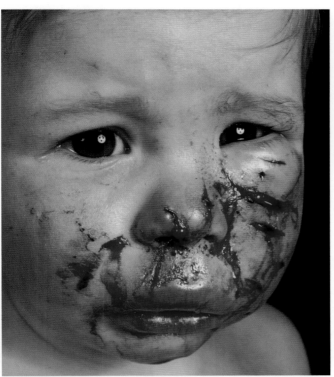

Fig. 10.29 Dog bite to the face in a toddler. Note the degree of facial swelling, particularly around the left eye and upper lip.

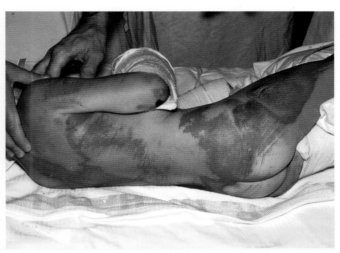

Fig. 10.30 Extensive superficial abrasions following multi-trauma. It is important that associated and more significant injuries are not overlooked (e.g. intra-abdominal injuries, pelvic trauma and limb fractures).

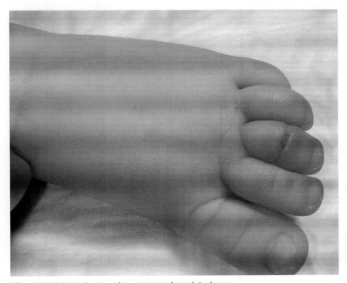

Fig. 10.31 Hair torniquet on the third toe.

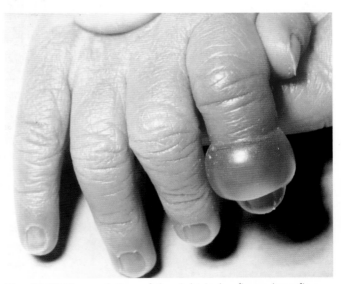

Fig. 10.32 Strangulation of the right index finger by a fine strand of wool.

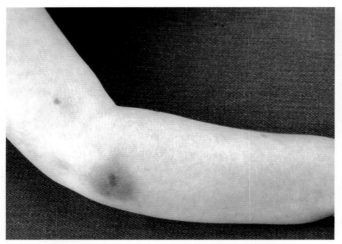

Fig. 10.33 Snake bite to the right forearm. The puncture marks of the fangs and surrounding bruising belie the potential seriousness of the injury. In Australia, for example, most snakes are highly venomous.

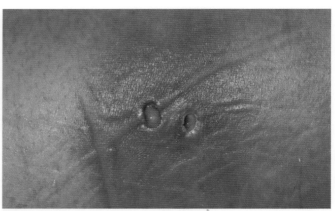

Fig. 10.34 Snake bite wound, in which secondary infection has occurred 4 weeks after being bitten by a tiger snake.

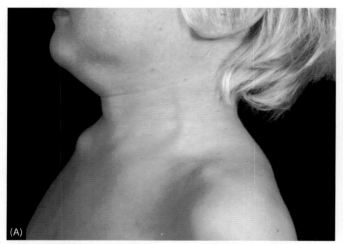

(A)

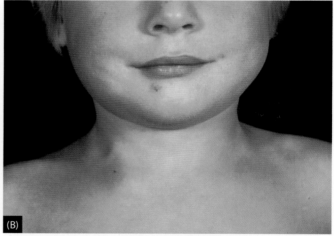

(B)

Figs. 10.35A, B (A) Fracture of the medial end of the right clavicle. This subcutaneous bone is one of the most commonly fractured in childhood. The fracture is visible clinically and accurate reduction of the fracture is not required. (B) Same patient: fractured right clavicle viewed from the front. Note the callus formation at the site of the fracture.

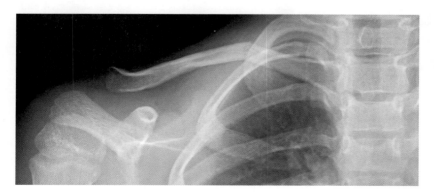

Fig. 10.36 Fracture of the right clavicle in a 4-year-old boy following a fall onto an outstretched arm.

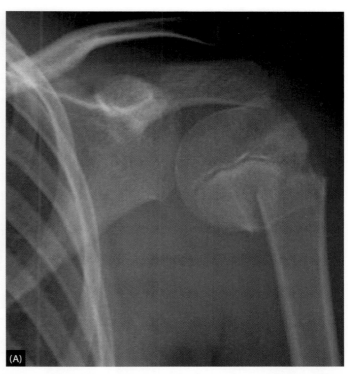

Figs. 10.37A–D (A) Fracture of the surgical neck of the humerus in a 12-year-old boy who fell off a roof onto his arm. Fractures through the neck of the humerus are less common in children than in the elderly. The axillary nerve is at risk of injury with this fracture. (B) Pathological fracture of the proximal humerus through a benign bone cyst (arrow). (C) Another child with a pathological fracture through a benign cyst in the upper humerus. (D) This 11-year-old child fell from a bouncy castle and sustained a spiral fracture of the mid shaft of the humerus. The radial nerve is endangered by this injury.

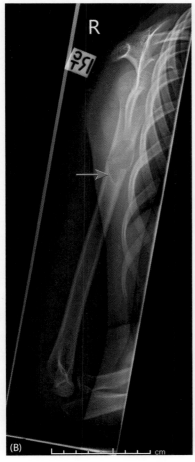

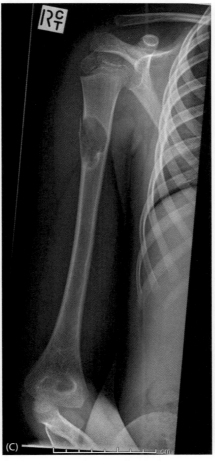

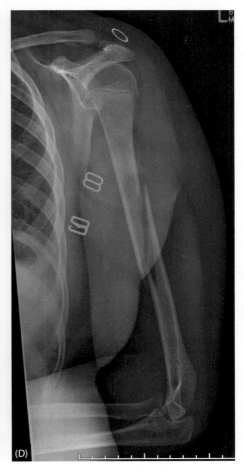

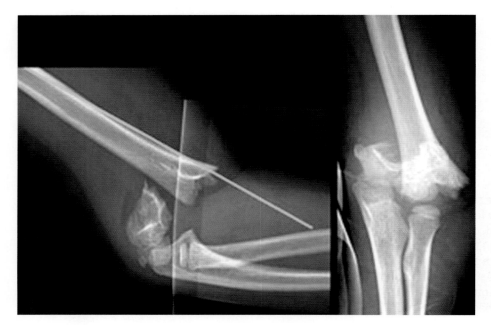

Fig. 10.38 Supracondylar fracture of the humerus. The distal fragment and elbow joint are displaced posteriorly with the distal humeral segment tilted backwards. The elbow joint is unstable. This injury may cause spasm or damage to the brachial artery, resulting in absence of the radial pulse. If unrecognised, persistent ischaemia may ultimately result in a Volkmann contracture. The yellow line indicates the malalignment of the humeral shaft.

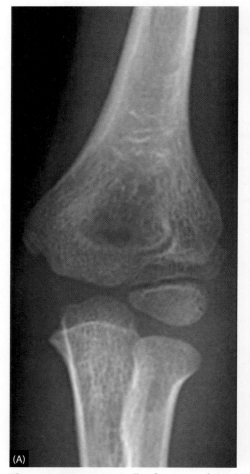

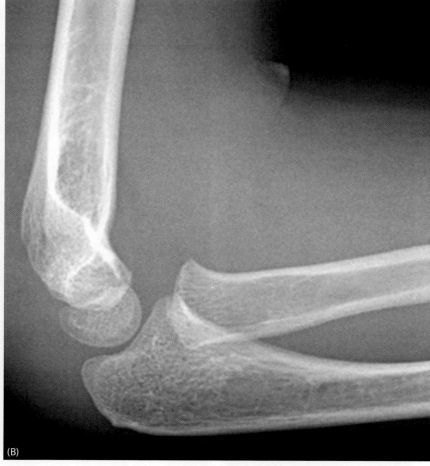

(A)

(B)

Figs. 10.39A, B Capitellar fracture of the humerus in anteroposterior (A) and lateral (B) projections. The lateral condyle of the humerus is displaced following an injury to the lateral side of the elbow caused by a fall on to the outstretched arm. The small flake of distal metaphysis indicates a fracture through the cartilage and the growth plate.

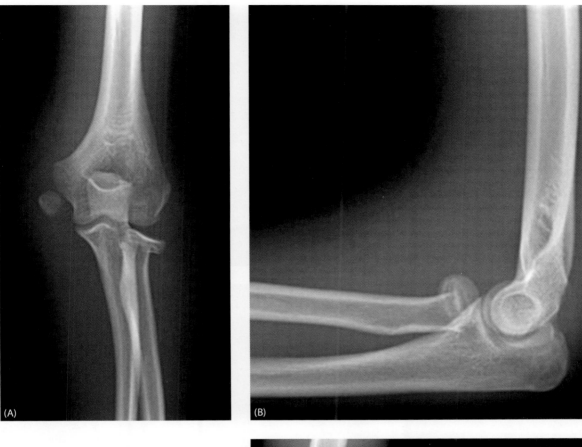

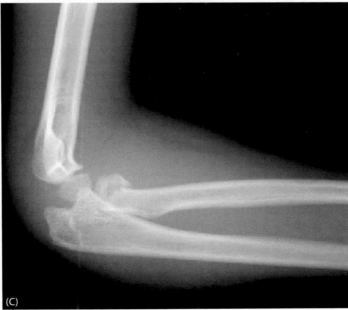

Figs. 10.40A–C Fracture of the head of the radius in an 11-year-old boy following a fall.

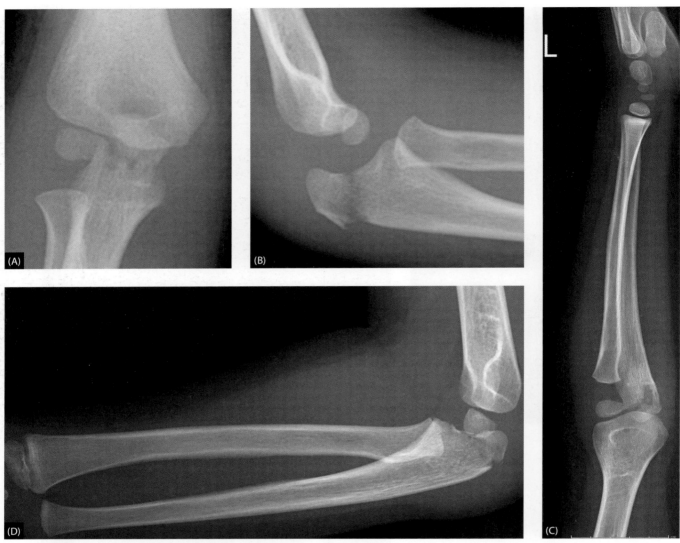

Figs. 10.41A–D (A, B) Fracture through the olecranon, presenting clinically as a tender swelling over the olecranon process. The lateral radiograph shows avulsion of the olecranon. (C, D) This 3-year old fell down the stairs, directly striking the elbow. The bony fragment of the olecranon is being pulled proximally by the attachment of triceps.

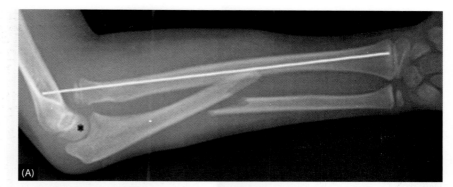

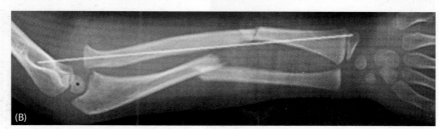

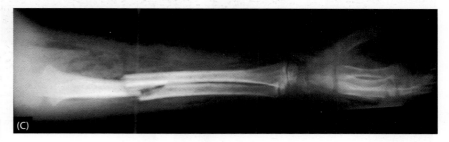

Figs. 10.42A–C (A) Monteggia fracture. A mid-shaft fracture of the ulna may be associated with dislocation of the radial head if there is a direct blow to the back of the forearm. The white line shows the alignment of the radius, demonstrating the concurrent displacement of the radial head. (B) A more severely displaced Monteggia fracture with associated mid-shaft fractures of both radius and ulna. (C) A compound fracture of the mid-shaft of the radius and ulna. This child developed gas gangrene, responsible for extensive gas inside and outlining the soft tissues of the forearm and hand.

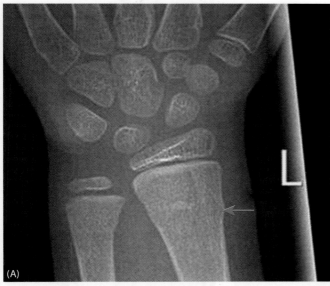

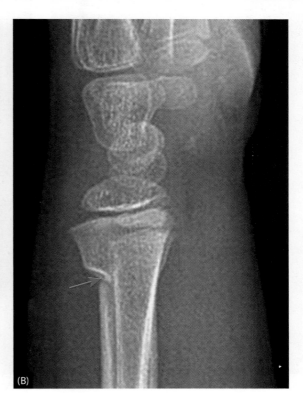

Figs. 10.43A, B (A) Greenstick fracture of the distal radius, with characteristic buckling of the cortex (arrow). (B) Greenstick fracture of the distal radius and ulna. This is a common result of a fall on to an outstretched arm in young children. One side of the cortex is split open (arrow) while the other side buckles.

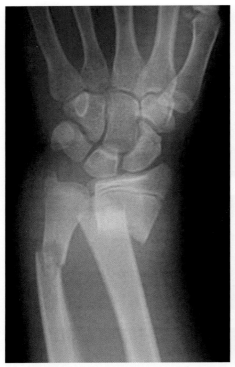

Fig. 10.44 Fracture of the distal radius and ulna with notable displacement.

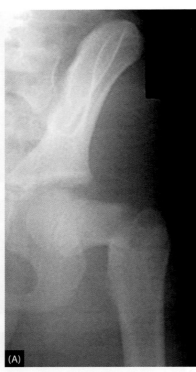

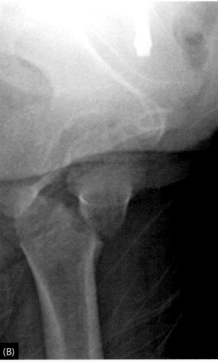

Figs. 10.45A, B (A) Neck of femur fracture, which is a less common injury in a child than in geriatrics and may reflect significant force. (B) Another example of a neck of femur fracture in a child.

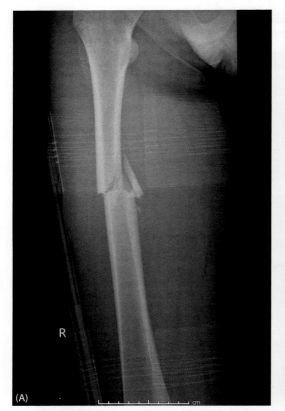

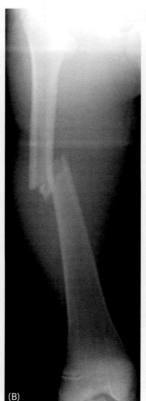

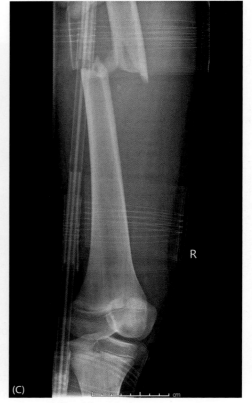

Figs. 10.46A–C Comminuted midshaft fracture of the right femur, which has been immobilised for transport in a splint.

Figs. 10.47A, B (A) Toddler's fracture of the tibia: the spiral fracture line is invisible in this view. (B) Another radiograph of a toddler's fracture showing the spiral fracture line and the periosteal reaction, highlighted by the arrows.

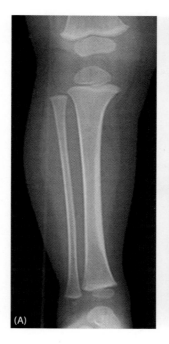

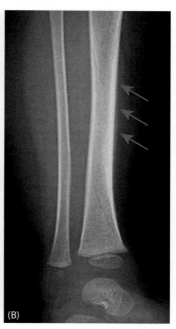

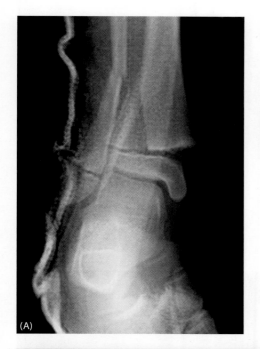

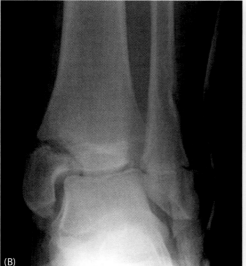

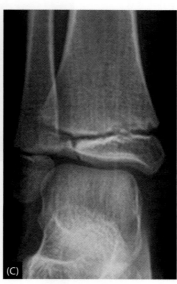

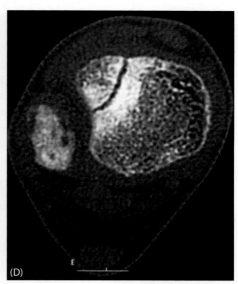

Figs. 10.48A–D (A, B) Severe injury to the lower leg with distal fracture to the shaft of the fibula and a fracture through the growth plate and up into the metaphysis of the distal tibia (i.e. Salter-Harris type II fracture). (C) Fracture along the growth plate and down through the epiphysis of the distal tibia: Salter-Harris type III fracture of the distal tibia (Tillaux fracture). This fracture has implications for both bone growth and the articular surface, with an associated poorer prognosis (e.g. premature secondary osteoarthritis). (D) Axial CT image of a Tillaux fracture in an adolescent, also demonstrating fusion limited to the central and medial aspect of the distal tibial growth plate. The aetiology of the Tillaux fracture is directly related to the interplay between the unfused lateral aspect of the growth plate and the fixed elements either side of this, namely the fused medial growth plate (medial) and tibiofibular ligament (lateral).

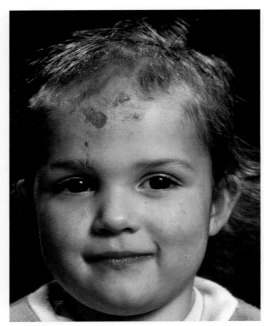

Fig. 10.49 The varied presentations of a child whose injuries may represent non-accidental injury. Note that the child has several small burns to the forehead, a healed scar above the right eyebrow and has had his hair cut in an uncontrolled fashion.

Figs. 10.50A–C Non-accidental injury to a 7-week-old boy who presented with subcutaneous air in the neck associated with fever and shortness of breath. There is a small left pneumothorax (A) but no obvious fractures on the left side on this chest radiograph. However, there are multiple healing fractures in the right chest wall. Callus formation can be seen. One week later, a repeat radiograph showed multiple healing fractures of both the left and right lower ribs (B). A bone scan performed at the same time demonstrated numerous fractures at various stages of healing (C). Other films not included here showed metaphyseal fractures of both femurs, both tibias and one ulna, as well as a fracture of the skull.

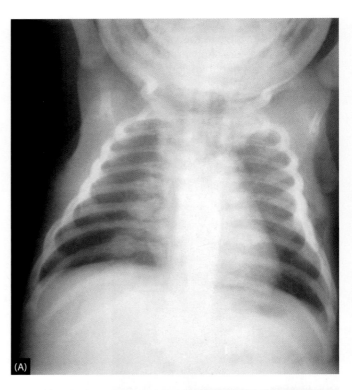

(A)

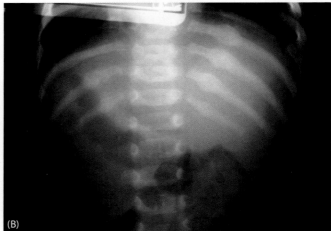

(B)

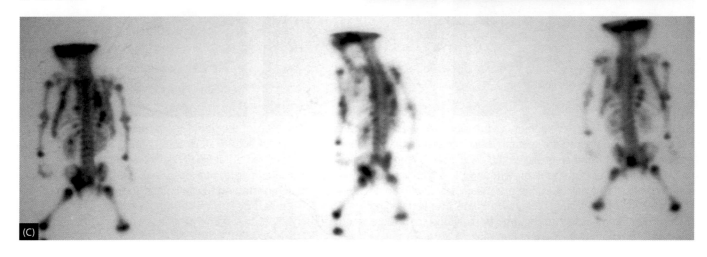

(C)

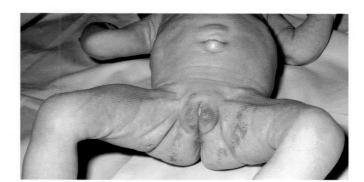

Fig. 10.51 Child abuse by neglect. This neglected and malnourished child presented with failure to thrive and severe nappy rash. She had appalling home circumstances.

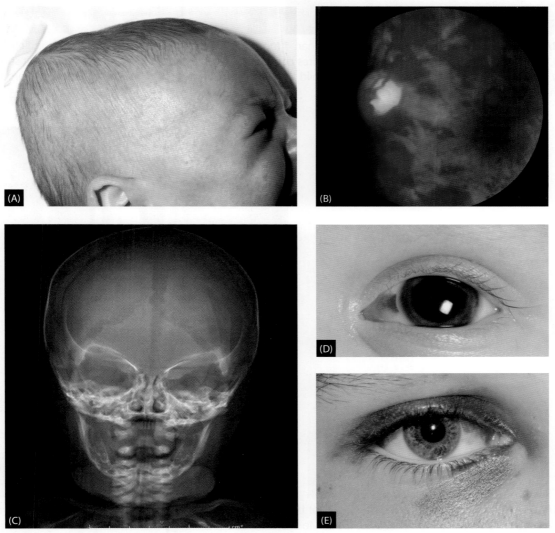

Figs. 10.52A–E (A) This infant was noted to have an occipital swelling, which was not midline, strictly spherical nor related to Ventouse delivery. Examination of the optic fundi revealed retinal haemorrhages, and it transpired the infant had been subjected to significant head injury. (B) Extensive intraretinal and pre-retinal haemorrhages, a common consequence of non-accidental injury in infants. This is caused by severe shaking and blunt trauma, often sufficient to cause a skull fracture as well. (C) Bilateral skull fractures were attributed to a single impact to the head in this child. (D) Outside the neonatal period, a subconjunctival haemorrhage in an infant should generate suspicion about non-accidental injury. (E) The yellow colour in this bruise suggests that injury occurred at least 18 hours previously. Any injury to the eyelids should prompt a thorough examination of the eyes (anatomy and visual function) including assessment for a blow-out fracture of the orbit. In this child the trauma was caused by a punch.

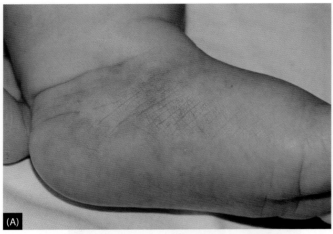

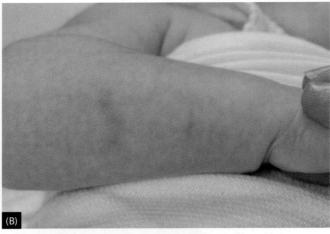

Figs. 10.53A, B (A) Any bruises on an infant aged less than 4 months should generate concern regarding inflicted injury. In this child, haemorrhagic oedema of infancy also requires consideration. (B) Even a single bruise on an infant should be carefully assessed in relation to child abuse. In this child the bruises might have been caused by a firm grip around the forearm.

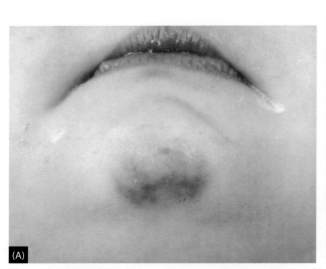

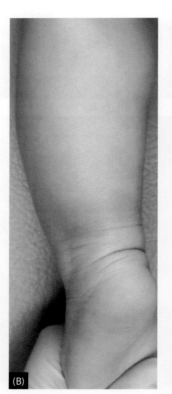

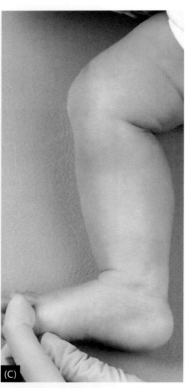

Figs. 10.54A–C (A) It is important to recognise mimics of bruising due to non-accidental injury. Bruises on bony prominences are more likely attributable to accidental causes. (B, C) Mongolian blue spots (congenital dermal melanocytosis) are an important differential for inflicted injury. These can occur in locations such as the limbs and anterior torso in addition to the more common locations such as the sacrum, buttocks and shoulders.

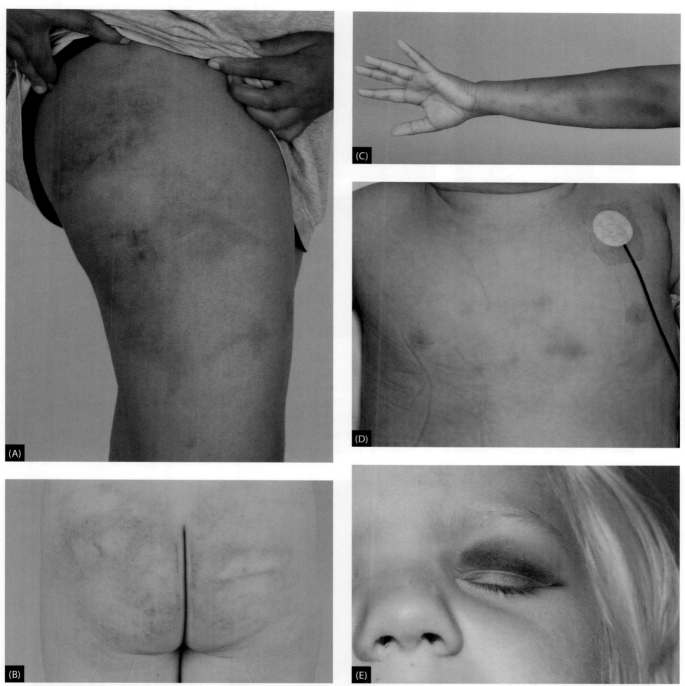

Figs. 10.55A–E (A) The buttocks and outer thighs are locations on the body where physical injury is commonly inflicted under the guise of discipline. Imprint bruising may result from forces transmitted unevenly through overlying clothing or as a result of impact with a patterned object, for example the sole of a shoe. (B) Extensive buttock bruising with sparing of the natal cleft and vertical lines of parallel bruises caused by 'crimping' of the skin. This is another pattern commonly caused by spanking inflicted under the guise of discipline. (C) When victims use their arms to shield sensitive parts of their body from blows during assaults, the pattern of bruising on the extensor surfaces of the arms may be termed 'defence wounds'. (D) Faint small bruises on the anterior chest wall overlay sternal injury, haemopericardium and haemothoraces. (E) Bruising to the upper eyelid may be the result of blood tracking along tissue planes, heralding an injury elsewhere.

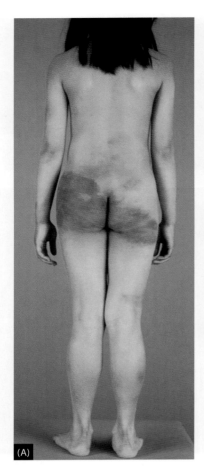

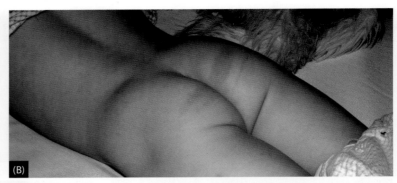

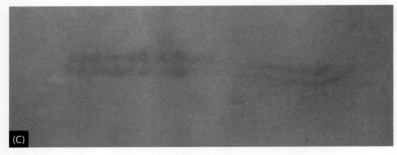

Figs. 10.56A–C (A) Repeated physical violence to a young girl. The inflicted trauma to the buttocks is striking, but do not overlook the bruises of varying ages on her arms, back and legs, indicative of previous abuse. (B) A recent buttock injury produced by beating with a rod. (C) Forceful contact with a linear object or edge can result in parallel linear bruises with central sparing. These are colloquially known as 'tram line' patterned bruises.

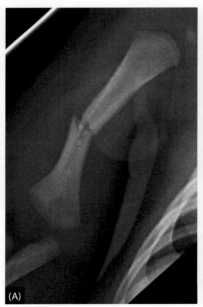

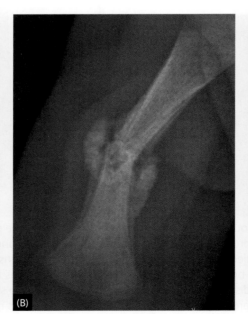

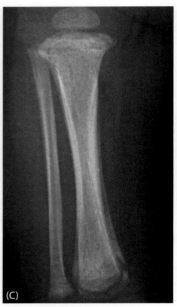

Figs. 10.57A–C (A, B) A time interval of 7 days has occurred between these two radiographs. The initial radiograph demonstrates clean fracture margins of a recent right humerus fracture. The second one reveals extensive soft callus, subperiosteal new bone formation along the humeral shaft and loss of clarity at the fracture site. Correlating the 'age' of a fracture with the history given is essential to recognising non-accidental injury. (C) Bucket handle metaphyseal fractures may be associated with subperiosteal new bone formation along the shafts of long bones.

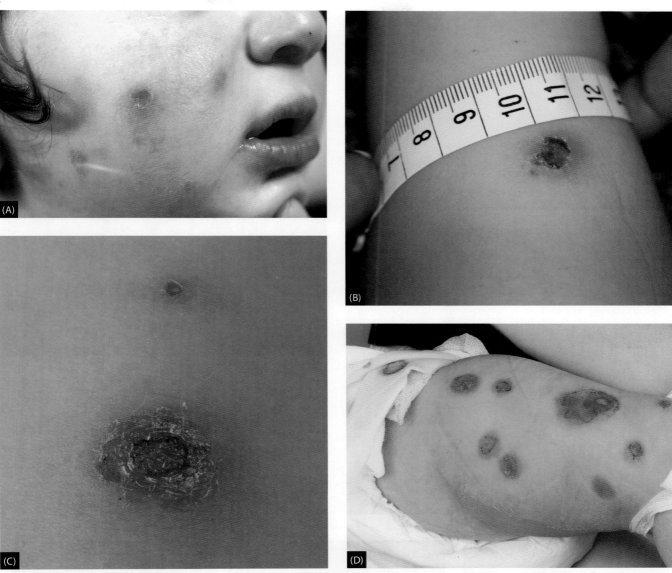

Figs. 10.58A–D (A) Cigarette burns to the cheek of a pre-school child. (B) Although features of this non-specific wound should generate suspicion about an inflicted cigarette burn, other causes should also be considered. (C) Small round craters with surrounding erythema and desquamation suggest possible causation by contact with the hot end of a lit cigarette. In this child the small superior 'satellite lesion' and the slightly yellow crusted overlying scab hint at the true cause, which is impetigo. (D) Dermatitis artefacta may present as unusual wounds that fail to heal in the usual time frame, and is an important differential for non-accidental injury.

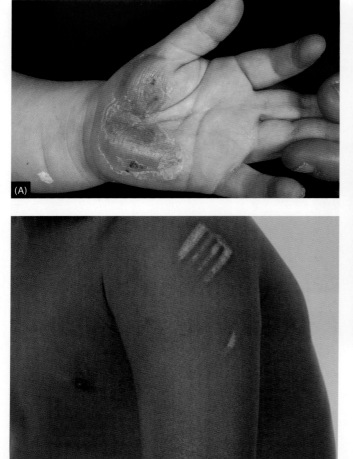

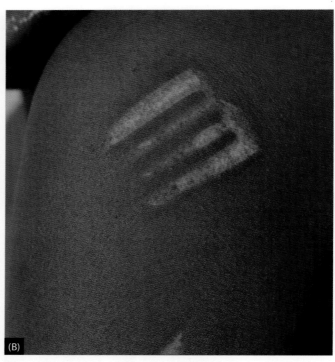

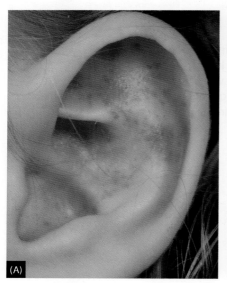

Figs. 10.59A–C (A) Burns to the palm of the hand in a toddler who had his hand forcibly held on a hot element as 'punishment' for a misdemeanour. Note the sparing of the fingers and palm, which is unusual for the 'exploratory' child who accidentally reaches out to a hot surface. (B, C) Scars resulting from fork-shaped contact burns were caused when this child's mother applied a heated fork to his skin.

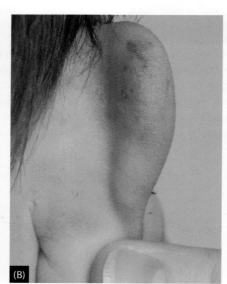

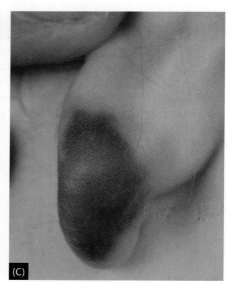

Figs. 10.60A–C (A, B) Children aged less than 4 years rarely injure their ears as a result of accidental trauma. A high degree of concern regarding child abuse should exist when bruising is noted to both ears. (C) Pinching and squeezing has resulted in localised bruising to the ear lobe.

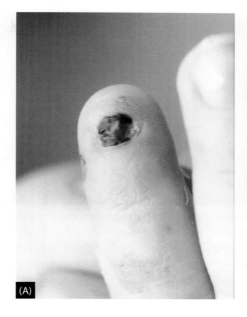

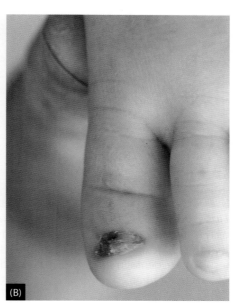

Figs. 10.61A, B Intentional avulsion of the nails is an uncommon manifestation of non-accidental injury, but one that should not be missed. The nail beds are healthy and nail regrowth has a normal appearance.

(A)

(B)

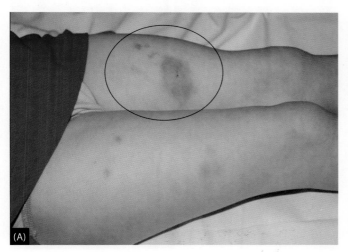

(A)

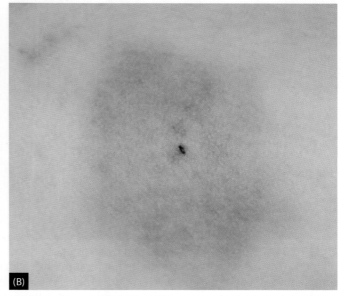

(B)

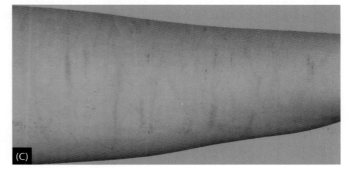

(C)

Figs. 10.62A–C (A, B) The elliptical shape of this gaping wound suggest that it is a puncture wound rather than an incision. (C) Self-inflicted incised wounds are often similar in appearance and of similar depth, are parallel or cross hatched, and are in easily accessible parts of the body such an the forearm of the non-dominant arm. Non-suicidal self-injury may be associated with prior childhood trauma, and adolescents demonstrating this behaviour are at greater risk of mortality than those who do not.

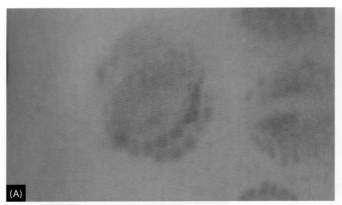 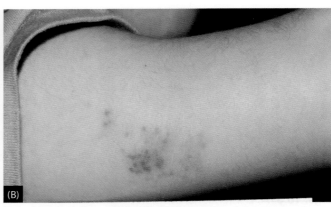

Figs. 10.63A, B (A) Human bite marks commonly result in a patterned bruise of two opposing arcs. In this child the overlay of two bite marks may be seen in addition to drag marks caused by teeth. The small size of these bruises suggests correctly that these bites were inflicted by another small child. (B) Petechiae (pin-point sized bruises) are more commonly seen as a result of accidental trauma and in association with medical conditions such as idiopathic thrombocytopaenia than as a result of inflicted trauma.

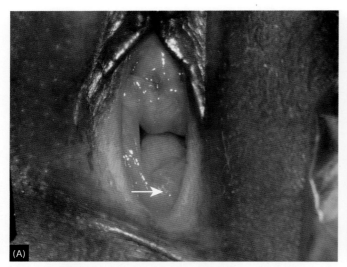 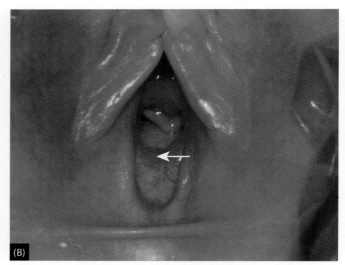

Figs. 10.64A, B (A) Vaginal penetration by an 'icy-pole' stick. In this girl, the hymen is deficient on the left side laterally and inferiorly. There is a lump of hymenal remnant at the six o'clock position (arrow) and erythema associated with new vessel formation between three and seven o'clock. There is a clear view into the vagina. (B) Vaginal penetration by a digit. The hymen has an irregular crescenteric appearance with a wide cleft at the six o'clock position (arrow). There is a condensation of tissue at four o'clock, with new vessel formation in the inferior aspect of the hymen.

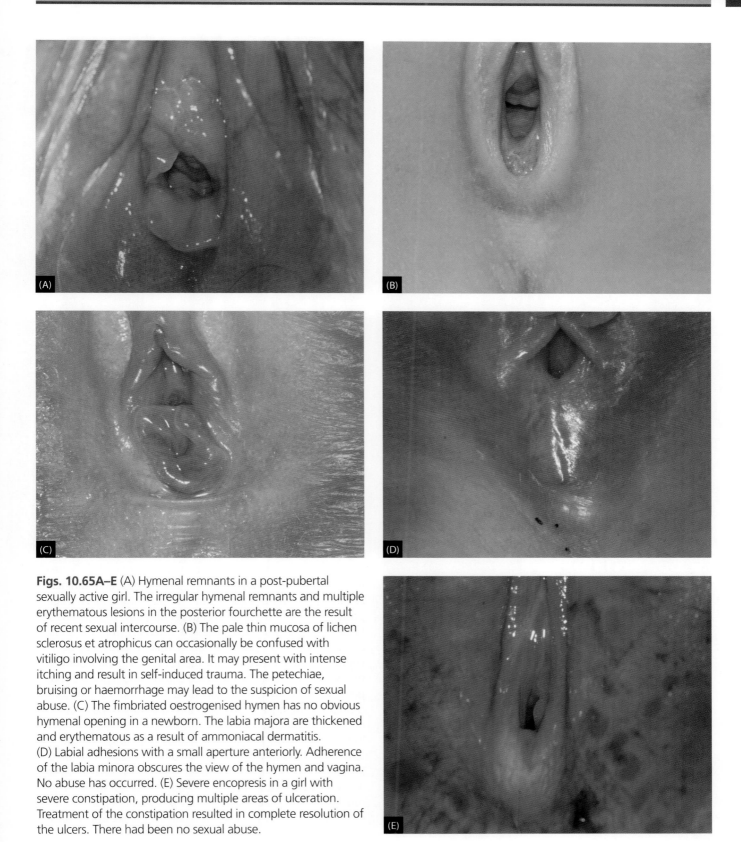

Figs. 10.65A–E (A) Hymenal remnants in a post-pubertal sexually active girl. The irregular hymenal remnants and multiple erythematous lesions in the posterior fourchette are the result of recent sexual intercourse. (B) The pale thin mucosa of lichen sclerosus et atrophicus can occasionally be confused with vitiligo involving the genital area. It may present with intense itching and result in self-induced trauma. The petechiae, bruising or haemorrhage may lead to the suspicion of sexual abuse. (C) The fimbriated oestrogenised hymen has no obvious hymenal opening in a newborn. The labia majora are thickened and erythematous as a result of ammoniacal dermatitis. (D) Labial adhesions with a small aperture anteriorly. Adherence of the labia minora obscures the view of the hymen and vagina. No abuse has occurred. (E) Severe encopresis in a girl with severe constipation, producing multiple areas of ulceration. Treatment of the constipation resulted in complete resolution of the ulcers. There had been no sexual abuse.

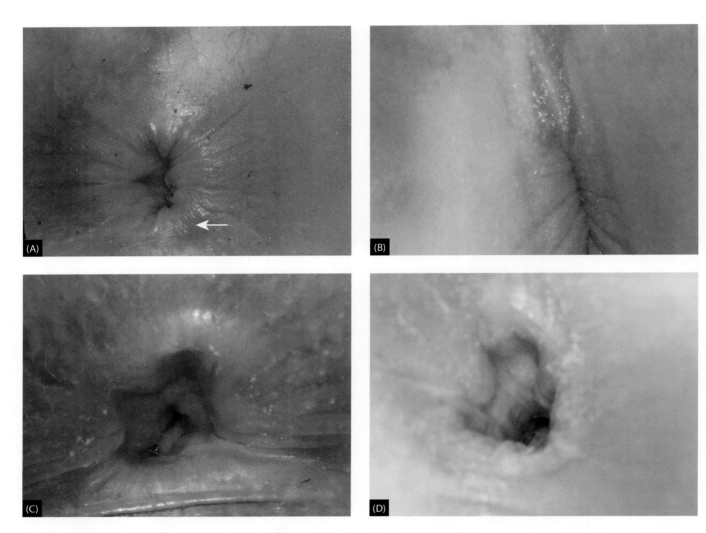

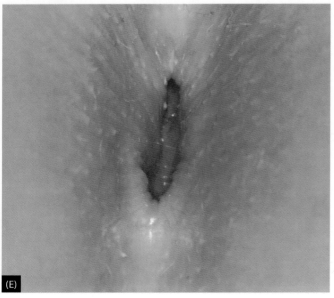

Figs. 10.66A–E (A) Recent anal penetration has resulted in an oedematous anal margin and irregular rugal folds. There is relaxation of the superficial part of the external anal sphincter. A blue area of venous congestion is visible at the five o'clock position (arrow). (B) Previous anal penetration. This girl has a healing midline scar, which extends anteriorly from the anus and is the result of anal penetration. Midline scars may be confused with a broad midline raphe or a congenital perineal groove. (C) This child has suffered chronic and repeated anal penetration. There are irregular rugal folds and a scar at three o'clock extending laterally. Note the 'tyre sign' of perianal oedema and venous congestion. (D) A pale scarred anus with loss of rugal folds. The 'funnelled anus' appearance is due to anal dilatation, which occurs on lateral separation of the buttocks. Faeces are visible in the rectum. This child has been abused repeatedly. (E) In this child there is loss of the anal rugal folds. Note the relaxation of the superficial part of the external anal sphincter. There is a narrow slit-like appearance on the lateral buttocks separation test.

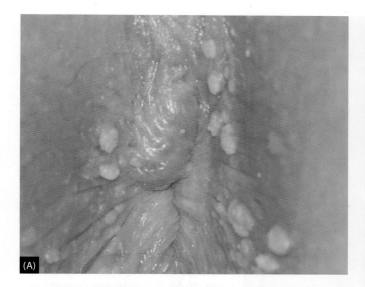

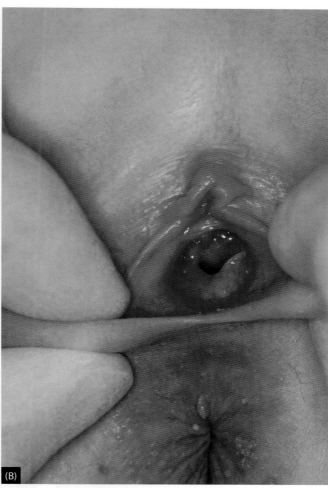

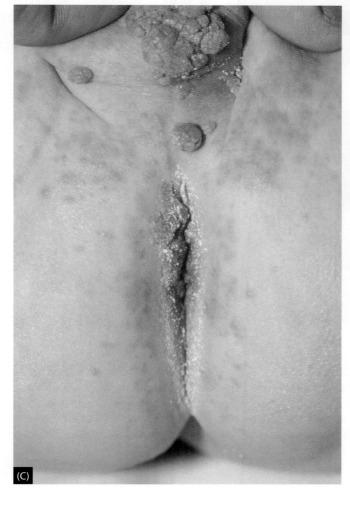

Figs. 10.67A–C (A) Anal warts. In addition to the obvious anal warts, there is a large anal rugal fold anteriorly to the right. (B) Perianal warts in a girl in whom sexual abuse was suspected and subsequently proved. The hymen is intact. (C) Perianal warts in another girl in whom sexual abuse was subsequently proved.

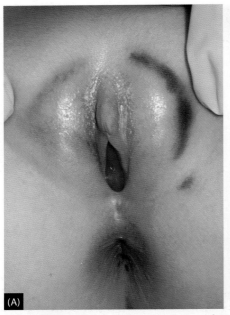

(A)

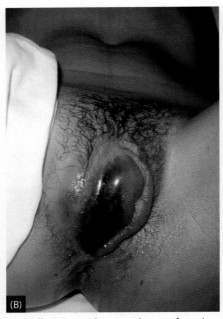

(B)

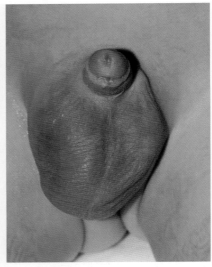

Fig. 10.69 Scrotal bruises caused by trauma should not be confused with idiopathic scrotal oedema. Bruising to a young boy's scrotum should generate significant concern regarding possible child abuse.

Figs. 10.68A, B (A) Perineal bruising after a straddle injury. This may be confused with sexual abuse. (B) Large labial haematoma following a straddle injury in an older child.

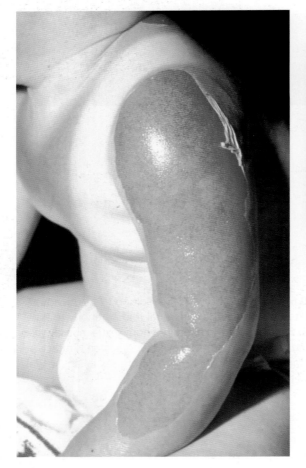

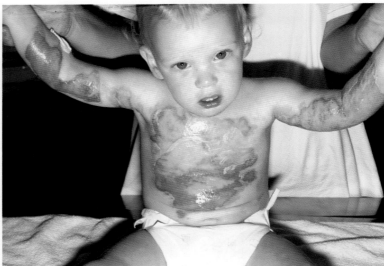

Fig. 10.71 An 18-month-old child who had pulled a saucepan of hot water off a stove, sustaining superficial dermal and mid-dermal burns. When examined, the broken blisters in the skin reveal eythematous, moist and tender underlying dermis with a brisk capillary return.

Fig. 10.70 Severe sunburn leading to a superficial dermal burn. The area exposed to the ultraviolet light shows a gradation from erythema to skin blistering. The protected area is white and undamaged.

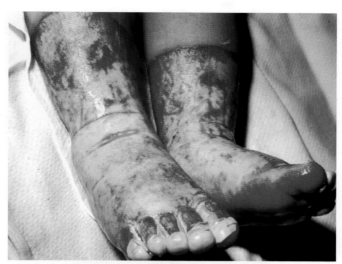

Fig. 10.72 Severe scald injury to both legs of a child who was immersed in an excessively hot bath. The 'tide mark' demaraction of injury is strongly suggestive of non-accidental injury. When examined, the burns demonstrated a mottled, dry eschar and decreased sensation, consistent with a deep dermal and/or full-thickness depth.

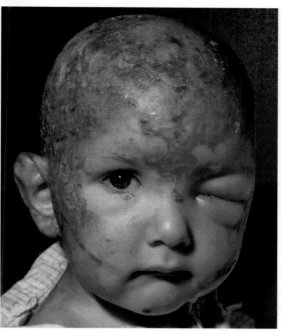

Fig. 10.73 Hot fat burn to the face causing deep burns to the scalp. The relatively greater heat and viscosity of hot fat when compared with boiling water contributes to a deeper burn in this setting.

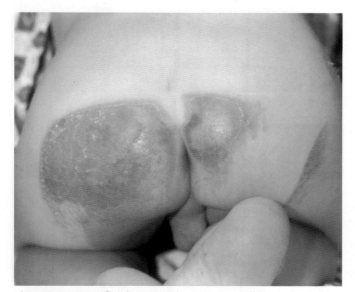

Fig. 10.74 Superficial contact burn in a small boy who sat against a wall heater.

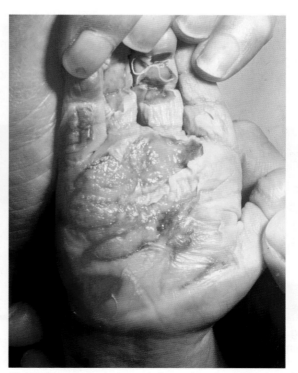

Fig. 10.75 Contact burn in an infant who placed his hand on the hot glass front of a combustion heater. This is a common accidental mechanism in childhood, but the possibility for non-accidental trauma should not be overlooked.

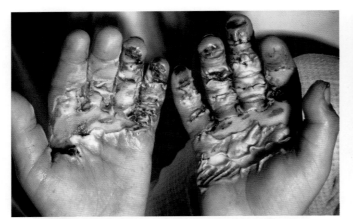

Fig. 10.76 Deep contact burns to both hands from a bar heater. Although the area is small, this is a serious injury because of the anatomical site and depth to which the burn has occurred.

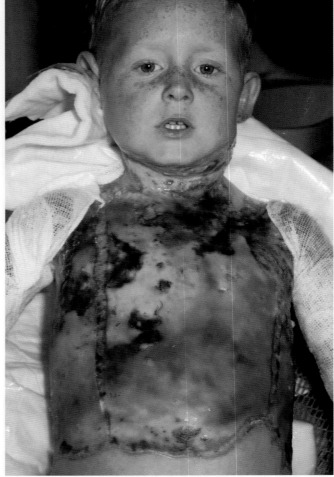

Fig. 10.77 This 6-year-old boy was igniting an incinerator with petrol and matches when his clothes caught fire, resulting in full-thickness burns to his chest and both arms. Circumferential full-thickness chest burns are life-threatening as they prevent chest expansion and so chest escharotomies have been performed. Unfortunately, the incisions have not extended into normal skin as they should, limiting the effectiveness of the intervention.

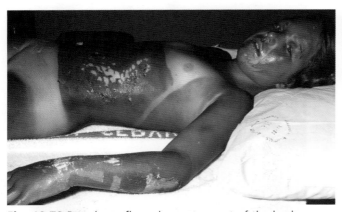

Fig. 10.78 Petroleum flame burns to most of the body. Flame burns tend to be deep on account of the high temperature, and both limb and chest escharotomies may be required in this case.

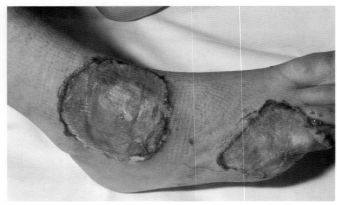

Fig. 10.79 High-voltage electrical burns in a boy who was lifting a metal pole, which touched high-tension wires. The resulting foot burns represent the exit point of the electrical current, with severe tissue injury including loss of the little toe.

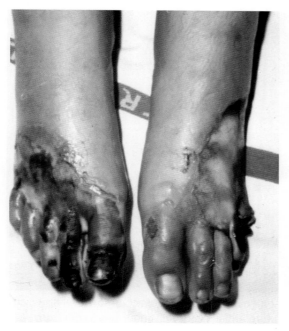

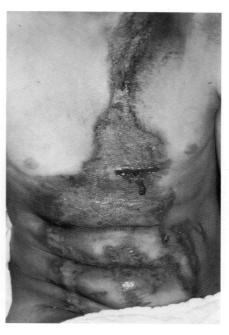

Fig. 10.80 Another high-voltage electrical burn showing extensive destruction of soft tissues. As a rule, the damage to underlying structures is more extensive than appears from the surface wounds.

Fig. 10.81 Lightning strike, producing deep burns to the chest and abdominal wall. Remarkably, the child survived.

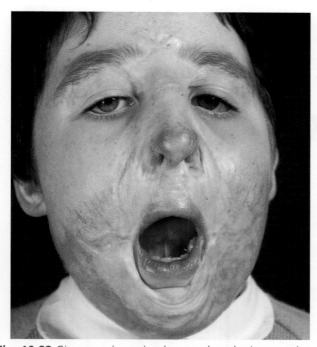

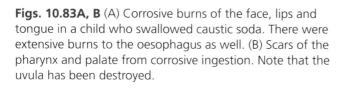

Fig. 10.82 Circumoral scarring has produced microstomia. This followed a flame burn to the lower half of the face.

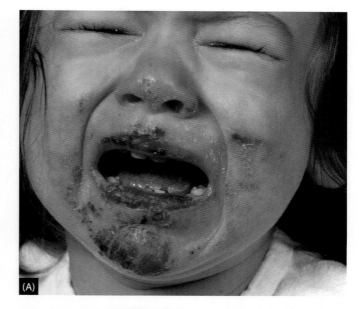

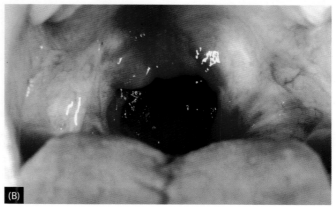

Figs. 10.83A, B (A) Corrosive burns of the face, lips and tongue in a child who swallowed caustic soda. There were extensive burns to the oesophagus as well. (B) Scars of the pharynx and palate from corrosive ingestion. Note that the uvula has been destroyed.

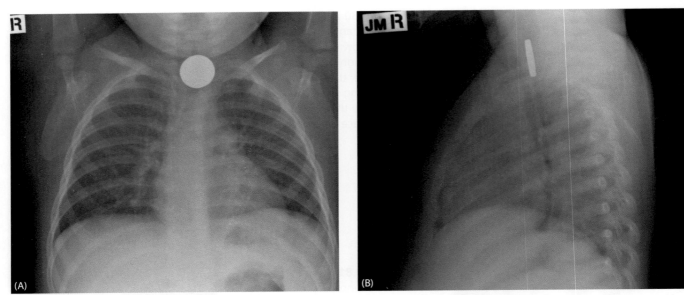

Figs. 10.84A, B (A) Arrest of a swallowed coin in the region of the cricopharyngeus. This is the most common level at which swallowed foreign bodies are arrested in the oesophagus. The lack of a circumferential lucency distinguishes a coin from the more sinister button battery (see also **Figs. 10.85A, B**). (B) The 'face-on' view of the coin in (A) informs the clinician that the coin is in the oesophagus and not the airway, as is attested to by this lateral view showing the anteriorly placed airway relative to the swallowed oesophageal foreign body.

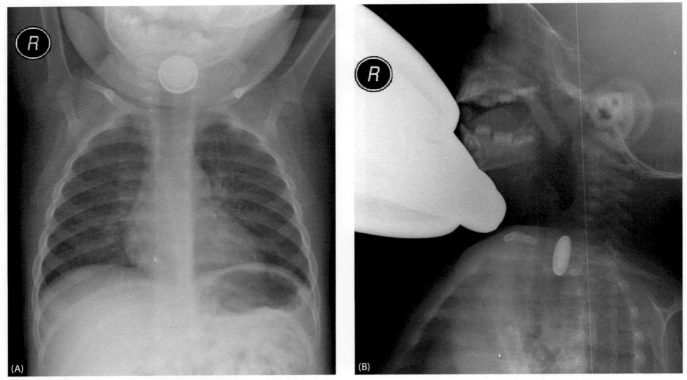

Figs. 10.85A, B (A) This child also has a foreign body in the upper oesophagus. The obvious circumferential lucency is pathognomonic for a swallowed button battery, which is a true surgical emergency. Without timely removal, the burns from oesophageal button batteries are highly morbid and can be fatal (e.g. from erosion into a major vessel). (B) The characteristic button battery appearance can also be appreciated on the lateral view, as can the relative increased thickness of the perioesophageal soft tissues indicative of the trauma (burns) from the button battery at this level.

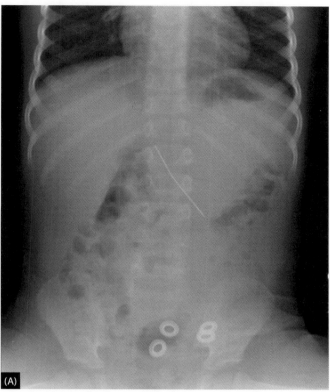

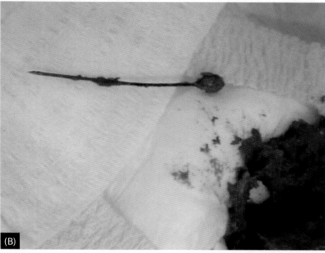

Figs. 10.86A, B (A) This child presented some hours after swallowing a hat pin. The circular lucencies over the pelvis are related to the child's clothing. (B) Same child: the hat pin was allowed to pass naturally and is evident in the child's nappy 3 days later.

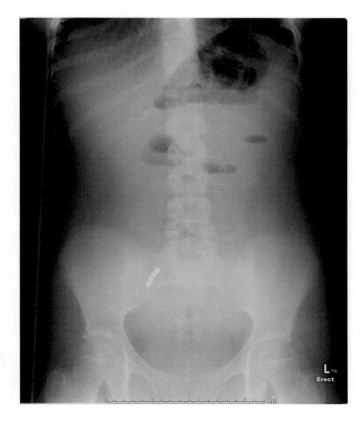

Fig. 10.87 Erect abdominal radiograph showing four swallowed magnets attracted to each other. It is not possible to tell whether the magnets are in the same or an adjacent bowel loop or, indeed, whether attraction has formed an enteroenteric fistula or perforation. However, the accompanying features of ascites and ileus (or obstruction) suggest a complicated course. Multiple perforations were evident at laparotomy.

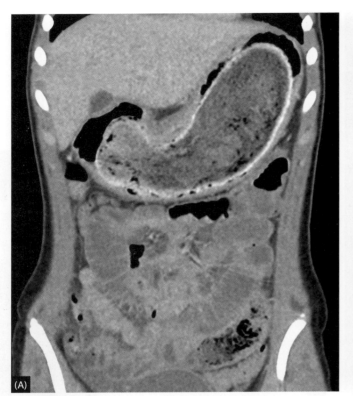
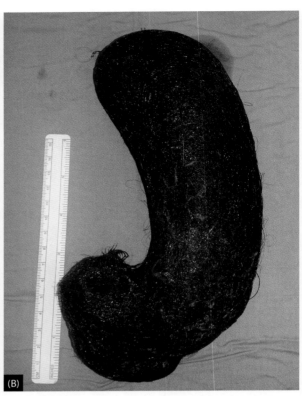

Figs. 10.88A, B (A) CT scan showing a trichophytobezoar in the stomach. (B) Photograph of the same trichophytobezoar after removal from the stomach. Trichobezoars and trichophytobezoars are caused by trichophagia, a compulsive behaviour characterised by eating one's own hair. They are usually seen in adolescent girls and may be a manifestation of an underlying psychiatric disorder or psychosocial problem.

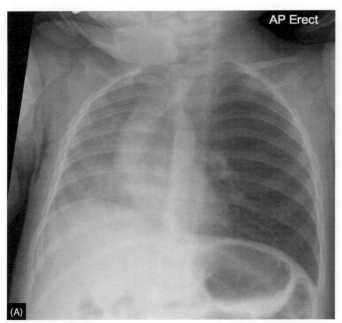
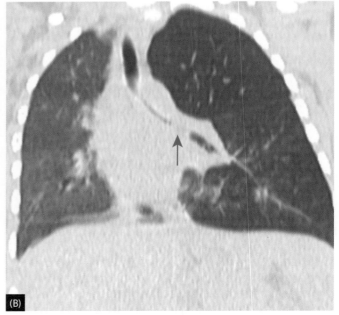

Figs. 10.89A, B (A) Chest radiograph of a toddler with overexpansion of the left lung and a history of peanut aspiration 3 weeks beforehand. The peanut was retrieved endoscopically from the left main bronchus. (B) CT of same patient showing the peanut impacted in the left main bronchus (arrow).

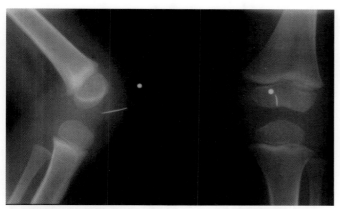

Fig. 10.90 Crawling or kneeling children may acquire a needle foreign body injury in the region of the knee. The exact location of the needle is determined using an image intensifier at the time of removal. The small ball bearing marks the entry wound.

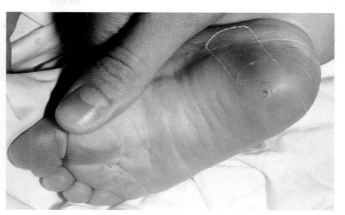

Fig. 10.91 Foreign body in the heel, initially thought to be a plantar wart.

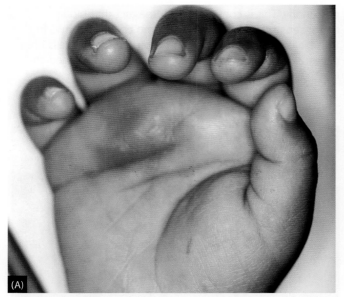

(A)

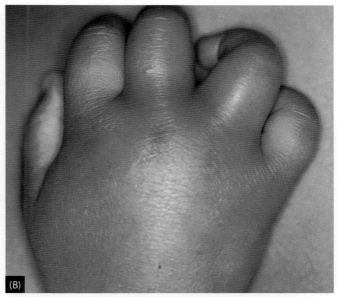

(B)

Figs. 10.92A, B Deep palmar abscess of the hand secondary to infection by a foreign body. Although the infection predominantly involves the palmar aspect of the hand, there is a marked swelling on the dorsum and separation of the middle and ring fingers.

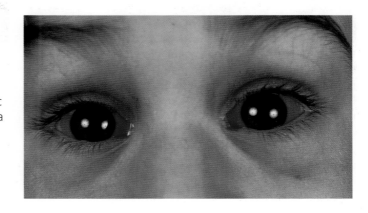

Fig. 10.93 A crushed chest with compression of the thoracic inlet produces temporary occlusion of the superior vena cava and rupture of the small veins in the region of the head and neck. This may manifest as subconjunctival haemorrhage. It can be differentiated from an orbital fracture because there is a posterior limit to the haemorrhage.

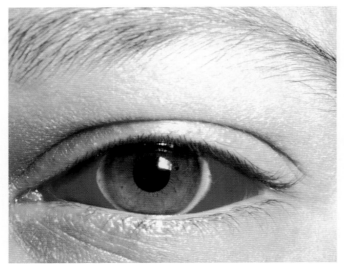

Fig. 10.94 Subconjunctival haematoma secondary to fracture of the orbital roof. The fracture has led to extravasation of blood into the orbital cavity behind the eye, which has tracked forward between the conjunctiva and the sclera. The anterior limit of the haemorrhage is at the limbus, where the conjunctiva is attached. There is no posterior limit to the haemorrhage, which is the major clue to the diagnosis. Local, direct trauma to the eye can be excluded by the clear anterior chamber and the lack of any trauma to the eyelids.

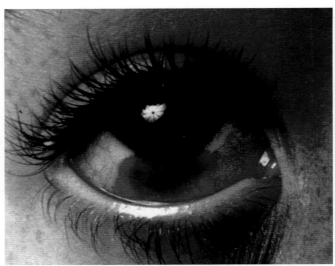

Fig. 10.95 Subconjunctival haemorrhage from a direct injury to the eye in a motor accident. The haemorrhage is maximal in the anterior part of the sclera and is less severe posteriorly. This is consistent with the fact that blood has arisen anteriorly, rather than from behind the eye. In these injuries, it is important to be certain that there is no penetrating injury to the globe, which requires immediate ophthalmological referral.

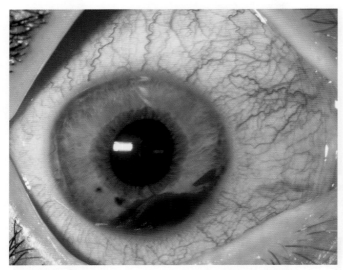

Fig. 10.96 Traumatic hyphema. The blood has settled into the lowest part of the anterior chamber and clotted. There is mild conjunctival injection. A sluggish pupillary reaction to light is common and is due to trauma to the iris constrictor muscle.

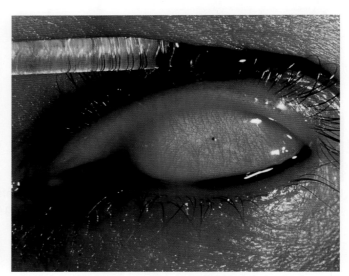

Fig. 10.97 A subtarsal foreign body causes discomfort on blinking. The pain is often out of proportion to the size of the foreign body.

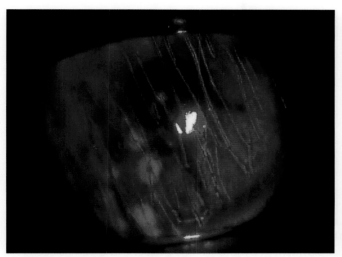

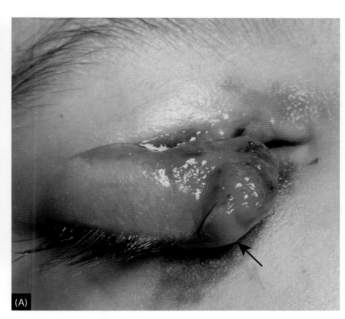

Fig. 10.98 Corneal abrasions following trauma from a velcro strap. Fluorescein staining shows the abrasions in green when viewed with a blue light.

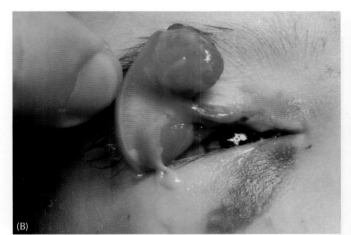

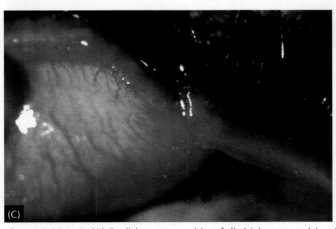

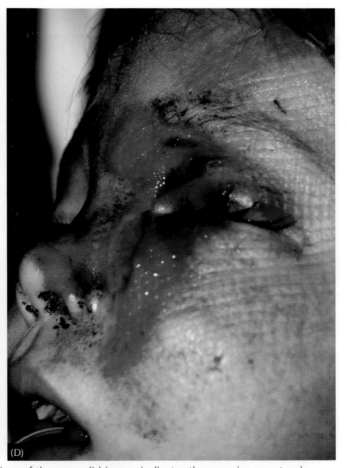

Figs. 10.99A–D (A) Eyelid trauma, with a full-thickness avulsion injury of the upper lid (arrow indicates the superior punctum). (B) When the torn eyelid is rotated the true extent of the lid avulsion is seen. The underlying globe was undamaged. (C) Eyelid showing the tear in the tarsal plate. The underlying globe was undamaged. (D) Extensive laceration of the medial aspect of the upper and lower lids, with division of the common canaliculus.

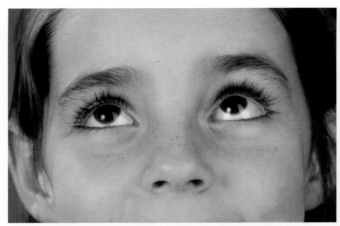

Fig. 10.100 Blunt trauma causing a blow-out fracture of the right orbital floor with limitation of upward gaze.

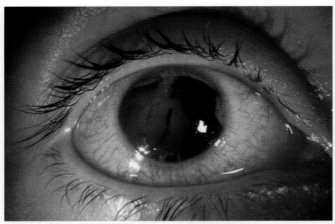

Fig. 10.101 Severe blunt injury to the eye following airbag deployment in a motor-vehicle accident. The iris has been avulsed almost completely, the lens is subluxated and there is total retinal detachment. Investigation revealed that the optic nerve had been avulsed from the globe. The other eye was ruptured by the impact of the airbag.

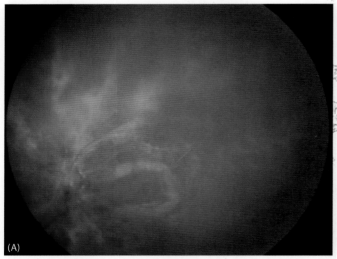

(A)

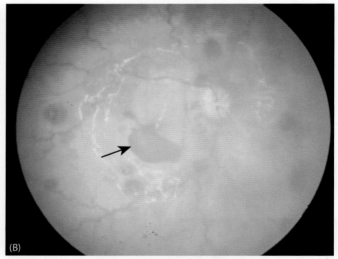

(B)

Figs. 10.102A, B (A) Retinal haemorrhage in a case of non-accidental injury (arrow). The haemorrhage is so extensive that almost no normal retina is visible. Note the pale C-shaped perimacular fold marked with an arrow. (B) Traumatic retinoschisis (arrow) secondary to non-accidental injury.

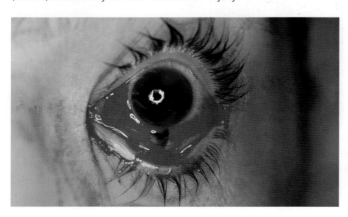

Fig. 10.103 Penetrating injury of the globe caused by an airgun pellet. Note the entry wound below the limbus with prolapsed choroid, extensive subconjunctival haemorrhage and hyphema.

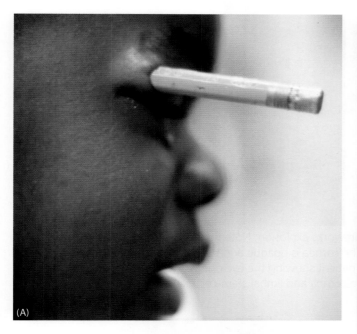

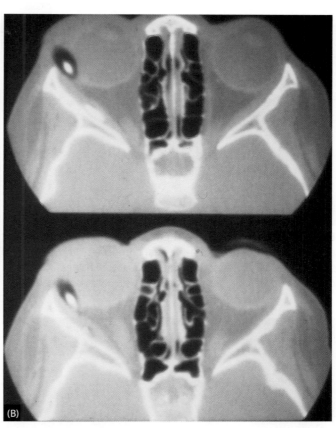

Figs. 10.104A, B (A) Penetrating injury of the orbit caused by a fall when running with a pencil in one hand. Despite the apparently severe nature of the injury, the globe was intact and vision returned to normal after the pencil was removed. (B) CT scan of the same patient showing the pencil in the lateral aspect of the orbit with an intact globe.

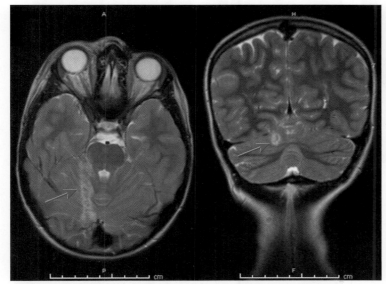

Fig. 10.105 This MR image demonstrates the importance of delineating the extent of any penetrating orbital injury. This child fell into a grass tree and a spike penetrated the right eyelid. He removed the spike and then collapsed with dizziness. Subsequent MRI revealed that the spike penetrated the orbit and into the cerebellum. The arrows indicate the track taken by the foreign body. A small amount of vegetable matter was removed at orbitotomy, and there were no long-term sequelae.

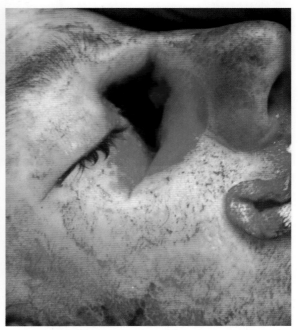

Fig. 10.106 Severe orbital and facial injury inflicted by a home-made compressed airgun. Associated brain injuries were fatal.

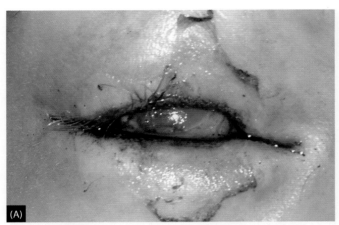
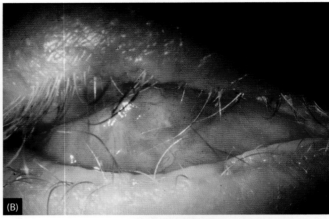

Figs. 10.107A, B (A) Severe chemical eye injury secondary to fireworks explosion. Note the eyelid swelling and singed eyelashes, which indicate a thermal component to the injury. The cornea is opaque and there is gunpowder residue on the skin, eyelashes and eye. This injury caused blindness. (B) Same patient showing the eye one year after injury. The cornea is opaque and vascularized as the result of stromal damage to the cornea and limbal stem-cell failure.

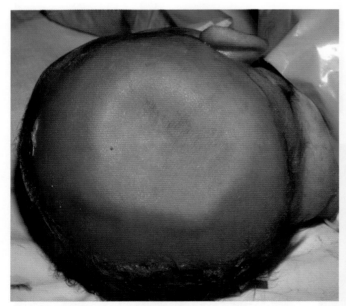

Fig. 10.108 This baby has a birth injury with a simple depressed fracture due to forceps application.

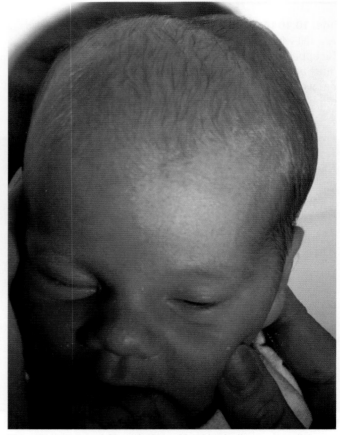

Fig. 10.109 A newborn baby with a cephalhaematoma in the parietal region, caused by subperiosteal bleeding.

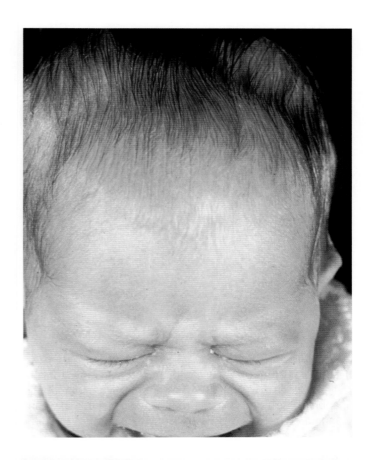

Fig. 10.110 Bilateral cephalhaematomas in an infant suffering a birth injury. Bleeding is limited by the coronal sutures anteriorly and the sagittal suture in the midline.

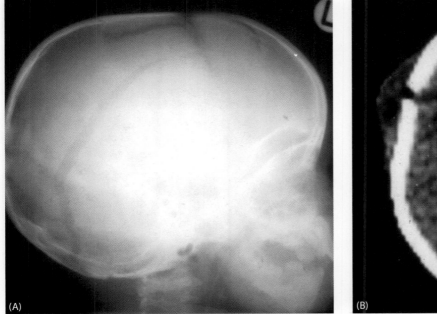

(A)

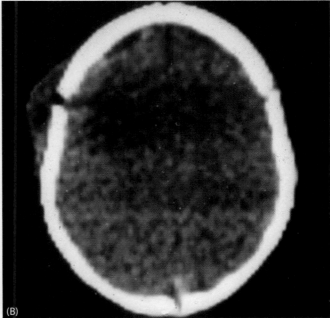

(B)

Figs. 10.111A, B (A) A fractured skull in a 2-year-old child with a very wide fracture line, which was associated with tearing of the underlying dura mater and the brain. This is the 'bursting fracture' of childhood. (B) A CT scan of the same child showing the wide fracture line and the superficial haematoma and CSF collection externally. There is also underlying injury to the brain.

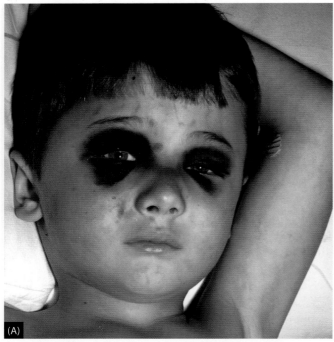

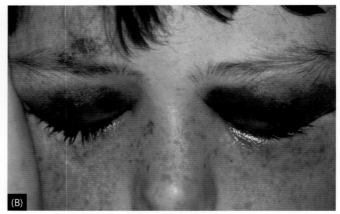

Figs. 10.112A, B (A) A child with an anterior cranial fossa fracture with secondary bruising around each eye – the so-called 'racoon eye' sign. (B) An older boy with an anterior cranial fossa fracture after a motor accident. The child was inappropriately sitting in the front passenger seat and wearing a loose lap-seat belt, which failed to prevent him from banging his head on the dashboard. The blood has tracked down from the fracture in the forehead to both eyelids.

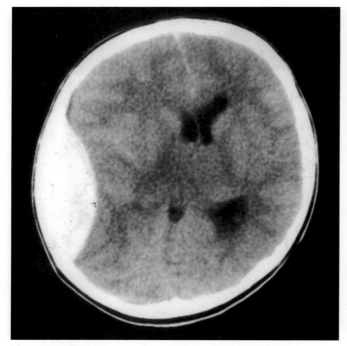

Fig. 10.113 A CT scan of an 18-month-old child who suffered a major head injury, with a large extradural haematoma causing significant distortion of the brain.

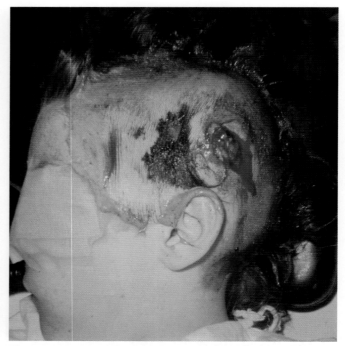

Fig. 10.114 This child was kicked by a horse in the side of the head and suffered a compound, depressed skull fracture with brain extruding through the wound.

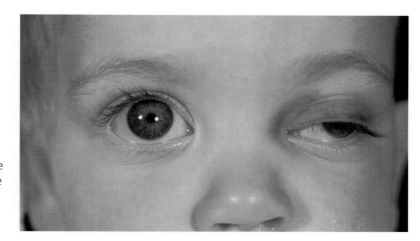

Fig. 10.115 This child suffered a head injury in the past and has a residual, post-traumatic third nerve palsy on the left side. The left eye is externally deviated, there is ptosis of the upper lid and the left pupil is dilated.

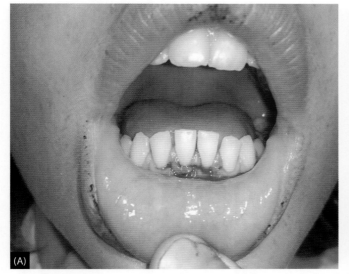

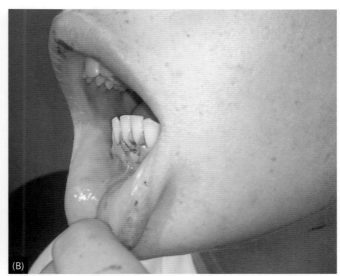

Figs. 10.116A, B Dental injury following a fall in which the child landed face down onto a very hard surface. (B) Viewed laterally, the injury to the gums is seen and there may be associated fractures of the mandible and/or loose teeth.

Further reading

Beasley SW, Hutson JM, Auldist AW (1996) *Essential Paediatric Surgery*. Edward Arnold Publishers, London.

Coran AG, Adzick NS, Krummel TM, Laberge J-M, Shamberger RC, Caldamone AA (2012) *Pediatric Surgery*, 7th edition. Elsevier Saunders, St. Louis.

Hutson JM, Beasley SW (2013) *The Surgical Examination of Children*, 2nd edition. Springer-Verlag, Berlin Heidelberg.

Hutson JM, O'Brien M, Beasley SW, King S, Teague W (2015) *Jones' Clinical Paediatric Surgery*, 7th edition. Wiley-Blackwell, Ames.

Puri P (2017) *Newborn Surgery*, 4th edition. CRC Press, Boca Raton.

Index